Critical Thinking
TACTICS
for Nurses

Achieving the IOM Competencies

SECOND EDITION

M. Gaie Rubenfeld, MS, RN
Associate Professor
Eastern Michigan University
Ypsilanti, Michigan

Barbara K. Scheffer, EdD, RN
Professor
Eastern Michigan University
Ypsilanti, Michigan

JONES AND BARTLETT PUBLISHERS
Sudbury, Massachusetts
BOSTON   TORONTO   LONDON   SINGAPORE

World Headquarters

Jones and Bartlett Publishers
40 Tall Pine Drive
Sudbury, MA 01776
978-443-5000
info@jbpub.com
www.jbpub.com

Jones and Bartlett Publishers
Canada
6339 Ormindale Way
Mississauga, Ontario L5V 1J2
Canada

Jones and Bartlett Publishers
International
Barb House, Barb Mews
London W6 7PA
United Kingdom

Jones and Bartlett's books and products are available through most bookstores and online book-sellers. To contact Jones and Bartlett Publishers directly, call 800-832-0034, fax 978-443-8000, or visit our website www.jbpub.com.

Substantial discounts on bulk quantities of Jones and Bartlett's publications are available to corporations, professional associations, and other qualified organizations. For details and specific discount information, contact the special sales department at Jones and Bartlett via the above contact information or send an email to specialsales@jbpub.com.

The authors, editor, and publisher have made every effort to provide accurate information. However, they are not responsible for errors, omissions, or for any outcomes related to the use of the contents of this book and take no responsibility for the use of the products and procedures described. Treatments and side effects described in this book may not be applicable to all people; likewise, some people may require a dose or experience a side effect that is not described herein. Drugs and medical devices are discussed that may have limited availability controlled by the Food and Drug Administration (FDA) for use only in a research study or clinical trial. Research, clinical practice, and government regulations often change the accepted standard in this field. When consideration is being given to use of any drug in the clinical setting, the health care provider or reader is responsible for determining FDA status of the drug, reading the package insert, and reviewing prescribing information for the most up-to-date recommendations on dose, precautions, and contraindications, and determining the appropriate usage for the product. This is especially important in the case of drugs that are new or seldom used.

Production Credits

Publisher: Kevin Sullivan
Acquisitions Editor: Emily Ekle
Acquisitions Editor: Amy Sibley
Associate Editor: Patricia Donnelly
Editorial Assistant: Rachel Shuster
Production Assistant: Lisa Cerrone
Marketing Manager: Rebecca Wasley

V.P., Manufacturing and Inventory Control: Therese Connell
Composition: Arlene Apone
Cover Design: Timothy Dziewit
Cover Image: © Bella D/ShutterStock, Inc.
Printing and Binding: Malloy, Inc.
Cover Printing: Malloy, Inc.

Library of Congress Cataloging-in-Publication Data
Rubenfeld, M. Gaie.
  Critical thinking tactics for nurses : achieving the IOM competencies / M. Gaie Rubenfeld, Barbara Scheffer.—2nd ed.
     p. ; cm.
  Includes bibliographical references and index.
  ISBN 978-0-7637-6584-2 (pbk.)
  1. Nursing. 2. Critical thinking. I. Scheffer, Barbara K. II. Title.
  [DNLM: 1. Nursing Process. 2. Clinical Competence. 3. Thinking. WY 100 R895c 2010]
  RT42.R78 2010
  610.73—dc22
                                                                    2009010210

6048

Printed in the United States of America
13 12   10 9 8 7 6 5 4

Contents

Foreword to First Edition

Ada Sue Hinshaw, PhD, RN, FAAN
Dean & Professor, School of Nursing
University of Michigan, Ann Arbor

Explicating and defining the characteristics or habits of the mind, and the skills or processes of critical thinking as used in nursing make a unique and valuable contribution to the profession and the discipline. *Critical thinking* has been a popular buzz phrase in nursing practice and education for a number of years. It has been a central theme for many staff nurse development workshops and for many nursing curricula, especially at the undergraduate level. Yet understanding and explaining the process was very complex and not easily accomplished. The authors started with this basic concern and through their conceptualization and research identified the crucial components delineating the habits or characteristics, and skills or processes required of the individual involved in critical thinking.

This text, *Critical Thinking TACTICS for Nurses*, makes a strong contribution to the profession, especially in the practice arenas. The explanations and relationships drawn with critical thinking are laid out in a user-friendly manner that draws on many examples. Through the TACTICS strategy, the professional is led through the critical thinking habits and processes from the perspective of nursing practice. The relationship of critical thinking to evidence-based practice is suggested to be equal—that is, a professional cannot practice integrating clinical evidence, the latest research, and a career of experience without being involved in critical thinking and all the processes and skills outlined in this text. Understanding these processes and skills empowers the professional nurse for tailoring interventions with clients and ultimately enhances the predictability of the positive outcomes sought for clients and families. Empowering nurses, in terms of their clinical autonomy and control over their practice, has been shown in magnet hospital studies and others to build a stronger, more positive work environment that in turn results in better client outcomes through a higher quality of care (McClure & Hinshaw, 2002; Institute of Medicine, 2004).

Critical thinking occurs within a context. To illustrate how critical thinking relates to several major contextual situations, its relationship to and use in patient-centered care, interdisciplinary team care, evidence-based practice, informatics, and quality improvement is outlined. These situations are the five healthcare competencies recommended by the hallmark Institute of Medicine report,

Crossing the Quality Chasm: A New Health System for the 21st Century. Understanding critical thinking as basic to the attainment of these futuristic competencies is crucial for all health professions, not just nursing.

Critical thinking habits and skills are basic to the conduct of high-quality nursing research. Without contextual perspective, creativity, inquisitiveness, intuition, open-mindedness, perseverance, and reflection, few exciting, unique questions would be raised in research. The development of a strong science foundation for nursing practice depends on habits such as contextual perspective, inquisitiveness, and creativity, while the processes and skills such as discriminating, analyzing, and logical reasoning are crucial for scientific inquiry. Transforming knowledge is the skill or process through which research findings are built into practice policies and procedures. Careful attention to critical thinking as part of the undergraduate and graduate nursing curricula prepares nurses for participating in or conducting nursing research, depending on their own career choices.

In both professional practice and nursing research, the clinical issues confronted and the clinical questions to be investigated are complex and diverse in nature. They require the knowledge and expertise of more than one discipline. Multiple federal reports have recommended interdisciplinary education for the health professions. Critical thinking is basic to all health professions, but a valuable contribution of this text is its explanation of how such thinking is not additive, but is greatly expanded when professionals function in interdisciplinary teams either as health providers or investigators.

Rubenfeld and Scheffer are to be commended for explicating what has been a central but conceptually fuzzy entity—that is, critical thinking. Their research enlightens the nature of both the characteristics or habits, and skills or processes involved in such reasoning. Their experience and expertise provide context and practicality. Their contribution to understanding critical thinking as part of, or basic to, professional practice, research, and education is impressive.

References

McClure, M. & Hinshaw, A. (Eds.). (2002). *Magnet hospitals revisited: Attraction and retention of professional nurses.* Washington, D.C.: American Nurses Publishing.

Institute of Medicine. (2004). *Keeping patients safe: Transforming the work environment of nurses.* Washington, D.C.: The National Academies Press.

Foreword to Second Edition

M. Elaine Tagliareni, EdD, RN
President, National League for Nursing
Professor/Independence Foundation Chair
Department of Nursing
Community College of Philadelphia

I have found my experiences in the nursing program to be very different
from my experiences in almost all other courses. I think it has taken, and
will take some time before I get my mind set on being a nurse. The questions we are asked and the process we learn combine rote learning with critical thinking, and critical thinking of a particular kind. I can honestly say
that combining these two things has been a real challenge. At times the lack
of clear answers to nursing care needs in situations has been hard to come
to grips with. But in truth, nursing has helped to change me from a trained
robot to an inquisitive one. I used to follow whatever guidelines I was given
without questioning. Now I think about how I can better the situation.

—First-year nursing student, 2008

As nursing practice and the entire healthcare enterprise continue to be characterized by uncertainty, unpredictability, new technologies, heightened ethical dilemmas, and constant change, students in undergraduate nursing education programs
(like the student quoted above) who are preparing to practice in a wide variety of
settings will be required to think in ways that reach far beyond current practice
realities. How will we, as nurse educators, prepare them for this lifelong journey?

According to the National League for Nursing (NLN), the national nursing
organization dedicated to excellence in nursing and nursing education that represents over 27,000 nurse educators in the United States from all types of nursing
education programs, the role of nurse educator is complex. The core values of the
NLN—caring, integrity, diversity, and excellence—create a foundation for the
NLN's mission to build a strong and diverse nursing workforce through excellence
in nursing education. Nurses assuming the role of academic nurse educator combine their clinical abilities with responsibilities related to designing curricula,
developing courses/programs of study, teaching, guiding learners, evaluating
learning, and documenting the outcomes of the educational process. In addition
to teaching, nurse educators are responsible for advising students, engaging in
scholarly work (e.g., research), being involved in their professional associations,
contributing to the university community through leadership roles, engaging in

peer review, publishing, maintaining their clinical competence, and being a change agent for continued improvement of the nursing program. Finally, nurse educators are future-oriented because they anticipate the role of the nurse in the future and design educational programs to prepare graduates to meet those roles. It is this component of the role—preparing nursing students for future work that will require inquisitiveness, clear problem-solving skills, and thinking critically about care situations in new and emerging health care settings—that has become a key issue for nurse educators as they plan for an uncertain future.

Certainly, the overriding purpose of nursing education is to prepare individuals to meet the healthcare needs of the public. This value, to serve the public trust, has consistently characterized reform in nursing education. From its earliest days, the NLN has been at the forefront of these reform efforts to transform nursing education (Ironside & Valiga, 2007). Most recently, the NLN's position paper, *Innovation in Nursing Education: A Call to Reform* (2003), asked nursing faculty to revise traditional definitions of innovation away from a long-held belief that innovation is synonymous with the addition of new content, and to embrace innovative practices and new ways to promote problem-solving and thinking critically using alternative pedagogies. In 2005, the NLN developed a second position paper, *Transforming Nursing Education*, and called for new models of nursing education to emerge, recognizing that we can no longer rely on tradition, past practices, and good intentions. The NLN recommended that proposed changes to nursing programs emanate from evidence that substantiates the science of nursing education and that provides the foundation for best educational practices for faculty to move away from a focus on content coverage and toward methods that promote student engagement in use of evidence-based practice and thinking in context. A third NLN position paper, *Preparing the Next Generation of Nurses to Practice in a Technology-Rich Environment: An Informatics Agenda* (2008), calls on faculty, deans, administrators, and the NLN itself to advocate that all students graduate with up-to-date knowledge and skills in each of three critical areas: computer literacy, information literacy, and informatics. The NLN recognizes that students need to have basic proficiency in informatics in order to practice safely and efficiently in a technology-rich environment and to integrate information literacy and informatics into the delivery of patient care. Within this context, the NLN has consistently understood and valued its mission to build a strong nursing workforce through excellence and innovation at all levels of nursing education.

Currently, driving forces in today's healthcare environment necessitate renewed energy directed toward significant reform. There is a renewed appreciation that healthcare education needs a redesign. What is reasonable to expect from nursing education? With increased errors, high turnover rates of new graduates in acute care, and concern that nursing graduates do not embrace decision-making that leads to accountability for the continuation of care, there is wide understanding that different and enhanced competencies are needed by nursing graduates at all levels of education (Institute of Medicine, 1996, 2006). The call to reform in nursing education is far reaching.

The authors of this book have called on nurse educators to reframe and redesign approaches to teaching critical thinking. They recognize that critical thinking is contextual and that it calls for renewed attention to quality and safety practices. They have incorporated the new approaches advocated by the Robert Wood Johnson-funded Quality and Safety Education for Nurses (QSEN) initiative. They have provided innovative ways to increase use of context-based pedagogies within our classrooms and clinical teaching environments. In short, they have provided data to validate that new approaches to teaching thinking are possible and essential in today's uncertain and unpredictable health care environment. It requires tremendous courage and energy on the part of nurse educators to embrace reform and to move toward a future of inquisitiveness and dialogue about teaching thinking. The NLN will join with its members to light the way and to promote reform. As the first-year nursing student quoted previously clearly articulates, thinking critically about nursing care situations is complex and requires practice, reflection, and more practice. It also requires new approaches to teaching and learning within our nursing programs. If you are reading this book, you are eager to approach teaching thinking in new ways, based on current research and up-to-date evidence-based practice. Congratulations as you move toward a future as yet undefined as you seek to enhance delivery of patient care through emerging standards of excellence in nursing education.

References

Institute of Medicine. (1996). *Crossing the quality chasm: The IOM health care quality initiative.* Retrieved April 23, 2009, from http://www.iom.edu/CMS/8089.aspx

Institute of Medicine. (2006). *Preventing medication errors: Quality Chasm series.* Retrieved April 23, 2009, from http://www.iom.edu/CMS/3809/22526/35939.aspx

Ironside, P., & Valiga, T. (2007). *On revolution and revolutionaries: 25 years of reform and innovation in nursing education.* New York: National League for Nursing.

National League for Nursing. (2003). *Innovation in nursing education: A call to reform (Position Statement).* New York: Author. Retrieved April 23, 2009, from http://www.nln.org/aboutnln/PositionStatements/innovation.htm

National League for Nursing. (2005). *Transforming nursing education. (Position Statement).* New York: Author. Retrieved April 23, 2009, from http://www.nln.org/aboutnln/PositionSTatements/transforming052005.pdf

National League for Nursing. (2008). *Preparing the next generation of nurses to practice in a technology-rich environment: An informatics agenda. (Position Statement).* New York: Author. Retrieved April 23, 2009, from http://www.nln.org/aboutnln/PositionSTatements/informatics_052808.pdf

Preface

This book is written for clinicians in various areas of practice, nursing students, and educators in clinical and academic settings who want to hone their critical thinking abilities and help others do the same. Although we come from a nursing perspective, our ideas are applicable in any healthcare discipline. Healthcare delivery is in dire need of critical thinkers, and all too often, books and articles note the need but provide few concrete suggestions for how to improve thinking. Most critical thinking resources are aimed at academic audiences and settings. Our aim is to bring *critical thinking* (called *CT* throughout this book) into the real world of healthcare delivery and education by offering practical suggestions for CT-promoting activities.

Because CT must be implemented within a context of problems or issues, this text addresses the CT needed to achieve five healthcare competencies outlined by the Institute of Medicine (IOM) in their *Quality Chasm* series. Those competencies—*quality improvement, patient-centered care, work in interdisciplinary teams, evidence-based practice,* and *using informatics*—will, in the IOM's vision, improve healthcare delivery in the United States. These and very similar competencies have been foci of healthcare improvement plans in many other countries as well. The international literature supporting moves in these directions is growing daily. Informatics has made our world accessible as it never has been before. Not only do we need to work in interdisciplinary teams in our own institutions, but teamwork now crosses borders as all nations strive to improve health for their citizens.

The conceptualization of CT throughout this book comes from our years of research in this area, most notably our Delphi Study to find a consensus description for CT in nursing. Through that research, an expert panel of 55 nurses from 9 countries and 23 U.S. states described 17 dimensions of CT in nursing—10 habits of the mind (affective dimensions) and 7 cognitive skills. The habits of the mind are *confidence, contextual perspective, creativity, flexibility, inquisitiveness, intellectual integrity, intuition, open-mindedness, perseverance,* and *reflection*. The skills are *analyzing, applying standards, discriminating, information seeking, logical reasoning, predicting,* and *transforming knowledge*. With those 17 dimensions, CT may be broken into manageable units as we describe thinking within the competency contexts.

Throughout this book, we often use the terms *critical thinking* (CT) and *thinking* interchangeably. We acknowledge that these terms are not synonymous in other contexts; however, within health care, we believe that all thinking is critical.

Keeping a focus on concrete, active learning strategies to promote CT, we have several strategies (called "TACTICS" to mirror our title) or practice activities throughout all chapters, except for the last two. These activities will help readers reflect on their personal and professional thinking styles while practicing CT-enhancing strategies. Some TACTICS are for educators to use in academic or practice settings; others are directed toward clinicians. Chapters 10 and 11 contain no TACTICS because, in a sense, each entire chapter focuses on tactics—to assess CT (Chapter 10) and to deal with complex change (Chapter 11).

We believe that you may now be able to see where the book's title comes from. Obviously, the idea of *tactics* comes from our desire to provide practical strategies. As an acronym, it stands for several activities important to promoting CT: *Tracking* alludes to following thinking paths, making them visible and therefore open for study and enhancement. *Assessing* denotes discerning the quality of thinking. *Cultivating* implies a growth-enhancing process; CT is not a concrete end point, but a process that may be enhanced. *Thinking*, as we described earlier, is defined as critical thinking with 17 dimensions. *Improve* is just what it says; we want to promote better CT. *Competency-based strategies* comes from the IOM competencies that serve as the context for our CT discussions. *Competency-based* implies performance of CT in the real world, as opposed to an academic checklist. *Strategies* are those means by which CT is practiced and enhanced so that healthcare quality may be enhanced.

Adding to what we hope are practical qualities of this book for busy clinicians, students, and educators, we have written in short segments and set off specific ideas in easily visible boxes, tables, and figures. Although our focus has been on thinking, we have needed to provide information on the contextual issues. Out of necessity, our descriptions of subjects such as informatics, evidence-based practice, and quality improvement are short and not meant to be primary references on those subjects. We hope that we have provided enough context for our readers to focus on the CT parts.

We appreciate the value of humor and visual variety to thinking and have therefore enlisted the aid of two superb artists, Mark Steele and Jesse Rubenfeld, to render cartoons here and there and make some of our ideas come alive. Our intention is to keep you visually stimulated so that your thinking stays at its peak and piqued.

We start this book with a chapter titled, "*Why* Critical Thinking?" in keeping with our belief that most CT journeys start best with questions. We also want you to appreciate, right from the start, why CT is so important. Unfortunately, the words *critical thinking* have become a bit hackneyed over the past few years. Because many groups have stated the need to address CT, it seems that everyone talks about it. We have found, however, that there are lots of things labeled *critical thinking* that really do not address thinking per se.

Chapters 2, 3, and 4 set the stage for understanding CT in a *what, who, why, how, where,* and *when* format. Chapter 2, "*What* Is Critical Thinking?" provides the framework of the 17 dimensions, how they were developed, and their special place as one of the few conceptualizations of CT that was based on evidence from nurses and linked to health care. Chapter 3, "*Who* Are the Critical Thinkers?" shows the importance of individual, cultural, and environmental factors that define us as thinkers. We specifically address our intended audience of clinicians and educators as we provide various strategies for CT self-reflection. Chapter 4, combines the "*How, When,* and *Where* of CT" because those factors are too intertwined to be addressed separately. This chapter introduces the five IOM competencies as the context for CT and becomes one of two bookends for the following chapters, each of which focuses on one competency. This chapter suggests specific strategies for educators to promote CT in their teaching, and strategies for clinicians to practice CT reflection in action.

Chapters 5–9 focus on the five IOM competencies. Chapter 5, "Critical Thinking, Quality Improvement, and Safety," describes the risk-laden state of affairs in health care, traces the history of quality improvement schemes, and justifies the need for reform. That reform is framed as a move toward enhanced CT. Chapter 6, "Critical Thinking and Patient-Centered Care," describes the shift from the old style of provider-centered care and explores patients' and significant others' CT as they interface with providers' CT. Chapter 7, "Critical Thinking and Interdisciplinary Teams," differentiates individual and team CT and shows how both are vital to quality health care. Chapter 8, "Critical Thinking and Evidence-Based Practice," demonstrates how important CT is to the various phases and tasks in this shift from basing practice on traditions and authority to practice based on the best evidence. Chapter 9, "Critical Thinking and Informatics," explores this burgeoning field and how various dimensions of CT are used to deal with information technology. We acknowledge the special challenges that the rapidly changing field of informatics holds for nurses like us who are "old"— primarily in their 40s and 50s.

Chapter 10 explores a popular, but frustrating, topic in nursing—that is, "Assessing Critical Thinking." Clinicians and health educators are being asked to show how their CT, and that of students, is improving. Because that assessment need has been so strong, especially in academic settings, most evaluation plans and instruments have been taken from other disciplines and have questionable validity in healthcare arenas. Or, they have been created without a clear description of CT or how it works. We offer suggestions for assessment methods, including one based on our research. Having established validity with our research-based 17 CT dimensions, we have shown respectable interrater reliability in limited testing of a method that is efficient, without compromising assessment of all the complexities of CT.

Chapter 11 is the other "bookend" for the previous chapters, which placed CT in the context of competencies and assessment. Originally, we envisioned this chapter as a look at the day-to-day realities, but as we finished with the previous chapters, we realized how strong the theme of complex change was throughout the book and titled the chapter, "Thinking Realities of Yesterday, Today, and Tomorrow." We described the dynamic nature of CT and how it fits perfectly with complex adaptive systems and their constant state of flux.

This book includes two appendixes. Appendix A is the CT Inventory that we developed; it has been updated for this edition based on responses from users in many classes and workshops. We have found that prompts, such as those in the inventory, help people think about their thinking, an essential prerequisite for improving CT.

We hope you will find this book practical and CT-stimulating. The complex healthcare system has no choice but to change to meet the needs of society today. Clinicians must use their CT to contribute their part to that change, and educators must change their teaching to prepare better critical thinkers Those changes, as outlined by many, including the IOM, must occur so that clinicians come to practice with visions of a future with higher quality care.

Because we are primarily educators these days, we enlisted the aid of our nurse practitioner colleague, Jane Duerr, to make sure we have well represented the clinician side of this book. Her stories from the "swampy lowlands" (to borrow a phrase from Schon) have counterbalanced our ivory tower views. We hope our clinician readers agree. For similar reasons and to capture day-to-day realities of CT in context, we have included several "stories" from nurses and others in practice arenas.

Enjoy your thinking journey as you read and reflect. We look to you to continue making CT a natural process within health care, today and tomorrow.

Acknowledgments

As with the first edition, this second edition would not have come to life without the assistance of many people. We would like to thank our nursing colleagues who gave us positive feedback on our previous writing projects, as well as the honor of the *AJN Book of the Year* award for the first edition. Thanks to Dr. George Allen, whose writing expertise we continue to envy; you taught us much about research on critical thinking assessment methods. To Drs. Margaret Lunney and Marsha Fonteyn, who have for years advocated for the importance of critical thinking in nursing and supported our work, you remain an inspiration to us. To Dr. Ada Sue Hinshaw, who gave us her valuable time and expertise by writing the foreword for the first edition of this book, we bow in admiration and thanks. And to Dr. Elaine Tagliareni, who agreed to write the foreword to this second edition in spite of her busy schedule as president of the National League for Nursing and Professor/Independence Foundation Chair of the Community College of Philadelphia, we are indebted. We are deeply honored to have such a distinguished pair of nursing leaders acknowledge the value of this work to the profession.

To our colleagues in practice, we again tip our hats in thanks. In particular, we are grateful to Marcia Hegstad, whose daily practice is the epitome of the power of nurses to effect positive change, and Judy Meyers, for whom evidence-based practice is as matter of fact as breathing. We sincerely appreciate your reviews for this edition.

We extend our sincere gratitude to our newest contributors: Diane DiFiore and Sandra Schmitt, who shared their groundbreaking work in patient-centered care, and Kate Kimmet, who provided examples of the thinking challenges of converting to electronic records. You are the nurses we want taking care of us. We are also indebted to Elizabeth Bucciarelli, Eastern Michigan University's health sciences librarian, whose patience and passion for helping students and faculty are unsurpassed. Thank you all for sharing your experiences with us so that your stories could inspire our readers.

We would also like to thank our nursing students at Eastern Michigan University, who are good natured about our frequent critical thinking discussions and our creative attempts to teach thinking in innovative ways. We especially want to thank David Caraballo for his reflection papers and Jose Valderrama for sharing his Hispanic cultural norms. Their contributions were kept in the second edition because they clearly demonstrated quality thinking. We would also like to acknowledge the RN-to-BSN students in Monroe, Brighton, and Livonia, Michigan, who shared numerous insights into their critical thinking during classes.

To Mark Steele, our cartoonist, who constantly amazes us with his ability to capture our ideas in humorous sketches, we say thanks for sharing your talents. And to our newest illustrator, Jesse Rubenfeld, we are grateful for his fresh, creative approach in capturing several of the new ideas in this edition.

To Jane Duerr, our colleague and dear friend who humbles us with her vast knowledge of nursing practice, we cannot find adequate words to express our gratitude. Her editing and help with developing new case studies were unbelievably generous, but most of all, we are grateful to her for cheering us on through the minutiae of editing.

Last, but not least, we'd like to thank our families, who again tolerated endless hours of viewing only the backs of our heads against the computer screen, who understood our absence from significant events, and who survived our mood swings. We love you and are so grateful that you do the household chores, feed us, run errands, and provide emotional support continually. Jesse and Tyler, thanks for the ongoing "Go Mom!" Rich, as always, thanks for your editing and re-editing; you are the expert final hurdle that allowed us to think this was good enough to give to the publisher. Nothing would get finished without your help and support. Dan and Anna, Amanda and Ryan, thanks for always asking how things are going with "the book." Kenn, thanks for ongoing support. Thank you Andrew and Allison, and Penelope, for just being you; your presence continues to put smiles on our faces.

Contributors

Jane Duerr, MSN, APRN, BC,
contributor of clinical scenarios and diligent reviewer.

Mark Steele, artist, contributor of cartoon art
(www.MarkSteeleArt.com).

Jesse Rubenfeld, illustrator, contributor of cartoon art
(www.jesserubenfeld.net).

Why Critical Thinking?

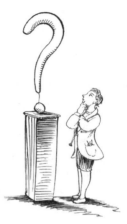

Healthcare delivery, and nursing in particular, is in dire need of critical thinkers. If you don't believe us, look at **Box 1-1** for the words of other authors. The ever-changing healthcare system is becoming increasingly complex and fraught with decision points where mistakes can occur. Clinicians make a jillion decisions every day. Most of those decisions are made in microseconds but can have very serious consequences. Some decisions allow for more thinking time, consultation with others, and a search of other resources before coming to a conclusion. But all decisions must be accurate and made in a timely manner.

There are many resources—books, articles, speeches—out there telling us what needs to be done to improve the quality of health care. Many of them allude to the need for critical thinking (CT), but few provide concrete suggestions for how to improve thinking. That's because it's not simple to improve thinking; it's not even simple to study it. Even a definition of nursing CT is hard to find. As complex as the healthcare system is, so too is CT.

The place of nurses in the healthcare system is also complex and getting increasingly so. Nurses are expanding their roles, taking on more responsibility, and learning to adapt to constant change. The kind of thinking that nurses do is convoluted and usually occurs in what Schon (1983) called the "swampy lowlands." The thinking of nurses is much more complex than most people realize.

BOX 1-1	*Why* Critical Thinking Is Essential in Nursing

"To provide quality care in this environment, nurses need to develop critical thinking (CT) skills that will provide them with expertise in flexible, individualized, situation-specific problem-solving." (Brunt, 2005, p. 60)

"Other reasons why nurses must be competent critical thinkers include the dramatic changes happening in health care related to information technology, fiscal cutbacks, human resource limitations, and the acuity of many patient care situations." (Carter & Rukholm, 2008, p. 134)

". . . critical thinking is an integral part of clinical decision making and therefore a routine part of nurses' work." (Daly, 2001, p. 121)

"To deal effectively with rapid change nurses need to become skilled in higher-level thinking and reasoning. . . . There is not always theoretical evidence to support practice, therefore, nursing needs to incorporate into its practice critical thinking processes to provide new answers to practical questions. . . . Every day nurses sift through an abundance of data and information to assimilate and adapt knowledge for problem clarification in an attempt to find solutions." (Edwards, 2007, p. 303)

"As health care systems become more complex . . . it is important for nurses to develop critical-thinking, problem-solving, and reflective practice techniques." (Rogal & Young, 2008, p. 28)

"Increasingly complex needs and expanding roles in the delivery of health care require professional nurses to be capable critical thinkers and self-directed learners." (Worrell & Profetto-McGrath, 2007, p. 420)

It is within this complex context that we explore CT in nursing. We want to impress on our readers why CT is so vital. We start this book with why, even before we tell you what CT is, because we want you to let your curiosity and questioning attitude lead the way into this exciting adventure.

Why Questions and Thinking

Why questions imply a search for reason, purpose, meaning, and value. The word *why* is frequently used to initiate inquiry, provide logic, justify conclusions, and find causes. *Why* demonstrates one of the first forms of thinking and exploration we used as children ("Why is the sky blue?"). Those of you with young children who constantly ask why might want the word banned from the dictionary on some of your tired days. But *why*, and the thinking connected with *why*, has triggered many important discoveries over the years. The discovery of penicillin, Einstein's theory of relativity, the exploration of space, and even the discovery of Viagra all followed *why*. (In fact, according to a personal communication with a pharmaceutical industry research scientist, it was a nurse who asked the question that led to the discovery of Viagra as a treatment for erectile dysfunction. During clinical trials of a pharmacological treatment of cardiovascular problems, she noticed that the volunteers were reluctant to return unused trial medications. She asked *why*, and the rest is history!)

For many, the natural tendency to ask *why* has diminished after years of traditional schooling. That is sad and also a bit frightening because *why* questions are powerful instigators of thinking. Even Albert Einstein emphasized the value of *why* questions when he said, "The important thing is to never stop questioning. Curiosity has its own reason for existing," and "I am neither especially clever nor gifted, I am only very very curious" (Famous Quotes and Famous Sayings Network, n.d.).

Why is also the favorite word of many educators who encourage students to provide rationales for their nursing interventions. *Why* is used by clinicians when they work as preceptors and mentors for new staff or when they question their own practice. Questioning why something is happening with a patient can be a life-saving inquiry. Clinicians and educators alike believe that *why* questions encourage critical thinking (Scheffer, 2001). We will tease your brain to consider why in this first stop at action learning, TACTICS 1-1. As discussed in the preface, TACTICS for clinicians and educators will be used throughout this text to engage you in activities that will stimulate your critical thinking and move thinking from abstract concepts to practical contexts.

TACTICS 1-1
_____

Exploring Your Use of *Why*

Clinicians and Educators

With a colleague or on your own, think about the last time you asked *why*. How many times a day do you ask it? Enough times to learn what you want to know? Too many? And what does it lead to? Are you simply asking out of habit, or do you then pursue the answers that prompt you to ask more questions and delve even deeper? How do colleagues react to your *why* questions? What motivates you to ask *why*?

Discussion

The answers to these questions should stimulate reflection. Are you satisfied with your answers? *Why* questions that stimulate reflection can prompt searches for purpose, meaning, and value. The great philosophers asked all these classic questions: *Why* are we here? *Why* do we exist? *Why* do we care? On a less esoteric level, reflection on *why* helps us understand and appreciate the value of thinking. So *why* does CT benefit health care? To answer, we will look at *why* there has been so much interest in thinking in recent years. We will also respond to *why* thinking is so important.

Asking *why* questions will inevitably lead one to ask more questions, such as *who, what, when,* and *where.* It is this questioning stance that is essential to studying CT. We'd like our readers to begin their CT journey with questions for two reasons. First, we know this approach works because that's how we began our travels through the CT maze. Many years ago, we knew why CT was important in nursing, and we asked how we could help nursing students become better thinkers; our exciting exploration of reading, researching, talking, and writing about CT took off. We want to share our discoveries so that you can build on what we have learned. Second, we'd like you to think about your questions, and the questions that they lead to, because they are the essence of great thinking.

The great educational philosopher Paulo Freire (1998) wrote,

> To stimulate questions and critical reflection about the questions, asking what is meant by this or that question, is fundamental to curiosity. Otherwise, all we have is the passivity of students in the face of the discursive explanations of the teacher and answers to questions that have not been asked. (p. 80)

Although we cannot hear your questions, we'd like you to imagine a dialogue with us. Think about your questions and jot down your reflections on them in the margins as you read along. Even though we have been immersed in the teaching of CT in nursing for two decades, we are frequently faced with new questions. What is your most burning question about CT in nursing? Write it here, and after reading the remaining chapters, look back and see if that question was answered. My burning question is:

_____

_____

_____

Why the Interest in CT in Health Care and Healthcare Education over the Last Two Decades?

Thinking has been a topic of discussion for philosophers for centuries, but other disciplines have also been concerned about thinking. Schon (1983) explored thinking in medicine, engineering, law, business, and education. Dreyfus and Dreyfus (1986) described the importance of thinking in the aviation industry.

Hundreds of thousands of articles and thousands of books have been written about CT in all disciplines. There are courses, whole curricula, and even institutes designed to improve thinking. We taught a required undergraduate nursing course called Critical Thinking in Nursing for several years. The National League for Nursing (NLN) highlighted the importance of promoting thinking in nursing curricula (NLN, 2006). An Australian Web site provides up-to-date information on colleges, universities, forums, and ongoing research on CT (Austhink, 2007). In health care, accrediting bodies, policy makers, and others promote CT. The Institute of Medicine (IOM; 2004) addressed CT across disciplines for improving national health care. Obviously, many people and organizations think critical thinking is very important; some of their statements about the benefits of thinking are shown in **Box 1-2**.

BOX 1-2	**The Benefits of CT**

"Professional knowledge is mismatched to the changing characteristics of the situation of practice—the complexity, uncertainty, instability, uniqueness, and value conflicts, which are increasingly perceived as central to the world of professional practice." (Schon, 1983, p. 14)

Problems encountered in practice are not in the book. (Schon, 1983)

"Knowledge is discovered by thinking, analyzed by thinking, organized by thinking, transformed by thinking, assessed by thinking, and most importantly acquired by thinking." (Paul, 1992, p. xi)

Thinking helps us recognize beliefs and assumptions that our minds consider to be facts. (Brookfield, 1995)

Knowledge, facts, and information are frequently equated with intelligence. But the ability to use knowledge in logical, ethical, and moral ways is not always equal to the quality of the knowledge, facts and information. Thinking provides the screening mechanism for converting knowledge, facts and information into practical application in the real world. (Schon, 1983)

". . . no way to create a neat and tidy step-by-step path to knowledge that all minds can mindlessly follow." (Paul, 1992, p. xi)

Pure logic and analytical reasoning is inadequate for expert decision making. Expert decision making is a blend of careful analysis, intuition and the wisdom and judgment gleaned from experience. Human thinking and decision making continues to exceed that of machines (artificial intelligence) because of three key factors: awareness of the environment, the ability to discriminate, and tolerance for ambiguity. (Dreyfus & Dreyfus, 1986)

"Only by changing how we think can we change deeply embedded policies and practices." (Senge, 1990, p. xiv)

"The deepest insight usually comes when they [people] realize that their problems, and their hopes for improvement, are inextricably tied to how they think." (Senge, 1990, p. 53)

Self-regulation, critical thinking, and creative thinking are probably the most important dimensions influencing learning. (Marzano & Pickering, 1997)

True understanding comes from the ability to think and act flexibly, distinguish nuance, appreciate context, and use reflection. (Wiggins & McTighe, 2001)

Our conceptualization of CT, the details of which are coming in Chapter 2, comes from years of practice and research in this area—most notably our Delphi study, which sought to find a consensus description for CT in nursing. Through that research, an expert panel of 55 nurses from nine countries and 23 U.S. states described 17 dimensions of CT in nursing—10 habits of the mind (affective dimensions) and 7 cognitive skills (Scheffer & Rubenfeld, 2000). The habits of the mind are *confidence, contextual perspective, creativity, flexibility, inquisitiveness, intellectual integrity, intuition, open-mindedness, perseverance,* and *reflection.* The cognitive skills are *analyzing, applying standards, discriminating, information seeking, logical reasoning, predicting,* and *transforming knowledge.* These 17 dimensions show CT broken down into manageable units. Because CT is complex, studying its pieces makes it more understandable, allowing you to see the thinking within various contexts. (Throughout the remainder of this text, every time we use one of the 17 dimensions, you will see them in italics to reinforce the language of thinking that you can begin to incorporate into your practice.)

So why has there been so much emphasis on CT in health care over the last few decades? One only has to pick up a newspaper or magazine or listen to the news to learn the answer. Some of the key matters that require more or better thinking are the information and technology explosions; dwindling resources; cost containment; third-party payer gatekeeping; demographics; morbidity and mortality data; patient safety and failure to rescue; and emergent ethical dilemmas such as the right to life, prolongation of life without quality, and stem cell research.

All healthcare disciplines are recognizing the need to pool their thinking to come up with better ways to deal with such complex issues. A notable example of such pooled thinking is the Institute of Medicine (IOM) project (IOM, 2003). The project's charge was to tap into the thinking energy of an interdisciplinary group—nurses, physicians, pharmacists, physical therapists, social workers, and others—to identify new directions for health care. Past solutions clearly do not address the growing complexity of our current problems. If it's not working today, it surely will fail tomorrow. To quote from Albert Einstein again, "The significant problems we face cannot be solved at the same level of thinking we were at when we created them" (Famous Quotes and Famous Sayings Network, n.d.).

One outcome of the IOM (2003) work was the development of five competencies—patient-centered care, interdisciplinary teams (IDTs), evidence-based practice, informatics, and quality improvement. These competencies were developed to help guide the thinking of all healthcare disciplines toward a unified plan of practice, education, and research to promote safe, effective, and efficient patient care. We will discuss these competencies fully in Chapters 5–9, but for now, let's look at some of the basic benefits of thinking in health care and who benefits from it. We'll start with a simple nursing situation and help Joyce, a novice clinician, who had trouble with a colostomy dressing.

TACTICS 1-2

Exploring Joyce's Thinking

> *Now wait a minute! I've done colostomy dressing changes a dozen times; I followed all the steps of the protocol exactly as I always do. Afterward I even checked out the textbook the nursing student left on the unit, and it says to do exactly what I did. So I'm asking myself, why didn't it work?*

Now refer to **Box 1-1** and **Box 1-2** and see if you can find any thinking clues that would help Joyce with her dilemma.

Discussion

The second statement in **Box 1-2**, "Problems encountered in practice are not in the book" (Schon, 1983), is a good match for what happened to Joyce. Do other statements also fit? "Not in the book" is the key here. One problem with a practice discipline such as nursing is that the real world seldom, if ever, looks like the book world. Nurses must rely on something else to deal with the many problems encountered in practice. Everything about nursing is contextual. Thinking is the one constant that will go from context to context.

The Context of Thinking

Studying CT by itself, outside context, is like studying how to take care of a colostomy without ever seeing a patient with a colostomy. There's only the abstraction of the idea, not the actual day-to-day reality of the concept. We can tell you why CT is important, but you won't fully appreciate that importance until you see CT in action. Studying CT by itself is a wonderful philosophical activity, but as nurses, we must look at CT in action. CT is a tool to be used in the muddy world of health care.

Because CT must be implemented within the context of specific problems or issues, this text addresses the CT needed to achieve five healthcare competencies outlined by the IOM in its Quality Chasm series. These competencies—patient-centered care, work in IDTs, evidence-based practice, using informatics, and quality improvement—will, in the IOM's vision, improve healthcare delivery in the United States (IOM, 2003). These and very similar competencies have been the foci of healthcare improvement plans in many other countries as well, and the international literature supporting movement in this direction is growing daily. Indeed, we have much to learn from clinicians, researchers, and educators in countries such as Canada, the United Kingdom, Australia, and the Netherlands, especially in the area of evidence-based practice. Informatics has made the world accessible as it never has been before. Not only do we need to work in IDTs in our own institutions, but teamwork now crosses borders as all nations strive to improve health for their citizens.

The Big Picture of *Why* Thinking Is Important

We've learned that the purpose of asking *why* is to find meaning and value or benefit. To focus on benefits, we need to explore who benefits and what is the benefit—*why* is thinking important to them? We will use the term *stakeholders* to describe the individuals and groups who have a "stake" (something to gain or lose) in some endeavor. Stakeholders may gain or lose power, control, money, and—yes—health. They are also thinkers who gain or lose from thinking or not thinking. And their thinking has an effect on the whole as well. See how complex this is?

To use a two-dimensional analogy, consider all the stakeholders in health care as being in a sequence of concentric circles. The innermost circle in the healthcare system contains the primary stakeholders. We classify them as primary because they benefit directly from the thinking of healthcare providers and, it is hoped, contribute their thinking as well. This primary group includes patients and their significant others.

The concentric circle of thinkers closest to the primary stakeholders includes clinicians, educators, and other providers in the IDT. The thinking of these people very directly affects patient outcomes. If done properly, the thinking of the individuals in this circle merges smoothly with the thinking of the primary stakeholders of the innermost circle. The results of that merged thinking are quality patient outcomes.

Moving outward, the next circle in this image would include unit managers, administrators, third-party payers, healthcare organizations, government groups, and healthcare professions. These stakeholders experience less direct effects of thinking in the "swampy lowlands of care" but are still essential stakeholders because their thinking has both positive and negative outcomes as well. Their impact has broader, long-lasting, and longer-term consequences as a result of legislation, policies and procedures, and guidelines.

Now let's take this two-dimensional image of concentric circles and make it three-dimensional. Visualize the primary stakeholders (patients and significant others), along with clinicians, educators, and the IDT, as the very center or nucleus. Take all those concentric circles full of other stakeholders' thinking and spin them around so they are on different planes. Picture the images from grade school of the rings of electrons rotating around the spinning nucleus of an atom. Are you getting the idea of the complexity and dynamic nature of thinking among the stakeholders?

Don't get overwhelmed by this complexity. We are going to help you dissect, or "up pack," things to get a better look at the thinking involved. Or, if you want us to sound more professional, we are going to do some *analyzing* to better understand the pieces of thinking and the impact that has on stakeholders.

Major Stakeholders and Critical Thinking

This next section focuses on CT with the major stakeholders. The major stake-holders in health care include two basic groups. Patients and significant others are the primary stakeholders group because they experience the direct consequences of thinking or nonthinking care. Clinicians, educators, and IDTs make up the second major group. This group is closest to the recipients of care and see and feel the "up-close and personal" results of thinking or nonthinking. These two groups and their thinking have the most impact on patient outcomes.

Quality patient outcomes require multiple levels of thinking from all stake-holders even beyond the major ones. Patients and significant others are thinkers themselves and often struggle to coordinate their thinking with that of the healthcare team.

Why *Is CT Important to Patients and Significant Others,*
the Primary Stakeholders?

Explaining why CT is important to patients and significant others is a bit of a no-brainer. Patients and significant others are at the center of the healthcare system. They are primary stakeholders in quality care. They are dependent on the thinking and actions of those who work in health care to receive quality care. In Chapter 6, we delve into CT and patient-centered care. For now, we will simply say that the delivery of safe, effective, and efficient care has always been the underlying goal of good nursing care. CT is essential to achieving these goals.

The following TACTICS exercise highlights how nursing staff using (or not using) CT affects the primary stakeholder, the patient. This exercise could be used by clinicians or educators to emphasize why thinking is important to safe, effective, and efficient patient care.

TACTICS 1-3

Exploring Safe, Effective, and Efficient Care for Mr. Stone

1. Read the scenario about Mr. Stone.
2. As you read, consider whether better thinking could have prevented the extended hospital stay.

Scenario 1-1: Mr. Stone

Mr. Stone is a 60-year-old male. He was admitted to the hospital 3 days before the Christmas holiday for emergency surgery after his left arm was severed midway between his wrist and elbow in an industrial accident. He was in good health prior to the accident but had smoked one to two packs of cigarettes a day for 40 years. The surgery to remove the severed portion of his arm and prepare for a prosthesis was successful. Nursing care included administration of pain medications, monitoring for infection at the wound site, and assistance with activities of daily living. Mr. Stone was expected to be discharged in two to three days. On day two after surgery, he developed pneumonia, and his hospital stay was extended six more days.

Discussion

Your answers about better thinking may be more general, but we'll start using the language of the dimensions of CT that we described earlier in this chapter, and about which we will give you details in the next chapter. Consider thinking dimensions that possibly were not used. If the nurses were *applying standards,* they would have designed care to include coughing, incentive spirometry, and precise assessment of respiratory status when developing their post-op care plan, not just medications and wound care. If the nurses were using *contextual perspective,* they would have more carefully assessed Mr. Stone's smoking habits and any history of respiratory problems. If the nurses were *discriminating,* they would have identified Mr. Stone as a very high-risk patient for post-op pulmonary complications because of his smoking. If the nurses were *predicting,* they would have recognized the serious consequences of not developing a rigorous plan for post-op coughing and deep breathing. They might even have made a referral to respiratory therapy to institute such a prevention plan.

Of course, Mr. Stone might have developed pneumonia in spite of all those nursing interventions; however, with better CT, the chances of this outcome would have been greatly reduced. Not only did Mr. Stone suffer the physical and emotional pain of the loss of an arm and early retirement, but because of his potentially preventable pneumonia, he also was hospitalized over the Christmas and New Year's Day holidays, a time of year that he would have enjoyed with family and friends at home.

In addition to safe care, CT is important for effective and efficient care. Effective care is individualized and accurate. It employs the correct interventions for the health situation at hand. Efficient care requires timely thinking so that resources are used appropriately. If Mr. Stone's nurses had been more effective in their thinking, they would have individualized their assessment, accurately diagnosed his risk for pneumonia right from the start, and implemented proper interventions. In addition, if Mr. Stone's nurses had used more CT, his hospital stay would have been shorter, thus saving time, money, and energy. In short, his care would have been more efficient. This scenario demonstrates the impact that thinking has on patients and their significant others. CT makes a huge difference in patient care outcomes!

The group of stakeholders in the next circle includes the clinicians, the educators, and the IDT. The stakeholders in this circle have the most direct impact on outcomes for patients.

Why *Is CT Important to Clinicians?*

Clinicians who think critically have more confidence in their reasoning. Confidence in reasoning allows nurses to speak their minds, to openly identify potential errors and "near misses," to contribute to team meetings, and to provide solid rationales for their decisions. Confidence empowers them to make valid contributions and decisions related to patient care and unit concerns.

CT is important to job satisfaction because it helps the clinician attain and maintain a professional nursing self-image. Even when parts of the nursing role are uncomfortable, good clinicians rely on professional ethics and intellectual integrity to reinforce their thinking. They derive job satisfaction from knowing that their thinking was actively engaged and the job was done to the best of their ability. One strategy to achieve such satisfaction is through reflection (Gustaffsson & Fagerberg, 2004). The scenario in TACTICS 1-4 illustrates how CT empowers decision making and enhances job satisfaction.

TACTICS 1-4

Enhancing Decision-Making Skills and Job Satisfaction Through Professional Integrity

1. Read Scenario 1-2.
2. Where did Juan use his best thinking?
3. How do you think Juan felt about the situation?
4. How did Juan's CT affect both decision making and job satisfaction?

Scenario 1-2: Juan's Home Visit

Juan is a community health nurse. His home-care patient load today included 17-year-old Jenny and her 3-week-old newborn, Billy. This was Juan's first home visit with Jenny, following up on a referral from the pediatrician's office because Billy had not gained weight since birth. Jenny was an unwed mother living with her parents in a spacious, professionally decorated home in an upper-middle-class neighborhood. Jenny looked tired and interacted only minimally with Juan, and she rarely looked at the baby, who was restless and fussy in his bassinet. Jenny's mother was home, and she did most of the talking, explaining how she expected Jenny to take full responsibility for Billy's care. In fact, Jenny's parents both worked and were frequently out of town on business, but because of Juan's visit, Jenny's mother stayed home to assure the nurse that though the visit was well-intentioned, it was certainly not necessary.

Juan examined Billy and found some disturbing data. Billy had lost another 3 ounces, and there were several dark areas on his back and legs. These markings had not been noted on the referral information.

Juan asked more questions. Jenny's mother assured him that Jenny was doing a fine job; they would be sure Billy got an extra feeding to gain his weight back; and all her children bruised easily, so Billy probably inherited that trait.

Juan, however, had to make a tough decision. He didn't want to believe the baby was being abused; this was a "normal"-looking family in a decent neighborhood. But he couldn't ignore the data: indications of ineffective maternal bonding, failure to thrive, and the apparent recent bruising all pointed to possible abuse. He also knew he was legally obligated to report suspected abuse. He was not comfortable with his decision to file a formal report, but he was confident it was the correct decision and that he could justify his reasoning. Juan found out later that the nurse at the pediatrician's office had similar concerns, but she only had the original weight loss data to go on. She told Juan that she didn't want to bias his thinking, so she didn't share her suspicions with him until after his visit.

Discussion

The key thinking areas that Juan used in this situation were *intellectual integrity* (although he did not want to believe that the infant was being abused, he had to consider the evidence), *applying standards* (he was legally required to report suspected abuse), *confidence* (he trusted his reasoning ability), and *logical reasoning* (he believed he had adequate evidence to support his suspicions).

Juan very likely also felt shocked, uncomfortable, and annoyed: shocked and uncomfortable that an upper-middle-class family might be abusing a child, and annoyed that the nurse in the pediatrician's office had not been open about her suspicions before the visit. He believed that he would have been *open-minded* enough to collect accurate information even if he had known of the nurse's "hunch."

When Juan reflected on the situation, he could justify and support his decisions. He knew his judgment was sound. As an individual and a professional, he derived satisfaction from knowing that he may have saved a life and provided an opportunity for a family to become more functional. He became a nurse because he wanted to help people, and that goal was accomplished. By doing his job with compassion and *intellectual integrity*, his behavior matched his role expectations, leading to job satisfaction.

Another way that CT benefits clinicians is by helping them move from novice to advanced beginner to competent to proficient and, ultimately, to expert (Benner, 1984). Throughout this process, the clinician moves away from the context-free rules of novice decision making to more sophisticated levels of thinking. Thinking is essential to expert nurses, who can imagine the whole of a situation from a few details. They use *reflection* in action; they have learned to trust their *intuition*. And they do all of this consistently. Expert nurses engage all CT dimensions so naturally and with such ease that their decisions look effortless. The hard work of the thinking behind their actions is rarely apparent unless they have recognized how important it is to think out loud. Many experts don't recognize how fine-tuned thinking is, but they couldn't be experts without it. This level of thinking benefits patients as well as nurses.

Why *Is CT Important to Educators?*

Nurse educators derive all the benefits that clinicians do from CT and more. CT helps novice (and experienced) educators accept the reality that they do not need to know everything. This acceptance usually comes harder to the novice educator. Most experienced educators come to realize that their brains do not have enough RAM to store all needed information and that the information they need to store keeps changing. With good CT habits of mind and skills, educators can be comfortable saying, "Let's go look that up," or "That's a good question, but I'll have to get back to you with an answer," or "Gee, I don't know, but let's see if we can figure it out." Thinking helps educators accept that they don't know it all, but because of their CT, they have effective strategies to search for the best information.

CT helps both service-based and academic-based educators promote learning processes. Notice that we said learning, not teaching. Teaching can be simply imparting information to a passive recipient. Learning requires active engagement among the learner, the content, and the educator. CT helps the educator design such interactive learning processes, illuminating the connection between pieces of information and allowing learners to discover answers through their own use of CT. For example, instead of simply sharing the latest evidence-based guidelines on the use of a new heparin-lock device with her staff, the staff development specialist provides the time and a place for focused dialogue, exploring the advantages and disadvantages of this new device. What are the challenges of using it? How is it best used in patient care? Does it meet guidelines? CT is important to create learning processes that maximize real behavior change and to transform information into useable knowledge.

CT also helps educators assess learning outcomes. For example, rather than selecting prepackaged assessment tools or educator-created competency check-offs for evaluation of learning, the critically thinking educator will examine existing tools to see how well they match with what needs to be learned. CT is needed to make those comparisons. For example, the nursing practice laboratory coordinator will anticipate how students should demonstrate competency in intramuscular injections. She will think about the answers to the following questions before she facilitates learning: What principles must the student articulate? What level of psychomotor skill must the student achieve? How can learning be designed to achieve the desired outcomes? What is the best way to assess that learning? These questions must be answered before the actual laboratory learning (and thinking) occurs with the students. This preteaching CT helps the coordinator design assessment tools that do the job they are intended to do. Without thinking about the assessment, as well as the learning, educators do only half of their thinking jobs. Thinking is the common denominator for service-based and academic-based educators if they want to promote learning that results in behavior change.

Why *Is CT Important to Interdisciplinary Teams?*

Effective IDTs (1) are made up of members from more than one discipline or professional group, (2) are expected to pool their CT skills and habits of the mind to expand on ideas, and (3) consider all members as equal partners in thinking, including patients and significant others. Current evidence indicates that functional interdisciplinary teams are the ideal for achieving desired health outcomes (IOM, 2003), and experts have noted the need to improve team thinking as well as actions (Halpern, 1998; Sanderson, 2003).

Other teams—multidisciplinary teams, for example—also benefit from CT, of course. But because CT is so important to IDTs, let us distinguish them from other healthcare teams: Multidisciplinary teams typically provide their discipline's perspective on patient situations but do not necessarily engage in collective problem identification and decision making. IDTs do all of this, and more.

So, what is different about CT in IDTs, and why is this thinking so important? We'll discuss the answers to these questions in Chapter 7, but to pique your interest, we have selected just three reasons why CT is so important to IDT.

First, the thinking of the individual team members provides a wide range of raw material on which team thinking can be built. Their CT, combined with their individual knowledge base and paradigms for problem identification and decision making, is an essential contribution to the team's overall functioning.

Second, the team can examine, discuss, and select options from a larger pool of information and "mix and match" options before making decisions. It is this pooling of ideas that leads to the synergistic thinking so valued in health care.

Third, team thinking is also important to group cohesion. Starting in the 1960s, the literature on group work and team work consistently identified group cohesion as essential to effective outcomes (Massello, 1998). Team thinking provides opportunities for developing trust and respect, both of which contribute to this group cohesion and, thus, to more effective outcomes—the goal of IDT work.

Why *Is CT Important to the Other Stakeholders?*

The thinking of stakeholders who are less directly involved in care also can have a profound effect on the care of patients. Their CT is also important to the stakeholders themselves because CT affects their more immediate goals, such as unit functioning, survival of the organization, social policy, and professional responsibilities. We have selected unit managers, healthcare administrators and third-party payers, and a collective of healthcare organizations, governments, and professions as examples of these indirect stakeholders. As you read, see if you can think of additional reasons why CT might be important to them and consider other such stakeholders who might be involved.

Why *Is CT Important to Unit Managers?*

Unit managers benefit from their own CT and the CT of others in many ways, including better use of resources, achieving unit goals, and demonstrating quality of care on the unit. The thinking unit manager (and thinking staff) might use *creativity* to rethink how clean linen is delivered to the unit in order to save money, or *flexibility* to schedule IDT meetings at convenient times to develop goals and strategies. He or she might model *inquisitiveness* by working with staff to identify new safety policies and procedures to improve quality on the unit. He or she might use *reflection* to mentor peers and improve consistency in management approaches (Hyrkas, Koivula, Lehti, & Paunonen-Ilmonen, 2003). Managers' CT abilities have a huge impact on all other stakeholders.

Why *Is CT Important to Healthcare Administrators?*

Administrators in charge of organizations such as hospitals, long-term care facilities, home care agencies, trauma centers, and outpatient clinics are primarily responsible for maintaining and developing their organizations and promoting quality service in a cost-effective way. CT is the only way to find solutions to what some view as polarized interests. For example, quality and cost-effectiveness are frequently viewed as opposites, yet CT can help reframe that perspective. Polarity management is one strategy for using CT to *analyze* commonalities and then find *creative* ways to deal with other issues (Yoder-Wise, 1995). *Transforming knowledge* is another CT essential for administrators whose organizations are moving toward more patient-centered care (Miller, Galloway, Coughlin, & Brennan, 2001). Hansten and Washburn (1999) noted that administrators must have "advanced abilities to think critically . . . to improve clinical systems, decrease errors and sentinel events, and engage staff involvement to refine patient care systems" (p. 39).

Administration in health care is not confined to the practice setting. Administrators in institutions of higher education that teach health providers also need and benefit from CT. The setting may be different, but the needs are the same; CT is important in finding the balance between quality education and its cost. We don't have to tell you that healthcare education—particularly in medicine, nursing, pharmacy, and dentistry—is expensive. Remember the bumper sticker, "If you think education is expensive, try ignorance!" Maybe we should make a bumper sticker that says, "If you think thinking time is expensive, try health care without it!"

Why *Is CT Important to Third-Party Payers?*

Speaking of cost, this is where thinking is important to third-party payers—the insurance companies, Medicare, and Medicaid. Remember Mr. Stone, who developed pneumonia because of inadequate CT? Fortunately, his insurance covered the cost of his prolonged hospitalization, but that cost was unnecessary and a waste of resources. According to data collected by the Michigan Nurses Association (MNA), "Hospital-acquired pneumonia among surgical patients may add between $22,390 and $28,505 per patient to hospital costs" (MNA, 2004, p. 8).

Third-party payers must rely on CT to maintain their ability to pay for health care and keep their stockholders happy. They particularly depend on *analyzing* and *predicting* to do their jobs. They also recognize the importance of changing their thinking from a focus on short-term goals to what will occur over the long term. Pronovost (2004) described a plan currently being used by Blue Cross and Blue Shield (BC/BS) in Michigan in which BC/BS works with interdisciplinary teams from 107 intensive care units to find ways to improve safety and save money. Other third-party payers will need to examine these problems more closely as the cost of health care, particularly of preventable conditions, rises.

Why *Is CT Important to Healthcare Organizations, Governments, and the Health-care Professions?*

The outermost circle of stakeholders contains the most complex organizations. CT at this level is very challenging and equally essential. Although at first glance these stakeholders may seem to have little impact on the day-to-day activities of healthcare organizations, in reality, their CT is very important to clinicians and educators. The CT of healthcare organizations, governments, and the healthcare professions influences the policies, legislation, and standards that guide both practice and education. It has long-term effects on the day-to-day activities and thinking of all stakeholders. Because these stakeholders have such a broad span of influence, they can use CT to see the "big picture" and the details, allowing them to design and implement policies that affect many people. Does this sound like *contextual perspective* or what?

Healthcare organizations need to use CT consistently to function effectively and achieve their missions and goals while maximizing their resources. For example, *creativity* helps them find better ways to organize staffing patterns. *Analysis* and *logical reasoning* help them examine infection patterns or track the rising costs of supplies. *Flexibility* helps them redirect services to meet changing customer needs.

All government organizations (both federal and state) that are mandated to protect the public welfare need at least *analysis, logical reasoning*, and *contextual perspective* to help accomplish their goals while balancing the demands of other activities, all competing for the same tax dollars. For example, *analysis* and *logical reasoning* can be used to determine why a state's mental health system is ranked lowest in the nation. *Contextual perspective* helps government groups understand how weather conditions affect the air conditioning needs of the growing numbers of citizens with chronic obstructive pulmonary disease.

Other healthcare professions also rely on all 17 CT dimensions to meet the criteria for their professional status. Those criteria will vary depending on the source you use, but the basics of any profession include a code of ethics, a body of knowledge, higher education, and self-regulation (Haynes, Boese, & Butcher, 2004). How could one achieve a code of ethics without *reflection* and *logical reasoning*? How could one develop a body of knowledge without *analysis* and *inquisitiveness*? How could a professional organization design guidelines for a university curriculum without *perseverance* and *information seeking*? How could one manage self-regulation and accreditation standards without *applying standards, discriminating,* and *intellectual integrity*? *Contextual perspective* is essential as healthcare professions move toward interdisciplinary teamwork, learning from each other while maintaining their autonomous bodies of knowledge. You can probably cite examples for all the remaining CT dimensions.

Summary of the Impact of Stakeholders' CT on Quality Patient Outcomes

That's a whole lot of folks who need to recognize the impact of their thinking (or nonthinking) and the aspects of their thinking dimensions. We have summarized why CT is important for these various stakeholder groups in **Box 1-3**. This is only a very brief overview that we hope you will be able to expand on as you continue your thinking journey.

BOX 1-3	*Why Is CT Important for Various Stakeholders?*

Why is CT important to:

1. Patients and significant others?
   Thinking promotes safe care.
   Thinking enhances effective care.
   Thinking increases efficient care.

2. Clinicians?
   Thinking empowers decision-making skills.
   Thinking enhances job satisfaction through professional integrity.
   Thinking achieves expertise in practice.

3. Educators?
   Thinking makes it OK to not know it all.
   Thinking promotes learning processes.
   Thinking enhances assessment of learning.

4. Interdisciplinary team (IDT)?
   Individual thinking provides the IDT with the raw material for problem identification and problem solving.
   Team thinking provides the synergy to create ideas that individuals would not achieve independently.
   Team thinking enhances group cohesion.

(continues)

BOX 1-3	(Continued)

5. Unit managers?

Thinking allows better use of resources.

Thinking promotes achieving unit goals.

Thinking demonstrates the quality of care on the unit.

6. Healthcare administrators?

Thinking promotes quality service in a cost-effective way.

Thinking is the way to find solutions to what some view as polarized interests, such as quality and cost-effectiveness.

Thinking promotes safe, quality patient-centered care.

7. Third-party payers?

Thinking maintains their ability to pay for health care.

Thinking keeps their stockholders happy.

Thinking keeps them in business.

8. Healthcare organizations, governments, and the healthcare professions?

Thinking allows them to see the "big picture" as well as the details.

Thinking allows them to design and implement policies that affect many people.

Thinking helps maximize resources.

Thinking forms professions' codes and bodies of knowledge.

What Else Is Needed to Emphasize *Why* CT Is Important?

Something is only important if we value it. Words on paper do not create value. As Fullan (1993) said, "You can't mandate what matters" (p. 21). CT can never be mandated; the only successful activity is using mandates "as catalysts to reexamining" (p. 24) the current state of affairs, which can lead to value changes. This applies to the nursing and healthcare sectors very clearly. Clinicians who are expected to promote CT but don't value it may give lip service to its importance and will not (1) commit the energy necessary for CT or (2) experience the role satisfaction that CT produces. Educators who expect to teach nursing and CT but do not value thinking will experience the same dilemmas.

So how can we help people learn to value CT? We start with Fullan's (1993) catalysts—words in mission statements, accreditation standards, and textbooks—and then we have to bring the words to life. We do this by talking about CT every day to nurture and cultivate our own CT and the CT of others. Consider the following scenario, in which a graduate student is explaining to his instructor how he modeled CT for a nursing student he was preceptoring on an inpatient medical surgical unit.

This scenario demonstrates why talking about your thinking makes it more real for your students (if you are an educator) or your staff (if you are a clinician). Because they cannot see your neurons firing, you have the responsibility to make CT overt. Once CT becomes overt through specific language, its value can be recognized.

Scenario 1-3: Modeling CT

A patient was admitted to an inpatient medical-surgical unit for evaluation of cardiac arrhythmia. She had a history of mental illness as well. Recent symptoms included nausea, diarrhea, and a low-grade fever. This was the reflection the graduate student teaching assistant shared with his instructor detailing how he had modeled his CT for an undergraduate nursing student:

I wanted the student to see how I was thinking through this problem and that it was OK to not have all the answers. The patient had a long history of bipolar disorder and had been taking lithium for several years, successfully managing her disease. The staff told us she was also a bit of a hypochondriac and that this was the second time this month she was complaining of the flu. I told the student, "We have to be careful and not let our perceptions affect our data collection; we have to be open-minded from the beginning. Let's use some inquisitiveness here and find out from the patient what is happening. We need a little more contextual perspective so we need to get some historical information, a sense of what has been going on in her life recently, food allergies, and so on. I'm also wondering about the possibility of lithium toxicity. Go grab a drug book and let's check that out. What do you think? How do her lab values compare to the norms? Let's do some analysis here and look at all the pieces and then think about how they do or don't fit together. Think about it for a minute and tell me what dimensions of our thinking will be needed next." We discovered that the patient was, in fact, having a toxic reaction to lithium. Her blood levels were over 1.5 mEq/L. She wasn't just being a hypochondriac. I really tried to use my CT words so that the student could see inside my brain. I had to figure this out all on my own—I want my student to have a head start.

The challenge is to really talk about thinking, not just talk about doing! It takes practice, *reflection,* and peer feedback to get things rolling. The TACTICS activity that follows was designed to help clinicians and educators stimulate, cultivate, and nurture their "talking about thinking."

TACTICS 1-5

Verbalizing CT So Others Will See the Value

Clinicians and Educators

This activity requires three people, paper and pencil, and maybe some colored highlighters. One person assumes the role of the educator, one person assumes the role of the staff member or student, and one person assumes the role of the observer. Ideally this activity could be videotaped, but it works equally well without taping. The activity can be repeated by exchanging roles after the first time around.

Part I (5–10 minutes)

EDUCATOR: Your job is to select a teaching situation that will help your staff or students learn some aspect of nursing care but will also allow you to model your thinking as you are modeling your explanation of care.

STAFF/STUDENT: Your job is to listen for the educator's CT messages and jot them down as you are learning.

OBSERVER: Your job is to listen for both the educator's and the staff or student's thinking. Take notes that can be shared with the others later. Note: What words were used that reflect thinking? How many thinking words (*open-mindedness, confidence, analyzing, predicting*, and so on) were used in comparison with action words ("Next I need to flush the tubing")? Be as specific as possible as you take notes.

Begin the exercise. After the 5–10 minutes, have each participant rate the educator, using the following scale of 1–10, with 10 being the total teaching activity.

What proportion of the teaching focused on doing?   1 2 3 4 5 6 7 8 9 10

What proportion of teaching focused on thinking?   1 2 3 4 5 6 7 8 9 10

Which specific CT descriptors were used? _____

What might the educator do differently the next time to more explicitly model thinking with CT words? _____

If you have highlighters, use them to mark the actual CT descriptors.

Part II (10–15 minutes)

OBSERVER: Share your notes and your rankings with the others.

STUDENT/STAFF: Share your notes and your rankings with the others.

EDUCATORS: Share your notes and your rankings with the others.

Discussion

How did everyone do? What did you discover about how your modeling of thinking can be used the next time you teach CT?

Educators in any setting are expected to teach thinking. Teaching CT, however, requires one to accept that CT is a process, not simply more content. For example, when teaching the process of communication, we don't simply lecture on it; we model it, provide lots of opportunities to practice it, and have students overtly identify skills such as restatement, clarifying, and open-ended questions. We use process recordings to help students see those skill labels and patterns of use. Teaching CT must also be process oriented. Reflection journals serve this purpose and are valuable tools to make thinking more overt.

Talking about thinking, as in the previous TACTICS exercise, helps us and others visualize thinking. Talking about thinking helps us recognize why CT is important to us and to our students, patients, organizations, and professions. Talking about CT using CT terminology can help us accomplish what organizational and professional mandates can only serve as catalysts for—valuing thinking.

PAUSE _____

and Ponder

Why *Do You Think CT Is Important?*

By now we hope you appreciate why CT is so important to the healthcare stakeholders, particularly why thinking is so important to clinicians and educators. CT is that important bridge that we will discuss further in Chapter 2, transforming information to useful knowledge on which patients and all the stakeholders can act. Without CT, any attempts for safe, effective, efficient health care are meaningless.

Reflection Cues

- *Why* questions imply a search for reason, purpose, meaning, and value.
- *Why* and the thinking connected with *why* have triggered many important discoveries over the years.
- Many disciplines believe that CT is important: medicine, engineering, law, business, education, aviation, and health care.
- Current healthcare situations that require more or better CT include the information explosion; dwindling resources; cost containment; third-party payer gatekeeping; morbidity and mortality data; patient safety and failure to rescue; and the emergent ethical dilemmas, such as right to life, prolongation of life without quality, and stem cell research.

- Many stakeholders experience the consequences of thinking and not thinking: patients and significant others, clinicians, educators and interdisciplinary teams, unit managers, healthcare administrators, third-party payers, healthcare organizations, governments, and healthcare professions.
- CT leads to safe, effective, and efficient care for patients.
- CT leads to empowered decision making, job satisfaction, and expertise in practice for clinicians.
- CT leads to realistic expectations and a focus on learning more than teaching.
- Clinicians and educators must begin to vocalize their CT to cultivate and nurture it in others.

References

Austhink. (2007). *Critical thinking on the web*. Retrieved November 7, 2008, from http://www.austhink.org/critical/pages/institutes.html

Benner, P. (1984). *From novice to expert: Power and excellence in nursing practice*. Menlo Park, CA: Addison-Wesley.

Brookfield, S. (1995). *Becoming a critically reflective teacher*. San Francisco: Jossey-Bass.

Brunt, B. A. (2005). Critical thinking in nursing: An integrated review. *Journal of Continuing Education in Nursing, 36*, 60–67.

Carter, L. M., & Rukholm, E. (2008). A study of critical thinking, teacher-student interaction, and discipline-specific writing in an online educational setting for registered nurses. *Journal of Continuing Education in Nursing, 39*, 133–138.

Daly, W. M. (2001). The development of an alternative method in the assessment of critical thinking as an outcome of nursing education. *Journal of Advanced Nursing, 36*, 120–130.

Dreyfus, H. L., & Dreyfus, S. E. (1986). *Mind over machine: The power of human intuition and expertise in the era of the computer*. New York: Free Press.

Edwards, S. L. (2007). Critical thinking: A two-phase framework. *Nurse Education in Practice, 7*, 303–314. doi: 10.1016/j.nepr/2006/09/004

Famous Quotes and Famous Sayings Network. (n.d.) *Famous quotes—Einstein quotes*. Retrieved August 1, 2004, from http://home.att.net/~quotations/einstein.html

Freire, P. (1998). *Pedagogy of freedom: Ethics, democracy, and civic courage* (P. Clarke, Trans). Lanham, MD: Rowman and Littlefield.

Fullan, M. (1993). *Change forces: Probing the depths of educational reform*. Bristol, PA: Falmer Press.

Gustaffsson, C., & Fagerberg, I. (2004). Reflection, the way to professional development? *Journal of Clinical Nursing, 13*, 271–280.

Halpern, D. F. (1998). Teaching critical thinking for transfer across domains: Dispositions, skills, structure training, and metacognitive monitoring. *American Psychologist, 53*, 449–455.

Hansten, R. I., & Washburn, M. J. (1999). Individual and organizational accountability for developing critical thinking. *Journal of Nursing Administration, 29*(11), 39–45.

Haynes, L., Boese, T., & Butcher, H. (2004). *Nursing in contemporary society: Issues, trends, and transition to practice*. Upper Saddle River, NJ: Pearson Prentice Hall.

Hyrkas, K., Koivula, M., Lehti, K., & Paunonen-Ilmonen, M. (2003). Nurse managers' conceptions of quality management as promoted by peer supervision. *Journal of Nursing Management, 11*, 48–58.

Institute of Medicine. (2003). *Health professions education: A bridge to quality.* Washington, DC: National Academies Press.

Institute of Medicine. (2004). *Keeping patients safe: Transforming the work environment for nurses.* Washington, DC: National Academies Press.

Marzano, R., & Pickering, D. (1997). *Dimensions of learning teacher's manual* (2nd ed.). Alexandria, VA: Association for Supervision and Curriculum Development.

Massello, D. J. (1998). Operations management: Administering the program. In K. J. Kelly-Thomas (Ed.), *Clinical and nursing staff development: Current competent, future focus* (2nd ed., pp. 337–364). Philadelphia: Lippincott.

Michigan Nurses Association. (2004). *The business case for reducing patient-to-nurse staff ratios and eliminating mandatory overtime for nurses.* Lansing, MI: Public Policy Associates. Retrieved February 5, 2009 from http://www.minurses.org/spc/MNA_Report_0607.pdf

Miller, J., Galloway, M., Coughlin, C., & Brennan, E. (2001). Care-centered organizations, Part I: Governance. *Journal of Nursing Administration, 31*(2), 67–73.

National League for Nursing. (2006). *Excellence in nursing education model.* New York: Author.

Paul, R. (1992). Critical thinking: *What every person needs to survive in a rapidly changing world.* Santa Rosa, CA: Foundation for Critical Thinking.

Pronovost, P. J. (2004, March). *Healthcare safety and quality revolution.* Paper presented at the American Association of Colleges of Nursing spring annual meeting, Washington, DC.

Rogal, S. M., & Young, J. (2008). Exploring critical thinking in critical care nursing education: A pilot study. *Journal of Continuing Education in Nursing, 39,* 28–33.

Sanderson, H. (2003). Implementing person-centered planning by developing person-centered teams. *Journal of Integrated Care, 11*(3), 18–25.

Scheffer, B. K. (2001). Nurse educators' perspectives on their critical thinking: Snapshots from their personal and professional lives (Doctoral dissertation, Eastern Michigan University, 2001). *Dissertation Abstracts International, 62, 02B,* 786.

Scheffer, B. K., & Rubenfeld, M. G. (2000). A consensus statement on critical thinking in nursing. *Journal of Nursing Education, 39,* 352–359.

Schon, D. A. (1983). *The reflective practitioner: How professionals think in action.* New York: Basic Books.

Senge, P. M. (1990). *The fifth discipline: The art & practice of the learning organization.* New York: Doubleday.

Wiggins, G., & McTighe, J. (2001). *Understanding by design.* Upper Saddle River, NJ: Merrill Prentice Hall.

Worrell, J. A., & Profetto-McGrath, J. (2007). Critical thinking as an outcome of context-based learning among post RN students: A literature review. *Nurse Education Today, 27,* 420–426. doi: 10.1016/jnedt.2006.07.004

Yoder-Wise, P. S. (1995). *Leading and managing in nursing.* St. Louis, MO: Mosby.

2

What Is Critical Thinking?

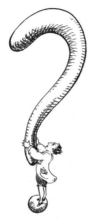

To emphasize the importance of this chapter's title question, we will pose some challenges for you. Consider how you would respond to these requests: (1) describe the thinking you use as a nurse, (2) improve your critical thinking, (3) tell us what critical thinking is, and (4) explain how critical thinking is supposed to be practiced in nursing. We would venture to guess that even though you consider yourself a good critical thinker, you'd be hard pressed to provide quick, simple responses. And, if you were then asked to describe how you became a nurse who thinks critically, it might be even more challenging. Don't be concerned: First, you're not alone, and second, that's what this book is designed to help you do—help you respond to requests such as those just mentioned.

Most people have difficulty describing their thinking processes, even expert clinicians and faculty who teach critical thinking (CT). That's not because they aren't good thinkers; it's just that, until recently, few people asked each other about their thinking, and we simply haven't developed a vocabulary to describe such heady things. When asked to describe their thinking, many people pause and say, "I just do!" When pressed to elaborate, you may get a variety of emotional responses. Many people will act frustrated because the request is unusual, they don't have ready answers, and they're too busy to think about it anyway.

If they're really frustrated, they might respond, "Why is it even important to try to describe thinking? Aren't actions more important in the big scheme of things?"

The answer is yes, but actions are only as good as their appropriateness to the problem or condition that prompted the action. In today's healthcare arena, those conditions change constantly. What you did yesterday might not work tomorrow or even an hour from now. You must keep abreast of new information and changing patient data and consistently make those things work together. And new information is being discovered and refined daily, if not hourly.

So what is a nurse to do? There's all this existing information, there's a constant flow of new information, and then there's the need to turn it all into a working knowledge so that you can provide safe, effective, efficient nursing actions. You need to bridge the gap between the ever-growing information and the actions it requires. You need a series of steps or a process to convert information into knowledge. Finally, you must translate that knowledge, which is very abstract, into practice actions, which are very concrete. That transition works best if you can recognize those steps or processes; otherwise, you are less likely to arrive at predictable and consistently successful actions.

We can't all be like Indiana Jones in the movie, *Indiana Jones and the Last Crusade*. He stepped off into the chasm as a leap of faith. After he found himself on firm footing, he threw pebbles back to define the bridge that was camouflaged by its surroundings. Think of CT as that bridge. We will provide some pebbles ahead of time; once you see that CT bridge, your mind will more easily transform information into knowledge, and that knowledge, albeit abstract, will be the basis of the best workable course of action. Why this is so important was addressed in Chapter 1, so we're hoping your curiosity is so stimulated, you are bursting to learn the details that we alluded to when we used the term *CT*.

The Critical Thinking "Bridge"

So CT is the metaphorical bridge between information and action, but what are those pebbles for? They're going to do for you exactly what they did for Indiana Jones: They're going to turn something that is invisible from one perspective into something visible from a new perspective. But first it might be helpful to look at the three reasons why the bridge (CT) is invisible in the first place. Reason Number 1: CT is intangible; you can't study it under a microscope, hold it, smell it, or examine it for a pulse. Reason Number 2: CT is very individual—no two people think in the same way, nor do they broadcast their thoughts, so it's impossible to learn how to think critically by watching only actions. Reason Number 3: CT requires effort. Many of us assume CT will just happen over time as we gain knowledge and experience, so we just wait and don't worry about it. This may have worked in the past, but time is a luxury these days. We need to use CT today, not tomorrow.

So how can you start to see this previously invisible CT? Can you do it without pebbles? To some extent, yes, you probably can. For example, think about the opposite of CT. We'll bet you can easily identify people who don't use CT. What do they do? Now think of a nurse you consider to be a great thinker. She's the person you want to work with, especially if you're a novice. If something new comes up, she's the one who can figure out how to deal with it. She's creative, open-minded, logical. Now, with this positive image, the next question is, Can you learn to get to that expert level of thinking? How and how quickly? Can you help other nurses get there too? The good news is yes, you can. However, this is where the pebbles come in. The pebbles are the three tools that will make the process of becoming a great CT nurse easier.

Pebbles on the Metaphorical Bridge

First, you need to be clear on just what CT in nursing is—for that, you need a definition. Second, you need to know how to describe what "it" looks like, using words to elaborate on the definition. Both of these tasks require a vocabulary. Once you can use specific words to describe your thinking processes, you can more easily discover what you're good at and where you need to improve. With a definition and words, you can also help others identify, describe, and improve their critical thinking. Third, you will need to visualize what CT words look like in action, particularly as CT is practiced in nursing. Addressing these three points—a definition, a vocabulary, and translating words to actions—will help us figure out the *what* of CT.

Pebble #1: Defining CT

Let's start by tackling the issue of defining and describing CT in nursing. We can't do justice to that task without some contextual and historical perspective. There are many descriptions of critical thinking in the literature; however, because many of those definitions are borrowed from other disciplines, they vary in terms of usefulness to nursing. We'll discuss some of the problems with those definitions in Chapter 10. For now, let's focus on the historical context of CT so that you can appreciate how essential this concept is to us, our patients, our students, and our society.[1]

In Western history, CT can be traced back to Socrates and his Socratic Method, or answering questions with questions. Actually, Socrates emphasized deep questioning of ideas that were accepted as fact but that may simply have been beliefs. For example, everyone then believed that the Earth was flat, but this did not make it a fact. Later, Plato and Aristotle expanded on Socrates' ideas to emphasize that things are not always what they seem and that sound reasoning takes into account objections to accepted ideas. During the Renaissance, Francis Bacon focused on empirical information gathering, establishing our modern research standards of

---

[1] With our apologies to the historians and philosophers in our audience who are already aware of this history, we will give only a quick overview of CT's philosophical roots. For those of you who yearn for more, check out some philosophy books or go to this Web site, which we used for much of the information in this section: http://www.philosophypages.com (Kemerling, 2001). Being Westerners, we will also apologize to other cultures, such as those from Asia, whose CT roots could be traced, for example, to the teachings of Lao Tzu and Confucius.

systematic study. That empirical, or fact, base was important to overcome the natural biases that our minds use to understand our world and our place in it. René Descartes promoted systematic doubt: All thinking should be questioned and tested. (It may be comforting to those who spend lots of time thinking about thinking that Descartes acknowledged our existence as thinking beings to be the most factual thing to know. Even if we doubt that anything else exists, we must exist to do the doubting. Now, think about that!) In the 18th century, Immanuel Kant's *Critique of Pure Reason* examined the conundrum of using principles for thinking that cannot be empirically tested. Consider this statement: We are "burdened by questions . . . prescribed by . . . reason itself . . . [which we] are not able to ignore, but which . . . [we are] also not able to answer" (Kant, 1787/1965, p. 7).

John Dewey, the often-cited CT promoter in educational circles, took CT into the 20th century with his pragmatic view of thought as part of human behavior. We'll revisit his ideas in Chapter 4. And Jean Piaget, cautioning about the dangers of egocentric and sociocentric characteristics of human thought, emphasized the need to be open to multiple points of view. In the 1980s, the aviation industry began designing strategies to help pilots progress from novice to expert levels more quickly (Dreyfus & Dreyfus, 1986). That industry was very interested in the CT of human pilots because an aircraft's autopilot could not be programmed to react to all the dynamic events that occur when taking off, flying, and landing an airplane. As advanced as artificial intelligence is, it cannot yet replace the human thinking required in emergency situations. Patricia Benner (1984), a well-known nursing theorist, collaborated with Dreyfus and Dreyfus in the development of her Novice to Expert Model of nursing care. It is not surprising that the aviation industry and professional nursing are equally concerned about critical thinking— both deal with split-second decision making to keep people safe.

Thinking, how the brain works, and how learning takes place became dominant themes in education in Western society in the early 1980s (Hart, 1983). Initially, the focus was on teaching CT in Kindergarten through Grade 12, with books such as *Developing Minds: A Resource Book for Teaching Thinking* (Costa, 1985). In the early 1990s, the movement to improve thinking spread to postsecondary education. Assessment of all students' CT skills is now part of college and university accreditation standards in the United States. For example, Criterion 4 of the Higher Learning Commission's Institutional Accreditation Guidelines (2007) cited the importance of "fostering and supporting inquiry, creativity, practice, and social responsibility" (p. 6).

Also during the 1990s, critical thinking became a focus in nursing education. The National League for Nursing (NLN; 2005a) listed CT among topics needed in educational programs preparing graduates for the demands of practice. The NLN also listed in its core competencies of nurse educators the need to facilitate learning. To facilitate learning, the educator "models critical and reflective thinking [and] creates opportunities for learners to develop their critical thinking and critical reasoning skills" (NLN, 2005b, Competency 1, bullet 7 & 8). The American Association of Colleges of Nursing's *Essentials of Baccalaureate Education for Professional Nursing Practice* (2008) listed the use of clinical/critical reasoning as one of its assumptions for a baccalaureate generalist graduate, and its accreditation arm— the Commission on Collegiate Nursing Education (CCNE)—required nursing programs to address all the components in the *Essentials* document, including CT (CCNE, 2008).

Thinking became a theme in healthcare delivery as well. The Joint Commission has, since the mid 1980s, focused on performance measurement or competency-based assessment and documentation in the healthcare arena (The Joint Commission, 2008). Competency-focused care requires clinicians and staff development specialists to hone their CT skills. In Case's (1998) "Competence Development: Critical Thinking, Clinical Judgment, and Technical Ability," staff development specialists were given practical strategies for nurturing CT. We will elaborate on the subject of competency and CT in Chapter 4. The American Nurses' Association also emphasizes CT in its *Nursing: Scope and Standards of Practice.* The language of CT is addressed in the Association's scope statement and incorporated throughout all the standards (2004). Nurse leaders have increasingly recognized the importance of thinking skills in nursing, but to guide this change, transformational leadership, supported by evidence-based management at all levels of administration, is needed (Hansten & Washburn, 1999; Institute of Medicine, 2004; Miller, Galloway, Coughlin, & Brennan, 2001; Schoenly, 1998; Thompson & Burns, 2004).

Outside of healthcare clinical settings, a seminal work by the American Philosophical Association (APA), under the direction of Facione, defined CT using a Delphi method to survey academicians. Philosophers composed roughly half of his 46-member panel; others were from fields such as education, physics, computer science, and psychology. They arrived at this consensus statement: "We understand critical thinking to be purposeful, self-regulatory judgment which results in interpretation, analysis, evaluation, and inference as well as explanation of the evidential, conceptual, methodological, criteriological, or contextual considerations upon which judgment is based" (Facione, 1990, p. 2). This definition of CT has been used extensively in nursing but, because no nurses or healthcare providers participated in the APA study, there is some question as to whether its findings are the best fit for nursing.

Because of the growing need for CT in nursing, some practitioners found it necessary to develop nursing-specific conceptualizations of CT so we could teach it better (e.g., Rubenfeld & Scheffer, 1999). In recent years, nurses have used research to describe CT and its components so that we have stronger evidence of CT in our profession. Of note is Fonteyn's (1998) work to describe thinking strategies for nursing practice. Using a "think aloud" method, Fonteyn and her team studied 14 expert registered nurses from a variety of specialty areas. Twelve predominant thinking strategies were identified. See **Box 2-1.**

BOX 2-1	Thinking Strategies of Expert Registered Nurses

- Recognizing a pattern
- Setting priorities
- Searching for information
- Generating hypotheses
- Making predictions
- Forming relationships
- Stating a proposition
- Asserting a practice rule
- Making choices
- Judging the value
- Drawing conclusions
- Providing explanations

Source: Fonteyn, 1998.

Following a method similar to that used by Facione for the APA, we conducted a comprehensive study to find consensus on a description of critical thinking in nursing in the mid-1990s (Scheffer & Rubenfeld, 2000). In this 3-year study, we also employed a Delphi method to gain consensus from a geographically disperse group of expert nurses through successive rounds of questions, answers, data analysis, and voting (Goodman, 1987). Our panel of 55 expert nurses was called from practice, education, and research settings and from nine countries and 23 U.S. states. During five rounds of questions and responses, we identified and defined 10 habits of the mind and seven cognitive skills of critical thinking in nursing.

We started our consensus rounds with a broad question: What are the skills and habits of the mind of critical thinking in nursing? Our choice of words was deliberate: We wanted to get at not only the cognitive skills but the affective component as well. Numerous authors (e.g., Tanner, 1997) have identified the importance of this affective component, which Facione (1990) named "dispositions." After a most helpful discussion with Dr. Pete Facione (a philosopher–scholar) and his wife, Dr. Noreen Facione (a nurse–scholar), we chose the label "habits of the mind" because we wanted to get away from some of the stereotypical views of traits or dispositions as being static. Because habits can be initiated and changed, this term seemed to be more dynamic.

For every round of our Delphi process, we "analyzed" data and returned reports to participants explaining what we had done with their information and asking a new set of questions based on the revised configuration of the data. By the end of five rounds, we were ready for voting on the final statement and definitions of the 10 habits of the mind and 7 skills. There was 88.2% consensus on the final statement and similar consensus on the definitions of the dimensions. (For the full report of the research method and consensus voting, see Scheffer & Rubenfeld, 2000.) The final consensus statement is:

> Critical thinking in nursing is an essential component of professional accountability and quality nursing care. Critical thinkers in nursing exhibit these habits of the mind: confidence, contextual perspective, creativity, flexibility, inquisitiveness, intellectual integrity, intuition, open-mindedness, perseverance, and reflection. Critical thinkers in nursing practice the cognitive skills of analyzing, applying standards, discriminating, information-seeking, logical reasoning, predicting and transforming knowledge. (Scheffer & Rubenfeld, p. 357)

See **Box 2-2** and the tear-out card on the inside cover of this book for definitions of the 10 habits of the mind and 7 skills. These dimensions of CT in nursing will be used as a framework for discussing CT throughout this text, so you will want to be able to refer to them frequently.

BOX 2-2	**Critical Thinking Skills and Habits of the Mind for Nursing**

Critical Thinking SKILLS

Analyzing: separating or breaking a whole into parts to discover their nature, function and relationships

Applying Standards: judging according to established personal, professional or social rules or criteria

Discriminating: recognizing differences and similarities among things or situations and distinguishing carefully as to category or rank

Information Seeking: searching for evidence, facts or knowledge by identifying relevant sources and gathering objective, subjective, historical and current data from those sources

Logical Reasoning: drawing inferences or conclusions that are supported in or justified by evidence

Predicting: envisioning a plan and its consequences

Transforming Knowledge: changing or converting the condition, nature, form or function of concepts among contexts

(continues)

| BOX 2-2 | (Continued) |

Critical Thinking HABITS OF THE MIND

Confidence: assurance of one's reasoning abilities

Contextual Perspective: considerate of the whole situation, including relationships, background and environment, relevant to some happening

Creativity: intellectual inventiveness used to generate, discover, or restructure ideas; imagining alternatives

Flexibility: capacity to adapt, accommodate, modify or change thoughts, ideas and behaviors

Inquisitiveness: an eagerness to know by seeking knowledge and understanding through observation and thoughtful questioning in order to explore possibilities and alternatives

Intellectual Integrity: seeking the truth through sincere, honest processes, even if the results are contrary to one's assumptions and beliefs

Intuition: insightful sense of knowing without conscious use of reason

Open-mindedness: a viewpoint characterized by being receptive to divergent views and sensitive to one's biases

Perseverance: pursuit of a course with determination to overcome obstacles

Reflection: contemplation upon a subject, especially one's assumptions and thinking for the purposes of deeper understanding and self-evaluation

Source: Scheffer & Rubenfeld, 2000, p. 358. Used with permission.

Comparison of the Nursing Delphi Study to the Philosophical Delphi Study

Box 2-3 compares the results of our study with those of Facione and his group. The definitions of CT skills are from Facione's 1990 Delphi study. The dispositions descriptions are taken from Facione, Sanchez, Facione, and Gainen (1995). In Facione's original work, he found 19 dispositions that fit into two types—approaches to life and living in general, and approaches to specific issues, questions, or problems. Those 19 dispositions were later consolidated to form seven dispositions in a factor analysis by Facione, Facione, and Sanchez (1994) as they began to develop a CT dispositions test.

BOX 2-3	Comparison of Nursing and APA Components of CT

NURSING SKILLS
(Scheffer & Rubenfeld, 2000, p. 358)

APA SKILLS
(Facione, 1990)

Analyzing:
"separating or breaking a whole into parts to discover their nature, function and relationships"

Analysis:
"to identify the intended and actual inferential relationships among statements, questions, concepts, descriptions or other forms of representation intended to express beliefs, judgments, experiences, reasons, information, or opinions" (p. 14) (Its subskills are identified as "examining ideas, identifying arguments and analyzing arguments" [p. 12].)

Applying Standards:
"judging according to established personal, professional or social rules or criteria"

Evaluation:
"to assess the credibility of statements or other representations which are accounts or descriptions of a person's perception, experience, situation, judgment, belief, or opinion; and to assess the logical strength of the actual or intended inferential relationships among statements, descriptions, questions or other form of representation" (p. 15)

Discriminating:
"recognizing differences and similarities among things or situations and distinguishing carefully as to category or rank"

Interpretation:
"to comprehend and express the meaning or significance of a wide variety of experiences, situations, data, events, judgments, conventions, beliefs, rules, procedures or criteria" (p. 13) (Its subskills are categorization, decoding sentences and clarifying meaning.)

Information Seeking:
"searching for evidence, facts or knowledge by identifying relevant sources and gathering objective, subjective, historical and current data from those sources"

Inference subskill:
querying evidence:
"to identify and secure elements needed to draw reasonable conclusions" (p. 16)

(continues)

BOX 2-3	(Continued)

NURSING SKILLS	APA SKILLS
Logical Reasoning: "drawing inferences or conclusions that are supported in or justified by evidence"	**Explanation:** "to state the results of one's reasoning; to justify that reasoning terms of the evidential, conceptual, methodological, criteriological and contextual considerations upon which one's results were based; and to present one's reasoning in the form of cogent arguments" (p. 18)
Predicting: "envisioning a plan and its consequences"	**Inference subskill:** conjecturing alternatives: "to formulate multiple alternatives for resolving a problem . . . to draw out presuppositions and project the range of possible consequences of decisions, positions, policies, theories, or beliefs" (p. 17)
Transforming Knowledge: "changing or converting the condition, nature, form or function of concepts among contexts"	**No comparable skill**
No comparable skill; see Habit of the Mind, Reflection.	**Self-regulation**

NURSING HABITS OF THE MIND (Scheffer & Rubenfeld, 2000, p. 358)	APA DISPOSITIONS (Facione, Sanchez, Facione, & Gainen, 1995)
Confidence: "assurance of one's reasoning abilities"	**CT Self-confidence:** "to trust the soundness of one's own reasoned judgments and to lead others in the rational resolution of problems" (p. 8)

BOX 2-3 (Continued)

NURSING HABITS OF THE MIND	APA DISPOSITIONS
Contextual Perspective: "considerate of the whole situation, including relationships, background and environment, relevant to some happening"	**Maturity:** "approach[ing] problems, inquiry, and decision making with a sense that some problems are necessarily ill-structured, some situations admit more than one plausible option, and many times judgments must be made based on standards, contexts, and evidence which preclude certainty" (p. 9)
Flexibility: "capacity to adapt, accommodate, modify or change thoughts, ideas and behaviors"	
Creativity: "intellectual inventiveness used to generate, discover, or restructure ideas; imagining alternatives"	**No comparable disposition**
Inquisitiveness: "an eagerness to know by seeking knowledge and understanding through observation and thoughtful questioning in order to explore possibilities and alternatives"	**Inquisitiveness:** "one's intellectual curiosity and one's desire for learning even when the application of the knowledge is not readily apparent" (p. 6)
Intellectual Integrity: "seeking the truth through sincere, honest processes, even if the results are contrary to one's assumptions and beliefs"	**Truthseeking:** "being eager to seek the best knowledge in a given context, courageous about asking questions, and honest and objective about pursuing inquiry even if the findings do not support one's self-interests or one's preconceived opinions" (p. 8)
Intuition: insightful sense of knowing without conscious use of reason	**No comparable disposition**
Open-mindedness: a viewpoint characterized by being receptive to divergent views and sensitive to one's biases	**Open-mindedness:** "being tolerant of divergent views and sensitive to the possibility of one's own bias" (p. 6)

(continues)

BOX 2-3	(Continued)

Perseverance:
pursuit of a course with determination
to overcome obstacles

Systematicity:
"being organized, orderly, focused
and diligent in inquiry" (p. 7)

Reflection:
contemplation upon a subject,
especially one's assumptions and
thinking for the purposes of deeper
understanding and self-evaluation

**No comparable disposition but
comparable to APA skill:
Self-Regulation:**
"self-consciously to monitor one's
cognitive activities, the elements
used in those activities, and the
results educed, particularly by applying skills in analysis and evaluation to
one's own inferential judgments with
a view toward questioning, confirm-
ing, validating, or correcting either
one's reasoning or one's results"
(Facione, 1990, p. 19)

No comparable habit of the mind.

Analyticity:
"prizing the application of reasoning
and the use of evidence to resolve
problems, anticipating potential
conceptual or practical difficulties,
and consistently being alert to the
need to intervene" (p. 7)

Although the comparisons are not direct, there are striking similarities between the two study results. However, a significant difference is also apparent. Two habits of the mind and one skill were not identified by the APA group—*creativity, intuition,* and *transforming knowledge.* Are these dimensions unique to nursing? Or are they unique to applied sciences or to health professions? We believe that our comparison shows that there are quite likely some discipline-specific dimensions of CT and some that are possibly universal.

Pebble #2: CT Language/Words

If these 17 dimensions represent CT in nursing, let's see how your thinking fits with them. Think about your thinking. Ask yourself, for example, how strong your CT *confidence* is or how you use *analyzing* in your clinical practice.

TACTICS 2-1

CT Self-Checklist

Look at **Box 2-4** and mark where you think you fall on each of those thinking continua.

This TACTIC can be used by both clinicians and educators.

BOX 2-4	Critical Thinking Self-Checklist

1. How confident am I in my reasoning ability?
   Not very confident   Very confident

2. Do I tend to look at situations with their context in mind, or do I tend to see things as separate compartments?
   Compartmentalized thinking   Contextual thinking

3. How creative am I in my thinking?
   Not very creative   Very creative

4. How flexible is my thinking?
   Rigid   Very flexible

5. How inquisitive am I?
   Not naturally curious   Innately inquisitive

6. How much intellectual integrity do I have?
   Go with my assumptions   Seek the truth no matter what

7. How intuitive am I?
   Not very intuitive   Always go with my gut

8. How open-minded am I?
   Quite biased   Open to all possibilities

9. How much perseverance do I have in my thinking?
   Once I have problems I'll stop   Keep at it no matter
                                                         what gets in the way

10. How reflective am I? Do I think about my thinking?
    Not very reflective   Always striving for deeper
                                                         understanding of self

11. How good am I at analyzing situations?
    I don't break things down much   I always pick things apart
                                                          to understand them

(continues)

BOX 2-4	(Continued)

12. How much do I pay attention to standards with my thinking?
Not used much for judgments   Always use criteria for judgments

13. How finely do I discriminate among things?
Don't recognize small   Always recognize small things
differences/similarities

14. How good am I at seeking out information?
I think about what's right there   I dig for all possible evidence

15. How strong is my logical reasoning?
I can't always justify my conclusions   I can always trace my
                                                               conclusions to evidence

16. How good are my abilities to predict consequences in situations?
Don't see much farther   I always think, What would
than my nose   happen if . . . ?

17. How well do I transform knowledge from one situation to the next?
Prefer textbook situations   Can adapt concepts to meet situation

Discussion

Are you beginning to see where your strengths and weaknesses lie? Let's take this further. At the beginning of this chapter, we asked how you would describe the thinking you use. Now how would you describe your thinking? Is it different now that you have the words to use? Is it easier to describe your thinking now that you know the words? Have you ever had to do this? In fact, most of us haven't been asked to describe our thinking—at least not until recently. These days, clinicians are being asked to show how they think because CT is recognized as being tied to quality of care. We need a new language of thinking—and a mutual understanding of what the words in that language mean.

Do you remember the first time you used a computer, ran into problems, and asked for help? If your helper was like most computer-literates, he or she probably used words like *booting, DOS, windows,* and *right-click.* Did you sit there with your mouth hanging open, feeling foolish? Were you at a loss as to what to say because you didn't know the language? Eventually, you probably learned enough computer lingo to function in today's technological world. Well, learning how to describe CT is a similar process. Without the words, it's impossible to even ask useful questions.

When we first started to teach CT, when we asked students to describe how they were thinking, they would tell us what they were thinking about. After trying several tactics to get our point across, we finally realized that the communication problem was very basic. Very few of our students had a vocabulary to use; they were not accustomed to describing something so abstract. As we used words to describe CT in nursing more and more in class, eventually it became clear that a list of descriptors would help students describe their thinking. Look at **Box 2-5** and see how many of those words and phrases you use and when and where you've heard or seen others using them.

BOX 2-5	**Words to Describe Critical Thinking**

DESCRIPTORS FOR CT HABITS OF THE MIND

Confidence
My thinking was on track, decisive; I reconsidered and still thought I made the best decision; I knew my conclusion was well-founded; My thinking was clear, unambiguous, trustworthy; I was secure in my thinking

Contextual Perspective
I could see the whole picture; I considered [reflected on, reconsidered] other possibilities; I took other things [surrounding issues] under consideration; I redefined the situation in view of. . .; Considering the circumstances, I . . . ; I broadened my view/perspective/mind

Creativity
I let my imagination go; I was inspired to think of. . . ; I stretched my mind; I took my thinking outside the box; I envisioned/dreamed up/invented. . . ; I tried to be visionary; My mind was fertile ground; I used the artistic side of my brain

Flexibility
I changed directions in my mind; I gave up on that idea and went on to. . . ; I moved away from my traditional thinking; I redefined the situation and started again; I questioned what I was thinking and considered another path; I tried to be adaptable in my thinking; I let my thinking go with the flow

Inquisitiveness
I had a strong desire for more knowledge; I itched to know more about. . . ; I was eager to know more; I took a lively interest in. . . ; I pricked up my ears, stuck my nose in. . . ; I burned with curiosity; I was really interested in. . . ; My mind was buzzing with questions

(continues)

BOX 2-5	(Continued)

Intellectual Integrity
I was not satisfied with my conclusion, so I. . .; Although it went against everything I believed. . .; I need to get at the truth; I tried to find the bottom line; I racked my brain; I questioned my biases; I asked myself difficult questions; I dug to the bottom; I reflected on my inferences; I examined why I thought that. . .

Intuition
I felt it in my bones; I couldn't put my finger on why, but I thought. . .; Instinctively I knew. . .; My hunch was that. . .; I had a premonition/inspiration/impression. . .; My natural tendency was to. . .; Subconsciously I knew that. . .; Without thought, I figured out. . .; Automatically I thought that. . .; While I couldn't say why, I thought immediately. . .; My sixth sense said that I should consider. . .

Open-mindedness
I tried to be receptive to new ideas; I tried not to judge; I listened to reason; I looked at both sides of the issue; I tried to be objective and unprejudiced; I questioned why I thought that. . .; I weighed the pros and cons; I tried to be neutral

Perseverance
I was single-minded in my determination to. . .; I persistently kept at it; I plodded on through my thoughts; I was stubborn and tireless in my pursuit; I kept going, trying this and that; I would not accept that for an answer; I had to overcome so many obstacles

Reflection
I pondered my reactions; I mulled it over in my mind; I ruminated over what I had thought and done; I had to reexamine/rethink/reconsider/review things; I evaluated my thoughts; I wondered what I could have done differently; I concentrated on my thinking process; I talked to myself about. . .; I deliberately meditated on what I was thinking

DESCRIPTORS FOR CT SKILLS

Analyzing
I dissected the situation; I broke things down so I could understand them better; I tried to reduce things into manageable units; I detailed a schematic of. . .; I sorted things out; I took the whole situation apart so I could see. . .; I looked for the parts; I made sure each component was addressed; I set it out, one, two, or three; I looked at each piece individually; I studied it bit by bit; I thought of it piecemeal instead of all together; I tried to see the trees instead of just the forest

Applying Standards
I knew I had to. . .; There are certain things you just have to account for; I thought of the bottom line that is always. . .; I know that some things are just right or wrong; As a professional, I knew I had to. . .; I knew it was unethical to. . .;

BOX 2-5	(Continued)

I considered what my license allowed and expected me to do; I thought of/studied the policy for. . . ; I compared this situation to what I knew to be the rule; I judged that according to. . .

Discriminating

I grouped things together; I put things in categories; I tried to consider what the priority was; I rank-ordered the various. . . ; I stood back and tried to see how those things were related; I wondered if this was as important as. . . ; I thought of the discrepancies in the story; I could distinguish the pieces; What I was hearing and what I was seeing was consistent [inconsistent]; I wondered what I should do first; When I focused on the finer details, I could see. . . ; This was different from [the same as] that

Information Seeking

I made sure I had all the pieces of the picture; I knew I needed to look up/study. . . ; I wondered how I could find out. . .; I went back to look more closely at. . . ; I asked myself if I knew the whole story; I kept searching for more data; I wanted [needed] to have all the facts [knowledge]; I looked for evidence of. . .

Logical Reasoning

I deduced from the information that. . . ; I could trace my conclusion back to the data; My diagnosis was grounded in the evidence; I considered all the information and then inferred. . . ; I could justify my conclusion by. . . ; I moved down a straight path from initial data to the final conclusion; I had a strong argument for. . . ; I made a good case for. . . ; There was sound evidence to support. . . ; My rationale for the conclusion was. . . ; Putting two and two together, I inferred. . . ; I brought reason to bear in the situation by. . .

Predicting

I could imagine that happening if I did. . . ; I anticipated. . . ; I was prepared for. . . ; I tried to be farsighted in my view; I made provisions for. . . ; I envisioned the outcome to be. . . ; I had a feeling that would happen; I could foresee. . . ; My prognosis was. . . ; I figured the probability of. . . ; I could tell that down the line. . . ; I tried to go beyond the here and now; The immediate plan was this, but the long term needed to be. . .

Transforming Knowledge

I knew I'd have to individualize; Although this situation was somewhat different, I knew. . . ; I wondered if that would fit in this situation; I thought this would be a textbook case, but it wasn't; I took what I knew and asked myself if it would work; I tried to translate that into this; I adapted my knowledge about. . . ; I could accommodate. . . ; I improved on the basics by adding. . . ; I figured if this was true, then that would be too; At first I was puzzled, then I saw that there were similarities, too; It was easy to cross over. . .

BOX 2-6	**CT Ironies to Ponder**

- If I teach you what CT is, I'm actually discouraging you from using CT to figure it for yourself.
- If I argue that CT is impossible or unnecessary, I'm actually being contra-dictory because posing such argumentation demonstrates CT.
- If CT truly requires a contextual perspective, then I must always adapt to the context to promote CT; does then CT itself change per context?

If you think you're ready, you can go to Appendix A and look at the CT Inventory. It's a more detailed version of the checklist in **Box 2-4** and can be used in a variety of situations. (You may find the descriptors in **Box 2-5** helpful when answering the questions it poses.) This inventory has been used to help nurses and nursing students describe their thinking and to evaluate growth in CT. Once you take the time to complete that inventory, we think you'll have a better sense of how you think, and you would really be able to answer some-one who asked, "How would you describe your thinking as a nurse?"

If, at this point, you are really excited by CT, you can tease your brain by considering the CT Ironies in **Box 2-6**. If you can spend enjoyable time pon-dering these more esoteric points, you have the makings of a philosopher!

Pebble #3: Visualizing CT in Action

And now for CT in action: What does it look like? Can you see it? Some argue that we cannot see or measure CT because it is only manifested in actions. That is some-what true, but there are problems with just looking at actions. Some "right" actions are pure luck; you can't count on them happening the next time. Some "right" actions are based on sloppy thinking. And some "right" actions are based on keen CT. Which kind of thinking do you want to count on? Sometimes it's easier to see the consequences of not thinking well than to see the results of well-thought-out actions. Things go wrong when nurses don't use CT. To fully appreciate CT in action, one really needs to combine descriptions of thinking with the actions that thinking produces. The following TACTICS illustrates that combined approach.

TACTICS 2-2

What Do Great Thinkers Look Like?

Clinicians

Think of the people you work with; rank them in terms of their thinking. One or two people probably stand out as great thinkers. What makes you put them in the great thinker category? It's probably their actions and their communication. Now, list those characteristics and see if you can picture great thinking in action.

Educators

Have your students or staff do the preceding exercise, writing down their descriptions of a great thinker they know personally, either as a formal paper or as an informal list of characteristics. Then have them share their descriptions and look for commonalities.

Discussion

In our workshops, students who do this exercise report the characteristics of great thinkers as follows: This person "always explains what he's doing . . . is always asking questions . . . can always stand up for herself when she's questioned . . . teaches every patient and family member he comes in contact with . . . rarely takes things at face value . . . rechecks everything . . . is the one we all go to for help with medication calculations . . . says what's on her mind . . . is the one we like to work with."

TACTICS 2-3

Talking and Thinking—A Patient Scenario

Clinicians

Consider this scenario.

You are working on a medical unit. Mrs. Franks, 79 years old with a history of alcoholism, was admitted 2 days ago for heart failure. Two hours before your shift began, she was moved to your unit from the telemetry unit. According to your shift report, she has been alert and oriented, has some minor lower extremity edema, has gone from many to a few crackles in her lungs, had her Foley removed this morning, and has urinated once in the past 6 hours. Her weight has decreased 4 kg since admission. She is not on a fluid restriction and has been eating and drinking small amounts. She has used her prn oxygen rarely. You walk into the room to find a very agitated Mrs. Franks trying to get out of bed, saying, "I have to get to the store before it closes because I have company coming for dinner." Speaking in a calm voice, you ask her to tell you how she feels. Meanwhile, you check her pulse and find it at 92 but regular. You remember that she's on a beta-blocker.

Now, finish this scenario. What would you think? What would you do and why?

Educators

Use this same case or find one that works with your setting and that matches the level of knowledge of your students or staff. Service-based educators should select a unit-specific case. Set up some parameters for responding to this scene; for example, if you are trying to promote better assessment skills among one unit's staff, have the nurses list their answers and place them in a centrally located box for a drawing later. Give a prize for the best answer, or post all the answers anonymously and have the staff rate them.

Discussion

So, what would exemplify best thinking in this situation with Mrs. Franks? We'll give you an idea of what an expert nurse would do. Obviously, novices would not necessarily come up with these responses.

We'd expect the nurse to assess respiratory rate, lung sounds, pulse oximetry, blood pressure, temperature, cognitive function, glucose (if there's any history of hypo- or hyperglycemia), hemoglobin level to consider if she's anemic, medications and side effects, and additional information about her alcoholism (e.g., how long since drinking last, amount consumed) and her past history of alcoholic behavior via her chart or family report, if possible. We'd also want the nurse to check patterns to see if her pulse of 92 is normal according to her baseline.

We'd expect each of those things to be assessed in just about that order. We'd expect the nurse to speak softly and confidently to the patient, ask her if she needs the bathroom or is in pain, orient her to her surroundings, help her stay in bed, and make sure she is safe before leaving her alone in the room.

That nurse should be entertaining reasonable hunches of what might be going on and ruling them in or out, such as decreased oxygen saturation, increased pulmonary congestion, cardiac event, infectious process (such as pneumonia or urinary tract infection), medication side effect, and anxiety over the new environment. We'd expect that nurse to be considering his or her knowledge of such things as normal aging, for example, and that responses are usually blunted in elders. Other knowledge would be in such areas as typical heart failure signs, symptoms, and complications. We'd expect that nurse to communicate with the healthcare team about this event. We'd expect a nurse who has worked in that environment for several months to have some intuitive response to this situation but not to jump to premature conclusions. Finally, we'd expect any nurse to take the situation seriously.

Some variations on this exercise would be to have staff or students discuss such scenarios in a group, write similar scenarios, and project what "wrong" things nurses might do in such situations.

PAUSE _____

and Ponder

Conclusions About **What** *CT Is*

This chapter was necessary to set the stage. Now, when someone asks you about CT, we hope you will have something more to say than, "That's a good question!" Understanding the concept of CT is essential to nursing practice, but the ideas and words that describe the concept are only building blocks. Now we need to use those building blocks to nurture and expand CT in nursing. The following chapters will help you continue this lifelong journey.

Reflection Cues

- CT bridges the gap between knowledge and actions.
- The Western history of CT can be traced as far back as Socrates up to recent nursing research.
- CT in nursing is exemplified by 10 habits of the mind (*confidence, contextual perspective, creativity, flexibility, inquisitiveness, intellectual integrity, intuition, open-mindedness, perseverance, reflection*) and 7 cognitive skills (*analyzing, applying standards, discriminating, information seeking, logical reasoning, predicting, transforming knowledge*).
- Dimensions of nursing CT not found in nonnursing descriptions are *creativity, intuition*, and *transforming knowledge*.
- Verbalizing one's CT requires descriptive language not commonly used in the action-oriented discipline of nursing.
- It is difficult to "see" the CT behind the actions. Actions must be combined with descriptions of thinking.
- Although most of us can identify colleagues who are good thinkers, it is very difficult to tease out the thinking behind their actions.
- Incorporating the language of thinking into our vocabulary increases our awareness of our own thinking, our awareness of the thinking of others, and our ability to describe our thinking to colleagues.

References

American Association of Colleges of Nursing. (2008, October 20). *The essentials of baccalaureate education for professional nursing practice.* Retrieved October 29, 2008, from http://www.aacn.nche.edu/education/pdf/BaccEssentials08.pdf

American Nurses Association. (2004). *Nursing: Scope and standards of practice.* Washington, DC: Author.

Benner, P. (1984). *From novice to expert: Power and excellence in nursing practice.* Menlo Park, CA: Addison-Wesley.

Case, B. (1998). Competence development: Critical thinking, clinical judgment, and technical ability. In K. J. Kelly-Thomas (Ed.), *Clinical & nursing staff development: Current competence, future focus* (pp. 240–281). Philadelphia: Lippincott.

Commission on Collegiate Nursing Education. (2008). *Standards for accreditation of baccalaureate and graduate nursing programs.* Retrieved November 19, 2008, from http://www.aacn.nche.edu/accreditation/

Costa, A. L. (Ed.). (1985). *Developing minds: A resource book for teaching thinking.* Alexandria, VA: Association for Supervision and Curriculum Development.

Dreyfus, H. L., & Dreyfus, S. E. (1986). *Mind over machine: The power of human intuition and expertise in the era of the computer.* New York: Free Press.

Facione, P. A. (1990). *Critical thinking: A statement of expert consensus for purposes of educational assessment and instruction.* Millbrae, CA: California Academic Press. (ERIC Document Reproduction Service No. ED315423)

Facione, N. C., Facione, P. A., & Sanchez, C. A. (1994). Critical thinking disposition as a measure of competent clinical judgment: The development of the California Critical Thinking Disposition Inventory. *Journal of Nursing Education, 33,* 345–350.

Facione, P. A., Sanchez, C. A., Facione, N. C., & Gainen, J. (1995). The disposition toward critical thinking. *Journal of Nursing Education, 44,* 1–25.

Fonteyn, M. E. (1998). *Thinking strategies for nursing practice.* Philadelphia: Lippincott.

Goodman, C. N. (1987). The Delphi technique: A critique. *Journal of Advanced Nursing, 12,* 729–734.

Hansten, R. I., & Washburn, M. J. (1999). Individual and organizational accountability for development of critical thinking. *Journal of Nursing Administration, 29*(11), 39–45.

Hart, L. A. (1983). *Human brain and human learning.* New York: Longman.

The Higher Learning Commission. (2007). *Institutional accreditation: An overview.* Retrieved November 24, 2008, from http://www.ncahlc.org/overview/2003overview.pdf

Institute of Medicine. (2004). *Keeping patients safe: Transforming the work environment for nurses.* Washington, DC: National Academies Press.

The Joint Commission. (2008). *Evolution of performance measurement at the Joint Commission 1986–2010: A visioning document.* Retrieved November 24, 2008, from http://www.jointcommission.org/NR/rdonlyres/333A4688-7E50-41CF-B63D-EE0278D0C653/0/SIWGProloguewebversion.pdf

Kant, I. (1965). *Critique of pure reason* (N. K. Smith, Trans.). New York: St. Martin's Press. (Original work published 1787)

Kemerling, G. (2001). *History of western philosophy.* Retrieved November 24, 2008, from http://www.philosophypages.com/hy/index.htm

Miller, J., Galloway, M., Coughlin, C., & Brennan, E. (2001). Care-centered organizations, Part 1: Governance. *Journal of Nursing Administration, 31*(2), 67–73.

National League for Nursing. (2005a). *Position statement: Transforming nursing education.* Retrieved November 24, 2008, from http://www.nln.org/aboutnln/PositionStatements/transforming052005.pdf

National League for Nursing. (2005b). *Core competencies of nurse educators with task statements.* Retrieved November 24, 2008, from http://www.nln.org/facultydevelopment/pdf/corecompetencies.pdf

Rubenfeld, M. G., & Scheffer, B. K. (1999). *Critical thinking in nursing: An interactive approach* (2nd ed.). Philadelphia: Lippincott.

Scheffer, B. K., & Rubenfeld, M. G. (2000). A consensus statement on critical thinking in nursing. *Journal of Nursing Education, 39,* 352–359.

Schoenly, L. (1998). Staff development programs: Strategic thinking applied. In K. J. Kelly-Thomas (Ed.), *Clinical & nursing staff development: Current competence, future focus* (pp. 192–212). Philadelphia: Lippincott.

Tanner, C. (1997). Spock would have been a terrible nurse (and other issues related to critical thinking in nursing). *Journal of Nursing Education, 36,* 3–4.

Thompson, D. N., & Burns, H. K. (2004). Public policy: Work environment for nurses and the impact on protecting patients from healthcare errors. *Journal of Professional Nursing, 20,* 145–146.

CHAPTER ——————— 3

Who Are the Critical Thinkers?

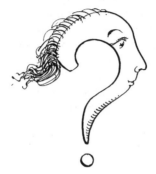

When characterizing people who work in health care, we usually focus on what they do, not how they think. However, people in the health professions, especially nurses, are some of the best critical thinkers in the world. Nurses have a wide breadth and deep depth of knowledge; they must apply that knowledge in a huge variety of contexts; and they must recognize and evaluate variations from the norm in every patient. As health care becomes increasingly complex, the thinking needed becomes even more sophisticated. Those who do the thinking must become even more cognizant of the thinking they employ to do the work of health care.

Who are you? Most of you are probably nurses or nursing students, but because these ideas are relevant to all healthcare providers, some of you may be from other disciplines. We hope so, because, as we will discuss later, we are big believers in the necessity of interdisciplinary practice (see Chapter 7 in particular). Are you a clinician or an educator, or does your position combine both roles? Perhaps you are a researcher, a manager, or an administrator in a practice setting. Nurses' roles and positions are often complex because they embrace multiple thinking tasks throughout the day.

We needed to develop an organized way to address you that also fits with our critical thinking–enhancing TACTICS. As we see it, you readers want to improve your critical thinking (CT) or help others improve theirs; therefore, we classified you as being in one of two categories—clinicians or educators. For clinicians, much of what we say focuses on how you can improve your CT; for educators, the focus is on strategies to promote CT in others. We're aware that in the real world, these two roles are not mutually exclusive. Clinicians often try to help others improve CT, and educators often work to improve their personal CT. Still, for ease of communication, we have divided you, our readers, into two groups, clinicians and educators.

A major reason why we've chosen to write to this audience is that we want to promote a unified view of CT as a vital but complex clinical and educational issue. We are quite aware that the literature on CT in nursing is primarily oriented toward those in academic settings—students and teachers. Indeed, most things we've written are academically slanted. However, the bottom line is that we all want to improve CT in clinical practice. If we don't start viewing this from both perspectives simultaneously, we'll be building an ivory tower version and a digging-out-a-trench version. Neither will be adequate to meet the thinking demands of health care today or tomorrow.

Clinicians

We envision clinicians at multiple points in their professional practice careers and in a variety of healthcare settings. Those multiple career points span from that of a novice who is learning in the clinical setting (i.e., nursing students or orientees) to that of a nurse who is considered an expert in practice. Many challenges tax your thinking skills in the practice arena, not the least of which is the seemingly constant change in the demands and responsibilities of your positions. Complex changes are occurring in all healthcare delivery systems (Erickson, Ditomassi, & Jones, 2008; Falise, 2007; Redman, 2006; Rossen, Bartlett, & Herrick, 2008). Kelly-Thomas (1998) referred to the "re-do" words typically heard in healthcare environments these days—reengineering, restructuring, retooling, revisioning. These re-do issues require, above all else, nurses to be *confident, contextual, creative, open-minded,* and *flexible* in their thinking strategies. We will return often to the subject of complex change, especially in Chapter 11, where we discuss the realities of thinking yesterday, today, and tomorrow.

Educators

We envision educators in various settings as well, primarily as service based (staff development specialists, preceptors, continuing education directors, and so on) or academic based (nursing school faculty). We expect that some of our clinicians and educators are graduate students pursuing one or both roles. Whichever kind of educator you are, you deal with many complex problems that affect how you see yourself as a thinker and how you'll be able to promote CT in your students and staff. Academic-based educators may be more familiar with CT language because much of what has been written about CT has been for traditional educational settings. We hope you will find this book to be helpful because it presents a practical view of CT, not just an academic view.

Other Thinkers Who Interact with Clinicians and Educators

Although for this discussion we've delineated two "who" groups and acknowledged that all people are thinkers, here is an important point: No one of us thinks in isolation. To view CT as an individual process will take us down a disastrous path where we waste time and money and possibly do harm. Other thinkers must also be considered, including patients, patients' significant others, and additional members of the healthcare team. We will address patient thinking in Chapter 6 and team thinking in Chapter 7, but for now, remember that everything we say about CT applies to all the thinkers around you—other nurses, students, healthcare providers, patients and their significant others, administrators, politicians, and many others.

Selected Factors That Affect Critical Thinkers

Many factors influence us as thinkers. For example, clinicians may be viewed as facing enormous challenges because their work is traditionally action oriented, taking place in settings that rarely sanction thinking time. Educators, on the other hand, are usually viewed as actively working when they sit with furrowed brows. In addition to these environmental factors, many other things influence one's thinking—genetics; self-concept; anxiety and other emotions; age; and culture, including family and cultural heritage, society, and organizational culture.

Genetics as an Influence on CT

Let's look at genetics, or basic "wiring," first. No two people think in the same way. (That's great, isn't it?) Whether those differences stem from genetics or one's upbringing is frequently debated. In reality, it's both, but we do know that some differences are inborn. Some people have the ability to remember numerous esoteric facts but can't figure out how to solve simple everyday problems such as how to boil water! Others never seem flustered when things go wrong but can't remember when they last went to the bathroom. Acknowledging differences in thinking without judging that one way is better than another is a challenge but a necessary one, especially for educators who are trying to individualize teaching strategies to nurture thinking.

If you haven't thought about your natural, inborn thinking abilities, do that now. Refer to the short inventory in **Box 2-4** or the CT Inventory in Appendix A to help you reflect on your thinking. If you can articulate your personal hard wiring, it will make you a better learner. Are you a visual thinker? (You need to see it to understand it.) Are you an auditory thinker? (Once you hear it, you remember it.) Do you have to do something with information—perform an action—before it stays in your brain? If you can describe to a teacher what works best for you, you will be a better learner. You will also be more sensitive to the learning and thinking styles of others and therefore be a better educator. Keep in mind that it is rare to have only one of these learning styles; most of us have combinations but find one that is our preferred style.

Consider this example from an author/educator:

My son has attention deficit disorder, and although his intelligence test results showed him to be above average, he could not learn how to add columns of numbers. When given a fourth-grade assignment to copy a list of numbers and add them, he would write the numbers in what seemed to be a random pattern so the tens or hundreds were never above and below each other. I kept saying to him, "Line them up!" and he would repeatedly do this random thing. Finally, in total frustration, I drew lines on the sheet of paper. Then he had no trouble at all. It made me realize that he has no patterning ability in his mind remotely close to what I have in mine. Once we moved to graph paper with big squares, he was fine with addition of long sets of numbers. (By the way, this boy moved to the advanced math classes in high school.)

This boy's situation, in addition to illustrating how vastly different thinking styles can be, shows us that intelligence is not a simple construct. Howard Gardner deftly illustrated thinking complexity in his description of multiple intelligences (Gardner, 1983, 1993, 1999, 2006). Refer to Gardner's list in **Box 3-1**. Can you relate to some of those intelligences more than others? We'd guess yes. Gardner believed that we have varying proportions of each of these intelligences but that some of them come more naturally to us than others. That may be due to genetics and/or because some groups and cultures value some traits over others. Our self-concept of our thinking style is largely based on our dominant intelligences.

Self-Concept as an Influence on CT

Think about this statement: I am a great thinker. Do you believe it? If yes, why? If no, why? You can probably imagine a philosophy professor saying this. That's because we traditionally associate "great thinking" with fields such as philosophy. Nursing is traditionally associated with doing and actions. Both of these traditional associations are too limited, especially the nursing one. Expert nursing care requires expert levels of thinking for actions to be safe.

Obviously, culture influences self-concept, but there's more to it than that, such as life circumstances and how much positive (or negative) feedback you get for your thinking ability. If your 10th-grade math teacher told you that girls are never any good at math (and yes, teachers still say such things), the girls in that class would need some other equally dramatic evaluation of their math skills to counter that attitude and develop a positive concept of themselves as mathematical thinkers. If you were always praised for your problem-solving abilities, you'd be proud of your analytical skills, thereby promoting a positive self-concept in that CT dimension.

The math example speaks to a very important point about the differences in how women and men think. Women and men are socialized differently, especially in relation to self-concept and thinking ability. This is not an all-or-nothing

BOX 3-1	Gardner's Multiple Intelligences

- *Spatial:* the mind's eye: preference for use of images, pictures, graphical representations
- *Logical-Mathematical:* use of an entire range of reasoning skills, preference for factual data, and both inductive and deductive reasoning
- *Linguistic:* embracing speaking and listening, reading, writing, and other forms of communication
- *Musical:* patterned rhythms of the mind, learning and knowing by sharing, expressing, perceiving, and creating pitch and patterns
- *Bodily-Kinesthetic:* using the body as a conduit for the mind, using action and motion
- *Interpersonal:* using the give and take of communication with intonation and punctuation with a goal of understanding, empathy, and learning from one another
- *Intrapersonal:* focusing on knowing self with a goal of internalizing learning through thoughtful connections and transformation of knowledge into meaning
- *Naturalist:* the ability to recognize and differentiate characteristics and phenomena of the plant and animal world as well as inorganic material immersion in a work of art.

Source: Gardner, 1983, 1999, 2006.

interpretation, however. Excellent research has been done on female thinking (Belenky, Clinchy, Goldberger, & Tarule, 1986; Gilligan, 1982), and there are many helpful suggestions for addressing gender differences in classrooms (Brookfield & Preskill, 1999). Though gender has a significant influence on self-concept and definitely is a force to be reckoned with in nursing, with its lopsided ratio of women to men, even the experts caution us not to assume that gender is the only factor that affects how we think.

Unfortunately, women are still trying to escape the negative connotations of descriptions like "she's really smart," which cause most of us to flash back to high school where that meant, "she's not pretty." The implication there was that looks were more important than brains. Think of how women are described in the media even today, and then consider how men are described; inevitably, women are described in terms of appearance, and men are described in terms of intelligence and accomplishments.

Although women have quite a few stereotypes working against them, men in nursing don't fare much better in how society views their thinking abilities.

Because these men are nurses, and not, for example, engineers, their thinking is considered less sophisticated. Unfortunately, people often judge a nontraditional career decision negatively, especially with respect to thinking ability. Why would a man be a nurse (when he could have been an engineer or doctor)?

So sometimes the world doesn't view us as great thinkers and sees us through gender-biased eyes. Let's stop buying into those notions and work on what we do have control over—our self-concept as great thinkers. Simply reflecting on your thinking can help you improve your self-concept. After completing such reflection assignments, our students have said, "We never thought about our thinking before. We really do think a lot, don't we?" If we accept the stereotypical beliefs that we're not great thinkers, is it any wonder that we have self-concept problems about our thinking?

Suzanne Gordon (2005), a reporter who has studied nursing extensively, had some interesting comments about our image. Her contention is that the usual descriptions of nursing as a calling and as a caring profession do us more harm than good. Such descriptions emphasize "virtue" and devalue our skill, knowledge, and thinking ability. "Updating the image of nursing will involve applying some critical thinking to the sentimentalized virtue script that nurses so often rely on today" (p. 440).

We need to value our brains and define ourselves as knowledge workers, not production workers. Kaeding and Rambur (2004) described knowledge work as

> based on assessment, judgment, problem-solving, and the generation of ideas. It is nonrepetitive, nonroutine, and dependent on cognitive activity. Manual work is integral but not dominant. Gender is valued equally. Professional knowledge is not hierarchical, and evidence of learning is important to safe and effective job performance. (p. 137)

Seago (2008) described how healthcare organizations are beginning to use the term *knowledge worker* as a new descriptor for healthcare providers to conceptualize the culture change needed for the 21st century. Maybe we should go back to wearing nursing caps, but this time we should make them in the shape of mortarboards representing the knowledge gleaned through education and experience.

Feelings, Especially Anxiety, as Influences on CT

Another major factor that influences thinking involves emotions. Intense feelings—love, hate, depression, elation—will always be factors shaping our cognitive skills. When we did our Delphi study to find consensus on CT, we specifically asked about habits of the mind in addition to cognitive skills. Most people, at least in nursing, acknowledge that CT has both affective (habits of the mind) and cognitive (skills) components. Those two components exist in tandem all the time. But, when we add an extreme emotional response to a situation, affective components of CT exert a stronger influence.

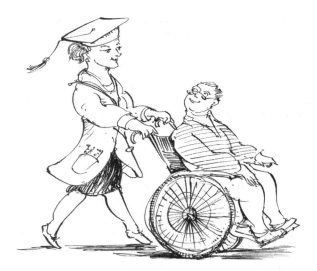

Many mood states affect thinking, but anxiety is particularly important in the healthcare sector, which has more than its share of anxiety-producing situations. Most older nurses (age 50 and older) can tell horror stories about how they were so terrified by nursing school teachers that they couldn't think at all. Hart (1983) called that "reptilian" brain functioning, meaning that the higher-order thinking skills of mammals shuts down, and only basic survival thinking takes over. Teaching through terror, we hope, has gone the way of our nursing caps. Nevertheless, doing a nursing task for the first time, even with a nurturing teacher to help, still makes our hearts race and our palms dampen. And some nursing tasks continue to make us anxious even after we've done them many times.

Many self-help books on how to deal with anxiety exist, so we're not going to give a short course here. However, we do encourage all of you to consider what happens to your thinking when you're anxious, and what circumstances, in particular, make you anxious. Also, consider what Margaret Carson (2003) called the "emotional burden" of nursing. Carson studied nurses who had been in combat situations, but she also cautioned nurses to consider the psychological toll of other high-stress nursing situations. In our experience, nurses do not do a good job of taking care of themselves; we need to think about our emotional responses more, value things like lunch and bathroom breaks, and consider the importance of decreasing anxiety to sharpen our thinking skills.

If you teach others, orient new staff, or function as a preceptor, we have a special message for you: If you expect your students and staff to be good thinkers, you must guide them gently, acknowledge their anxiety, and employ teaching and mentoring strategies, such as humor, that reduce anxiety. It is both humbling and helpful to remember your first lecture or your first attempt to catheterize an uncooperative patient. Telling students about your fears or relating to new staff how you botched simple jobs in your first weeks on the unit can do wonders to help them relax and reassure them that they also will gain mastery. Most of all, we must approach teaching as a collaborative effort, not a game of one-upmanship in which you are the all-knowing expert and your students have blank slates for brains. Anxiety is a day-to-day reality of nursing. We need to acknowledge it, remember its influence on thinking, and constantly work to lessen it to help ourselves and others.

Generational Influences on CT

The nursing profession contains four generations of workers; those age-related differences affect many important attributes—attitudes, beliefs, communication, work style, and, of course, thinking. There are several classifications of generations. Oblinger and Oblinger (2005) described them this way: "Matures," born between 1900 and 1946; "Baby Boomers," born between 1946 and 1964; "Generation X," born between 1965 and 1982; and the "Net Generation," born between 1982 and 1991. Having four generations working together is a new phenomenon because nurses now remain in the workplace longer than they once did (Sherman, 2006). It behooves clinicians and educators to reflect on the significance of generational differences to avoid conflict and misunderstanding.

Some believe that generational differences are more related to technology exposure than to age itself, so when reflecting on implications of those differences, an open mind is crucial. Although any generalizations will inevitably be incorrect in specific instances, it is helpful to consider how these generalizations could affect thinking. Continuing with Oblinger and Oblinger's (2005) descriptions, Matures were described as self-sacrificing, respectful of authority, and intolerant of waste and technology. Putting that in a thinking frame of reference, we might expect our older nurses' *information-seeking* and *applying-standards* CT skills to be manifested as seeking answers from authorities whom they respect. They may have less *flexibility* in their thinking, but they will have *perseverance*. They will not be *confident* when dealing with technology, but from their years of experience, they may have a larger *contextual perspective* and will likely be strong on *intuition* and *confident* in their logical reasoning in a wide range of situations. (We discuss issues of age and technology more in Chapter 9 on informatics.)

Baby Boomers were seen as optimistic workaholics with a strong work ethic and sense of responsibility; they are intolerant of laziness and believe they can do most things well (Oblinger & Oblinger, 2005). We might expect them to be *confident* in their thinking and have strong *predicting* and *discriminating* abilities. Like the Matures, they have years of experience to draw on as they think through situations and may do well with *transforming knowledge*. They may be less *open-minded* in their thinking, especially when they deal with Generation Xers, who are not workaholics.

Generation X was characterized as independent, free, skeptical, and comfortable with multitasking and as valuing a balance of life and work. They are intolerant of red tape and hype (Oblinger & Oblinger, 2005). They may be more *flexible* in their thinking and *open-minded* to divergent views as long as those views aren't seen as restrictive. They will likely *seek information* from a variety of sources, not necessarily from authorities. Because they are skeptical, they may be more independently *inquisitive*. When *applying standards*, they may use more personal standards than work-related standards.

The Net Generation, also called Millennials, are hopeful, determined, into the latest technology, and intolerant of anything slow (Oblinger & Oblinger, 2005). They don't know a world without the Internet, and so their *information-seeking* skills are first and foremost oriented there. They may be impatient with the older workers who are less adept at surfing, but they may work and think well in teams because they are used to networking. They are likely *creative* in their thinking, seeking their own approaches to knowledge rather than doing what they're told. They may have a wider *contextual perspective* because they are used to visual communication and experiential learning, but they may miss things that are not of interest to them.

Obviously these generalizations are simplistic, but what is important to consider is that we cannot expect a young, recently graduated nurse to think in the same way that the older nurse would. Weston (2006) called this the generational "mental model." "Based upon world events that framed their youth and initial work experiences, members of each generation have develop [sic] somewhat unique mental models . . . logical and consistent with their lived experience" (electronic, para 1, "Sources of Multigenerational Misunderstandings"). We must promote tolerance of the differences among us and tailor teamwork and teaching/learning to the thinking style of each person. In the practice arena, we must acknowledge the strengths and contributions of each generation and link people together based on how they can help each other (Sherman, 2006).

Teaching and learning issues are especially challenging; because teachers, both in academia and in clinical settings, are primarily Baby Boomers, the teaching approaches that fit with their characteristics are a misfit for the learning needs of Generation X and the Net Generation. Faculty who are used to sequential knowledge building, recall of information, and repetition must learn to know the new generation of learners who are used to digital, interactive, and fast-paced learning (Skiba & Barton, 2006).

Cultural Influences on CT

Unquestionably, we are influenced by our native culture and by the culture in which we live and work. Depending on your level of ethnocentrism or your exposure to different cultures, you may not realize how deeply cultural norms affect your thinking and that of people around you.

Culture, as defined by Giger and Davidhizar (2004), is

> a patterned behavioral response that develops over time as a result of imprinting the mind through social and religious structures and intellectual and artistic manifestations. Culture is also the result of acquired mechanisms

that may have innate influences but are primarily affected by internal and external environmental stimuli. Culture is shaped by values, beliefs, norms, and practices that are shared by members of the same cultural group. Culture guides our thinking, doing, and being and becomes patterned expressions of who we are. (p. 3)

Culture is not static; it changes with time as cultural groups change definitions of their parameters. Although we can trace almost everything we think and do back to some cultural influence, there are some aspects of culture that are especially relevant when it comes to CT, particularly communication and time orientation. We will also discuss the organizational culture of the healthcare work environment and how it affects CT.

Communication, Culture, and CT

Communication is the most obvious area where culture could affect CT. The term *communication* covers a broad range of topics about which numerous books are written. In this section, we focus on two: language and translation of meaning across cultures, and one's style for communicating thinking.

First, consider what language a person speaks. Is it the language of the majority? If not, consider what implications translation can have on the various components of CT. Words to describe thinking are complex and abstract and often have no direct translation in other languages. On a recent trip to Japan to present a paper on CT, we found that the phrase *habits of the mind* caused the most complex translation problem. There was no direct translation, so we tried to think of a synonym. In our research, we chose that phrase—*habits of the mind*—deliberately because we wanted to get across these finer points: The word *traits* often connotes static qualities, and we wanted to stay away from that. *Characteristics* was too broad, and *dispositions* was closely aligned with *traits*. As the translator tried these and other words, she became very frustrated. *Tendencies toward* seemed to work, as did *affinity for*, but ultimately, the complete meaning of habits of the mind was probably never effectively translated.

What did this do to our discussion about CT? In this case, the idea that habits of the mind can be enhanced and our suggestions on how to do that may literally have gotten lost in translation. Because language is the basis of understanding, the very words used to describe CT and its dimensions need to be clarified at the outset of any discussion. If we aren't using the same descriptors, we may not be talking about the same thing.

Second, consider the different styles of communication that exist among cultural groups. To study CT requires questioning, but how is questioning viewed in other cultures? Is it considered an impolite or a desirable activity? Group activities to enhance CT usually involve sharing thoughts about thinking style; such sharing can be seen as a very intimate process. Do some cultures have "rules" that prohibit such personal exchanges?

I (Gaie) will switch to singular first-person writing here for a moment because this observation is personal. I can think of two extremes to illustrate the differences in communication style among cultures. One occurred in my native Newfoundland, a small maritime province in Canada. The other occurred in Japan, where I recently did the presentation on CT to which I referred earlier. I have not lived in Newfoundland for many years, but I visit frequently. It seems that there is open debate on everything in my home province. I have never seen a place with so many radio talk shows! Everyone has an opinion on everything, and people freely express their opinions through whatever medium is available. Several people talking at once, using emphatic gestures, is more the norm than the exception. While doing a presentation on CT to nurses there several years ago, I had to stop frequently for discussion and questions from the audience. To someone unfamiliar with the culture, the questions might have seemed confrontational. I felt right at home!

In Japan, on the other hand, the large audience of nurses was extremely quiet. I was a bit intimidated when I walked into the auditorium to find 3,000 nurses who were so silent, it reminded me of how the room sounded the day before while I rehearsed—but then it was completely empty. I'm used to the din that American and Canadian audiences make as they wait for programs to begin. In Japan, when I asked for questions, there were few. Those who spoke did not use hand gestures and began each interaction with a deferential comment, such as "excuse me." Japanese nursing faculty, who are very interested in promoting CT, told me they have to repeatedly encourage students to discuss issues and ask questions; students there are much more comfortable with lectures.

Extremes such as these, and all kinds of examples in between, occur in nursing practice and schools throughout North America as well. What do such differences mean to the educator or clinician? Because questioning is considered a desirable part of CT, the tendency is to believe that the assertive communicator is a better critical thinker. However, we must consider just what it is that we most value. Is it the communication of questions or the questioning itself that is important? Perhaps we need to think of ways beyond verbal means to encourage questioning. Perhaps quiet people are more comfortable sharing their questions in writing. Smaller group discussions that are not teacher led or Web caucuses might be more appropriate for those from cultures in which open questioning is seen as impolite.

Time Orientation, Culture, and CT

If communication styles seem culturally bound, what about other things, such as the cultural influence on time orientation? There is a certain expectation of a "futuristic view" in nursing descriptions of CT. Speaking generally, certain groups have one of three dominant time perspectives—past, present, or future. Of course, there are many exceptions to these broad generalizations, but we usually view Eastern cultures as more focused on the past, Hispanic and Native American/Aboriginal cultures as more focused on the present, and European American cultures as more focused on the future.

A Hispanic nurse once told us that he asks Hispanic patients if they'd like him to record appointment times on their cards half an hour earlier so they'd be on time for their appointments. He initiates that question with a comment about his own tendency for tardiness because he's not very future oriented.

Another example from Gaie: A friend and I recently stopped to visit a basket maker on a Mi'kmaq reservation in Cape Breton, Nova Scotia. We were so fascinated with her exquisite weaving of a quill basket that we stayed longer than planned. Upon realizing the time, we jumped up, saying, "We'll be late getting to our friend's house. We need to get going." The basket maker looked at us, smiled, and said, "Just tell them you were on the res' and you're on Indian time." Clearly, her present-oriented perspective was so much a part of her culture that she was very comfortable making humorous references to it. Later I thought about what it would be like if she were a student in my CT class. What would she think when I stressed the importance of "predicting" (one of the CT skills we identified in our study) as part of CT? Would she adopt a futuristic thinking mode because it was expected? How would that affect other parts of her thinking, honed by years of her own culture's influence?

Another issue relative to time is the predominant U.S. value of time-is-money. Along with time-is-money comes time-equals-action. For vivid examples of this in health care, we only have to look at managed care approaches in which nurse practitioners and physicians are required to see large numbers of patients each hour to meet income quotas. Home healthcare nurses are given similar quota directives—ones that make quality care difficult. What happens to CT in a culture that clearly values the tangible results of work but not the process of improving quality through thinking? It takes time to think; some things take longer to think about than others, and some people think faster or slower than others.

TACTICS 3-1

Cultural Influences on Thinkers

Clinicians

Using the checklist in **Box 3-2**, reflect on your culture and how it might affect your CT habits of the mind. Then think of someone you work with who comes from a culture different from yours. Think of a patient from a different culture. How do you think those persons would answer the questions?

Educators

Use the checklist in **Box 3-2** as the basis for a group discussion. Consider whether your students and staff gain an awareness of other cultures.

Discussion

Did you learn anything about your culture? Other people's cultures? You've probably considered such things before, but have you put them into a CT frame of reference? We tend to think of cultural norms in terms of such things as eating, holidays, and dress, but we don't often associate them with our thinking.

BOX 3-2	Cultural Influences on Thinking Habits of the Mind

Directions: Place an X on the line to indicate your self-rating.

My culture:

- values

  limited questioning of authority ⟵————————————————⟶ open debate

- is primarily focused on the ❏ past.

  ❏ present.

  ❏ future.

- values

  contemplation ⟵————————————————————————⟶ actions

In my culture I am encouraged to:

- be confident of my reasoning ability

  never ⟵————————————————————————⟶ always

- consider where someone is coming from when I interact

  never ⟵————————————————————————⟶ always

- be as creative as possible

  never ⟵————————————————————————⟶ always

- be flexible, even if it means changing my expectations

  never ⟵————————————————————————⟶ always

- be openly inquisitive

  never ⟵————————————————————————⟶ always

- seek the truth, even if it differs from my beliefs

  never ⟵————————————————————————⟶ always

- be sensitive to my gut feelings

  never ⟵————————————————————————⟶ always

- reflect on my biases

  never ⟵————————————————————————⟶ always

- stick to something until I accomplish it

  never ⟵————————————————————————⟶ always

- spend time reflecting on my thinking and actions

  never ⟵————————————————————————⟶ always

Organizational Culture and CT

This brings us to a significant cultural influence on you as a thinker—the organizational culture of your work environment. We discuss organizational cultures more in Chapter 4 in the section about how, when, and where to think; in Chapter 7 with interdisciplinary teams; and again in Chapter 11, where we discuss day-to-day realities. Here we consider how much your employment environment defines you as a thinker. Much has been written about the influence of work environment on thinking (e.g., Chan, 2001; Senge, 1990). In her study of nursing preceptorship, Myrick (2002) identified the work climate or environment as a key variable enabling CT.

Organizational cultures can be very powerful. There is a strong tendency to assume that behaving in accordance with one's organizational culture is the "correct" way to do things and avoids role conflict. Such assumptions generally lead to a status quo environment that precludes thinking. After all, it's easy. Status quo thinking, however, is not healthy and eventually leads to the decline, entropy, and ultimate demise of the organization (Higgins, 1995).

Organizational cultures that promote a status quo existence are potentially dangerous to critical thinkers. Brookfield (1993) recognized this situation and warned critically thinking nurses about "cultural suicide" (being ostracized by coworkers as a result of challenging the status quo). Many critically thinking nurses are thought of as being on the fringes of mainstream thinking because they question, challenge, and annoy those who prefer to keep things the same.

Although few would admit to this, today's complex systems of healthcare practice and education often blatantly discourage CT. Mohr, Deatrick, Richmond, and Mahon (2001) addressed organizational values conflicts, painting a picture of troubled organizations. Some unhealthy traits they mentioned were over-control, distraction with minutiae, repression, intolerance for new members and diversity, territorial behaviors, depression, submissiveness, and horizontal violence (passive-aggressive behavior). This is a culture that will certainly not contribute to the growth of its members' CT.

Organizational cultures that encourage CT and acknowledge the inevitability of change are called "learning organizations," and they use "systems thinking" (Chan, 2001; Senge, 1990). Their members exhibit traits of trustworthiness, autonomy, responsibility, and reflection (Mohr et al., 2001). They rely on resources such as books, computers, links to libraries, and librarians. They provide think time and emphasize language/description and sharing of thinking. They give verbal "credit" and reward the thinking process, not just the end product. They welcome debate. If you are fortunate enough to work in that kind of environment, it is bound to positively influence you as a thinker. People like us, who spend a lot of time thinking about thinking, define such places as heaven, nirvana; we dream about such organizational cultures and hope to see them as the norm in nursing.

TACTICS 3-2

Environmental Factors Influencing Thinkers

Clinicians

Think about your environment. Generally speaking:

1. Where does it fall on the continuum from status quo thinking to our description of thinking heaven?
2. What is your position in that environment?
3. Can you influence the working culture?
4. How could you influence it?
5. Make a list of things you can influence in your environment that would make it more thinking-friendly.

Educators

Think about your teaching style.

1. Complete the checklist in **Box 3-3**.
2. How would you rate yourself as a positive influence on the thinking of your learners?
3. Review one of your teaching plans; do you see evidence of thinking–promoting strategies?
4. Can you or should you change anything in your plan?

BOX 3-3	**Thinking–Promoting Teaching Style Checklist**

In my teaching I:

- evaluate and give credit for thinking processes (e.g., "good thinking!").
- use multisensory techniques.
- encourage lots of questions.
- do not get defensive when questioned or challenged.
- help students find information resources.
- describe to students how I think.
- model my thinking.
- use deliberate methods to decrease anxiety.

(continues)

BOX 3-3	**(Continued)**

- develop teaching objectives/expected competencies that go beyond recall of information and require transforming information into usable knowledge.
- use humor.
- create a thinking-friendly environmental culture that accepts "mistakes" as opportunities to grow.
- vary teaching methods and strategies throughout each session.
- engage students in peer review activities.
- provide written reflection time in class.
- ask students to expand on their answers (e.g., "tell me more").
- promote students' positive self-concepts.
- emphasize collaborative learning between teacher and student (as opposed to authoritarian style).
- allow/encourage the student to be the teacher.

Discussion

How does your environmental culture stack up? Are you doing a good job of promoting CT in your organization? Cultures that promote CT have members who think individually and collectively. Such organizations are not neat; indeed, they appear rather chaotic. They are in a constant state of change. We'll discuss this change process in Chapter 11, but for now, think about what kind of thinker you are and how much that part of you is defined by your work culture. What can you do to make your environment more conducive to CT?

This reflection process helps to identify who in your organization are potential CT mentors. Not all members of an organization strive to be great thinkers. The larger the numbers of critical thinkers in an organization, the better the quality of health care.

PAUSE _____

and Ponder

Defining Ourselves as Critical Thinkers

In this chapter, we have focused on clinicians and educators who are the keys to promoting CT in nursing. Once again, let us caution you: CT is not just an individual phenomenon. Our CT is influenced by all the thinkers around us, and we influence their thinking, too. Repeatedly throughout this book, we assert the importance of this point. Today's healthcare delivery and educational systems are enormously complex. If clinicians and educators don't define themselves as critical thinkers, we will have unsolvable problems.

Reflection Cues

- This chapter specifically speaks to clinicians and educators about their identities as thinkers.
- Clinicians include everyone from beginning nursing students to expert nurses in the practice arena.
- Educators include everyone in all areas of teaching, from staff development to continuing education to the academic settings.
- Many factors influence one's development as a critical thinker.
- Genetics, or your natural thinking processes, influences *who* you are as a thinker.
- Gardner's multiple intelligences increase our awareness of different styles of thinking and processing information.
- Self-concept as an influence on CT is shaped by many factors, such as gender and social mores.
- Nurses are great thinkers, even though the world doesn't always see them as such or acknowledge their thinking as essential to their actions.
- Nurses are knowledge workers, not production workers.
- All emotions, especially anxiety, exert a huge influence on one's CT.
- The values, attitudes, and beliefs of different generations impact the teaching, learning, and thinking of healthcare providers.
- Both our native cultures and the cultures in which we live and work influence us as thinkers.
- Cultural differences in communication and time orientation affect *who* we become as thinkers.
- Organizational cultures can help or hinder one's development as a thinker.
- Cultures that discourage CT have traits such as intolerance, territorial behaviors, and repression.
- Organizational cultures that promote CT are called learning environments and use more systems thinking.
- We need to reflect on *who* we are as thinkers and how we promote a culture of thinking.
- Clinicians and educators must promote a unified view of CT as being vital to both practice and educational settings.

References

Belenky, M. F., Clinchy, B. M., Goldberger, N. R., & Tarule, J. M. (1986). *Women's ways of knowing: The development of self, voice, and mind.* New York: Basic Books.

Brookfield, S. (1993). On impostorship, cultural suicide, and other dangers: How nurses learn critical thinking. *Journal of Continuing Education in Nursing, 24,* 197–205.

Brookfield, S. D., & Preskill, S. (1999). *Discussion as a way of teaching: Tools and techniques for democratic classrooms.* San Francisco: Jossey-Bass.

Carson, M. (2003, November). *There to care: A lesson from nursing history.* Paper presented at the 37th biennial convention of Sigma Theta Tau International, Toronto, Ontario, Canada.

Chan, C-P. C. A. (2001). Implications of organizational learning for nursing managers from the cultural, interpersonal and systems thinking perspectives. *Nursing Inquiry, 8,* 196–199.

Erickson, J. I., Ditomassi, M. O., & Jones, D. A. (2008). Interdisciplinary institute for patient care: Advancing clinical excellence. *Journal of Nursing Administration, 38,* 308–314.

Falise, J. P. (2007). True collaboration: Interdisciplinary rounds in nonteaching hospitals—It can be done! *AACN Advanced Critical Care, 18,* 346–351.

Gardner, H. (1983). *Frames of mind: The theory of multiple intelligences* (10th anniversary ed.). New York: Basic Books.

Gardner, H. (1993). *Multiple intelligences: The theory in practice.* New York: Basic Books.

Gardner, H. (1999). *Intelligence reframed: Multiple intelligences for the 21st century.* New York: Basic Books.

Gardner, H. (2006). *Multiple intelligences: New horizons.* New York: Basic Books.

Giger, J. N., & Davidhizar, R. E. (2004). *Transcultural nursing: Assessment and intervention* (4th ed.). St. Louis, MO: Mosby.

Gilligan, C. (1982). *In a different voice: Psychological theory and women's development.* Cambridge, MA: Harvard University Press.

Gordon, S. (2005). *Nursing against the odds: How health care cost cutting, media stereotypes, and medical hubris undermine nurses and patient care.* Ithaca, NY: Cornell University Press.

Hart, L. A. (1983). *Human brain and human learning.* New York: Longman.

Higgins, J. M. (1995). Innovate or evaporate: Seven secrets of innovative corporations. *The Futurist, 29*(5), 42–48.

Kaeding, T. H., & Rambur, B. (2004). Recruiting knowledge, not just nurses. *Journal of Professional Nursing, 20,* 137–138.

Kelly-Thomas, K. J. (1998). *Clinical and nursing staff development: Current competence, future focus* (2nd ed.). Philadelphia: Lippincott.

Mohr, W. K., Deatrick, J., Richmond, T., & Mahon, M. M. (2001). A reflection on values in turbulent times. *Nursing Outlook, 49,* 30–36.

Myrick, F. (2002). Preceptorship and critical thinking in nursing education. *Journal of Nursing Education, 41,* 154–164.

Oblinger, D. G., & Oblinger, J. L. (2005). Is it age or IT: First steps toward understanding the Net Generation. In D. G. Oblinger & J. L. Oblinger (Eds.), *Educating the Net Generation* (Chapter 2). Retrieved November 24, 2008, from www.educause.edu/educatingthenetgen/

Redman, R. W. (2006). The challenge of interdisciplinary teams. *Research and Theory for Nursing Practice, 20,* 105–107.

Rossen, E. K., Bartlett, R. B., & Herrick, C. A. (2008). Interdisciplinary collaboration: The need to revisit. *Issues in Mental Health Nursing, 29*, 387–396.

Seago, J. A. (2008). Professional communication. In R. G. Hughes (Ed.), *Patient safety and quality: An evidence-based handbook for nurses* (pp. 2-247–2-269). Rockville, MD: Agency for Healthcare Research and Quality. (AHRQ Publication No. 08-0043)

Senge, P. M. (1990). *The fifth discipline: The art & practice of the learning organization.* New York: Doubleday.

Sherman, R. O. (2006). Leading a multigenerational nursing workforce: Issues, challenges and strategies. *Online Journal of Issues in Nursing, 11*(2). Retrieved November 25, 2008, from http://www.nursingworld.org/MainMenuCategories/ANAMarketplace/ANA Periodicals/OJIN/TableofContents/Volume112006/No2May06.aspx

Skiba, D. J., & Barton, A. J. (2006). Adapting your teaching to accommodate the net generation of learners. *Online Journal of Issues in Nursing, 11*(2). Retrieved November 25, 2008, from http://www.nursingworld.org/MainMenuCategories/ANAMarketplace/ANAPeriodicals/OJIN/TableofContents/Volume112006/No2May06.aspx

Weston, M. J. (2006). Integrating generational perspectives in nursing. *Online Journal of Issues in Nursing, 11*(2). Retrieved November 25, 2008, from http://www.nursingworld.org/MainMenuCategories/ANAMarketplace/ANAPeriodicals/OJIN/TableofContents/Volume112006/No2May06.aspx

Institute of Medicine Competencies as a Context for Thinking: The *How, When,* and *Where* of Critical Thinking

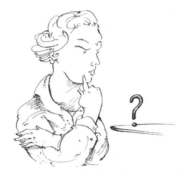

You can probably tell that our scheme of the *why, what, who,* and so on, looks good to start with but gets very muddy as we move along. We gave up trying to keep them separated and have combined the last three of the six—how, when, and where—together. It was difficult to keep *who* separated from *what* and *why,* but it is virtually impossible to discuss these last three out of the context of the others. If nothing else, critical thinking (CT) is contextual in nature. No matter what crosses our minds, it does so because something (*what*), somewhere (*where*), at some time (*when*), triggered that thought. *How* one thinks about anything, therefore, is influenced by the context (*when* and *where*) of that thought. That thinking, in turn, affects *what* happens relative to that issue or problem. The process is dynamic and convoluted. CT must have a context; otherwise it's just an academic abstraction. CT is a "tool in search of a job" (Scheffer & Rubenfeld, 2006, p. 195).

Current Challenges and Solutions for Healthcare Delivery

Nowhere is the *how* of CT more needed than in the healthcare arena, and the *when* is definitely now. Health care is faced with many challenges these days. People are living longer and therefore acquire more chronic conditions. Increasing numbers of specialists have made great strides in helping people deal with these many conditions, but at the same time, care has become fragmented. The healthcare system is fraught with politics. In the United States, there are many citizens with no health care because they have no insurance. A nursing shortage of heretofore unseen proportions looms with no coordinated plan to correct it. We could go on and on; most of you could add issues that would make the list continue for pages.

The Institute of Medicine Quality Chasm *Series*

The challenges facing the U.S. healthcare system have been made very public by the U.S Institute of Medicine (IOM), which, in 2000, produced the first of several reports: *To Err is Human: Building a Safer Health System*. The report's startling statement that perhaps as many as 98,000 Americans die yearly from medical errors drove home a picture of the healthcare system's dire situation. The IOM advocated an acceptance that error is inevitable and that blaming individuals is not the way to deal with those errors, and recommended that errors be analyzed to determine ways to prevent them in the future.

In its 2001 report, *Crossing the Quality Chasm: A New Health System for the 21st Century*, the IOM called healthcare professionals to action to improve patient care quality and safety. Six aims were described: Health care should be safe, effective, patient centered, timely, efficient, and equitable. One recommendation was to convene an interdisciplinary summit to recommend approaches to accomplish these aims. The culminated ideas from that summit, which met in 2002, were reported in *Health Professions Education: A Bridge to Quality* (IOM, 2003). The summit found that one major way we can affect practice is to change how we prepare healthcare practitioners. We need to lay better groundwork.

"All health professionals should be educated to deliver patient-centered care as members of an interdisciplinary team, emphasizing evidence-based practice, quality improvement approaches and informatics" (IOM, 2003, p. 3). The relationship among those five areas is shown in **Figure 4-1**.

We will return to this statement shortly because we have chosen it as the core of the next five chapters of this book. However, it is important to note that the IOM has continued to produce reports that describe potential solutions to the dilemmas in health care. In 2004, *Patient Safety: Achieving a New Standard for Care* expanded on earlier ideas for studying and preventing errors (IOM, 2004a). The critical role of nurses in patient safety was the focus of another 2004 report, *Keeping Patients Safe: Transforming the Work Environment of Nurses* (IOM, 2004b). Sources of threats to safety in which "bundles of change" were needed were identified in "each of the four fundamental components of all organizations: (1) management and leadership, (2) workforce deployment, (3) work processes, and (4) organizational culture" (IOM, 2004b, p. 48). In a description of what nurses do, an important distinction was made between visible and invisible activities. Those "invisible" activities were thinking activities.

The invisible or cognitive work incorporates knowledge learned from formal education and subsequently acquired expertise. It includes such processes as assessing a patient's health condition, monitoring and detecting when a change in therapy is needed, and integrating an individual patient's health care needs with the interventions of a variety of different health care providers to formulate a plan of care tailored to the particular patient. While certain assessment, monitoring, and care planning actions may be visible (e.g., a nurse watching a cardiac monitor or listening to a patient's chest), these cognitive processes are not. Often when a nurse appears to be carrying out a visible activity . . . he or she is actually performing numerous invisible tasks. (IOM, 2004b, p. 89)

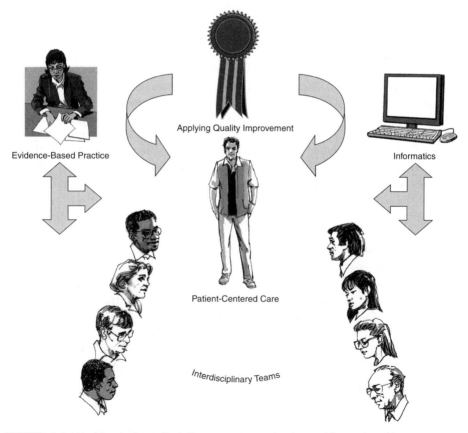

FIGURE 4-1 Working in interdisciplinary teams and using evidence-based practice and informatics for patient-centered care and quality improvement.

We strongly recommend that our readers visit the IOM Web site (http://www.iom. edu) periodically to view the important work that is being done to promote a safer, higher-quality American healthcare system.

Nursing has risen to the challenges posed by the IOM. More and more publications are making reference to the IOM ideas in proposals for change in nursing. For example, Finkelman and Kenner (2007) gave suggestions for how to incorporate the IOM reports into nursing education. Recently, the Agency for Healthcare Research and Quality (AHRQ) and the Robert Wood Johnson Foundation developed a handbook for nurses on patient safety and quality (Hughes, 2008). That three-volume set is a wealth of information for nurses, and indeed all health providers, providing background research and tools for improving the quality of care.

In 2008, the American Association of Colleges of Nursing (AACN) revised its *Essentials of Baccalaureate Education for Professional Nursing Practice*; early in the discussion of background influences on this document was reference to the IOM reports and the necessity of building a safer healthcare system (AACN, 2008). Many of the IOM recommended revisions to health education can be seen in the nine essentials.

In the next five chapters, we will show how many of the IOM suggestions are being, and could be, incorporated into nursing. We focus on the thinking processes that must accompany any attempts for reform. We've chosen the 2003 report on reforming health professions education to be a contextual scaffold for our thoughts on thinking. And that's our cue to go back to the 2003 IOM statement we quoted earlier: "All health professionals should be educated to deliver patient-centered care as members of an interdisciplinary team, emphasizing evidence-based practice, quality improvement approaches and informatics" (IOM, 2003, p. 3). Those five areas of education were envisioned as competencies that healthcare providers should reach.

Core Competencies to Improve Health Care

To live up to the vision of necessary changes in health professions education, the IOM advocated a set of five core competencies for all health professions. *Competency* was defined as "the habitual and judicious use of communication, knowledge, technical skills, clinical reasoning, emotions, values and reflection in daily practice" (Hundert, as cited in IOM, 2003, pp. 3–4). **Box 4-1** includes the definitions of the five competencies. As you can see, specific actions outlined in each definition fall into the communication, technical skills, clinical reasoning, emotions, values, and reflection categories of competence.

What Are Competencies?

We want to make sure that everyone understands what constitutes competencies or competency-based performance, because there are many misconceptions about these terms. By using the word *competencies*, the IOM was focusing on summative behaviors that they want, even expect, to see in practice. Competencies are very

BOX 4-1	Core Competencies for a New Vision for Health Professions Education

1. *Provide patient-centered care*—identify, respect, and care about patients' differences, values, preferences, and expressed needs; relieve pain and suffering; coordinate continuous care; listen to, clearly inform, communicate with, and educate patients; share decision making and management; and continuously advocate disease prevention, wellness, and promotion of healthy lifestyles, including a focus on population health.
2. *Work in interdisciplinary teams*—cooperate, collaborate, communicate, and integrate care in teams to ensure that care is continuous and reliable.
3. *Employ evidence-based practice*—integrate best research with clinical expertise and patient values for optimum care, and participate in learning and research activities to the extent feasible.
4. *Apply quality improvement*—identify errors and hazards in care; understand and implement basic safety design principles, such as standardization and simplification; continually understand and measure quality of care in terms of structure, process, and outcomes in relation to patient and community needs; and design and test interventions to change processes and systems of care, with the objective of improving quality.
5. *Utilize informatics*—communicate, manage knowledge, mitigate error, and support decision making using information technology.

Source: Institute of Medicine, 2003, p. 4.

specific endpoints that can be assessed; they are more than just a general list of areas for improvement. The use of competency language in the IOM's recommendations makes a stronger statement than a mere focus shift in healthcare delivery and education. They expect providers to be consistently competent in their performance in these five areas. Note the phrase *habitual and judicious use* in the preceding quote.

Bargagliotti, Luttrell, and Lenburg (1999), citing Lenburg's earlier work, provided this definition: "Competency-based performance evaluation is defined as a criterion-referenced, summative evaluation process that assesses a participant's actual ability to meet a predetermined set of performance standards under controlled conditions and protocols." They noted the difference between this type of evaluation and traditional checkoff methods in which a set of steps is demonstrated. Competency-based evaluations focus on evidence of effective implementation of specified skills; critical elements are demonstrated, but not necessarily in a step-by-step format. It's a bottom-line, real-world view, not a set of textbook steps. In short, it's all about performance.

Critical Thinking and Competencies

Although the actual term *critical thinking* is never used in the IOM competencies, words that are close cousins certainly appear in these performance ideals. The definition of *competency* cited previously speaks directly to clinical reasoning, knowledge, values, and reflection. Looking at all competencies, we see phrases such as *sharing decision making for patient-centered care; integrating best research when employing evidence-based practice; understanding quality and designing interventions in applying quality improvement; managing knowledge and supporting decision making with informatics* (IOM, 2003). In short, CT seems to be a necessary prerequisite to meeting the core competencies and is threaded throughout each of the five. We will link specific dimensions of CT to these five core competencies as we explore the thinking needed to make them a reality in Chapters 5–9. For now, let's consider some underlying approaches that will need to change for the IOM competencies to become a reality.

A Picture of Changes in Healthcare Delivery and Education

Clearly evident in the IOM's vision is a move away from status quo behavior in healthcare education and practice and toward a focus on context-bound thinking (the how, when, and where). The quality of clinical practice will improve, and there will be more collaboration among providers and with patients. Decisions will be based on evidence found through current informatics rather than on tradition. In the IOM view, these practice changes will occur through changes in health professions' education practices. We will begin our discussion of the *how* and *where*, then, with changes in education, but we'd like you to take a broad view of education. The education of health professionals doesn't just occur in educational institutions; it occurs in the practice setting as well. Because nursing and other health professions deal with a rapidly changing body of knowledge, all professionals must be lifelong learners.

There are many driving forces for change in practice arenas, such as cost containment, consumer demands, and new information. However, without a concomitant change in health professions education, that change will take longer (an important *when* consideration) and be less embedded in the values of clinicians. In addition, because of the immediate demands of the practice arena, service-based educators will very likely feel the pressures to change more quickly than academic-based educators.

Changes in Teaching and Learning Within a Thinking Framework

Let's consider how teaching and learning are approached in service settings as compared with academic settings because, although teaching/learning principles and approaches are used in both, the nature of the settings (*where*) sometimes makes a difference to the related issues. **Box 4-2** compares some of those key differences.

BOX 4-2	Differences Between Academic-Based and Service-Based Education	
Factor	Academic-Based	Service-Based
Time blocks for teaching	Structured	Variable
Amount of time in blocks	Hours	Minutes
Mix of novice to expert	More homogeneous	More heterogeneous
Mix of students	Nursing students	Nursing and unlicensed personnel
Focus on knowledge	Knowledge more than practice	Practice more than knowledge
Context	More noncontextual	More contextual
Teaching environment	Mostly classrooms	Variable spaces

Service-based educators often have to fit their teaching of required updated information into short, variable time slots to accommodate various shifts of nurses. Academic-based educators generally have structured class or clinical time that lasts anywhere from 1 to 8 hours. Time and schedules certainly make a difference in the techniques used to teach clinicians as compared with nursing students.

Service-based educators often deal with very heterogeneous groups—experienced nurses, novice nurses, and unlicensed assistive personnel. This creates additional challenges, because the language used in teaching and the expectations of the group must be modified, and leveling information must play a part. In spite of these differences, both practice- and academic-based educators use some similar teaching/learning approaches; thus, change in educational offerings, as well as delivery, will occur in both settings. Service-based educators, with their less structured teaching situations, may find these changes easier to deal with. Educators in academic settings may experience more challenges because of traditions.

How these changes in education occur is where CT comes in: We must change our thinking. To meet the five core competencies, education cannot be carried out in the tradition of educators handing down information to learners. Instead, academic faculty and service-based educators will need to help students become active knowledge seekers rather than passive information receivers. This type of teaching and learning is a collaborative effort, not the one-up, one-down configuration of the traditional authoritarian teaching. Giddens and Brady (2007) advocated a change from our traditional content-saturated nursing education to a concept-based approach. In the latter, students are active learners instead of passive recipients of content.

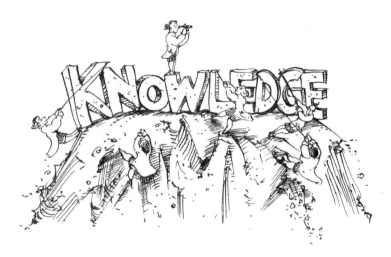

Minds for the Future

Howard Gardner (2006), whom we cited in an earlier chapter as describing multiple intelligences, had some interesting thoughts on what he called "five minds for the future." His contention was that the future will demand "capacities that until now have been mere options" (p. 2). Those five "minds" are *disciplinary, synthesizing, creating, respectful,* and *ethical.* The disciplined mind has to do with mastery and continual honing of the skills of a profession or specialty. The synthesizing mind is particularly relevant to the health professions in that it is concerned with pulling together several sets of information and making an amalgam of that information. The creating mind is able to clarify and solve problems in innovative ways. The respectful mind appreciates the differences among people, and the ethical mind focuses on responsibility as citizens.

Gardner (2006) encouraged us to look at these minds relative to changes in today's world and how we educate future generations. He saw those without one or more disciplines as "being restricted to menial tasks," and those "without synthesizing capabilities . . . as overwhelmed by information and unable to make judicious decisions." Those without creativity "will be replaced by computers and will drive away those who have the creative spark." Those without respect "will poison the workplace," and those without ethics "will yield a world devoid of decent workers and responsible citizens" (pp. 18–19).

Gardner's (2006) views are focused on needed changes in education, not just in formal settings, but in today's workplace.

We should be concerned with how to nurture these minds in the younger generation, those who are being educated currently to become the leaders of tomorrow. But we should be equally concerned with those in today's workplace: how best can we mobilize our skills—and those of our coworkers—so that all of us will remain current tomorrow and the day after tomorrow? (p. 10)

As we anticipate changes in society, we must think of those changes as they are and will be mirrored in healthcare systems. Gardner's (2006) ideas are particularly relevant to helping health professionals learn differently than they have in the past and to focus on thinking. We need to reform nursing education, and we need a drastic change in our views of the workings of the mind. We're not sure what Gardner would say specifically about nursing education, but he had this to say about education in general: "current formal education still prepares students primarily for the world of the past, rather than for possible worlds of the future . . ." (p. 17). Perhaps closer to home for an applied science such as nursing is this comment: "We acknowledge the importance of science and technology but do not teach scientific ways of thinking, let alone how to develop individuals with the synthesizing and creative capacities essential for continual scientific and technological progress" (p. 17).

Although Gardner's labels—synthesizing in particular—are not identical, they are very similar to "integrative learning" advocated by the Association of American Colleges and Universities and the Carnegie Foundation for the Advancement of Teaching (2004), which had this to say:

Integrative learning comes in many varieties: connecting skills and knowledge from multiple sources and experiences; applying theory to practice in various settings; utilizing diverse and even contradictory points of view; and, understanding issues and positions contextually. Significant knowledge within individual disciplines serves as the foundation, but integrative learning goes beyond academic boundaries. Indeed, integrative experiences often occur as learners address real-world problems, unscripted and sufficiently broad to require multiple areas of knowledge and multiple modes of inquiry, offering multiple solutions and benefiting from multiple perspectives (2nd para).

We think these descriptions sound very much like CT. Perhaps a change of labels, from CT to integrative learning, will help make the case that we must look closer at how we teach and learn thinking in nursing. Tanner (2007) made important links from integrative teaching to CT and nursing education. "*Integrative teaching and learning* may well become the buzz phrase for this decade, replacing the ubiquitous, yet conceptually fuzzy, emphasis on *critical thinking*" (p. 531).

How change in teaching/learning will occur will not be easy. Frederic Moore Binder, former president of Hartwick College (Gaie's excellent alma mater), recently cited this old adage: "Changing a college curriculum is like trying to move a cemetery" (2000, para. 5). Perhaps service-based educators have less "buried" patterns, but we'll bet you can relate. As educators who have struggled through curriculum changes, we can attest to the truth of that cemetery analogy.

We have a long tradition of teachers being authorities and all-knowing. Students come through an education system that largely uses this hierarchical model of teaching; they expect to be takers of information. When changes occur in practice, they are used to someone handing them the new information. How, then, can nurse leaders and educators promote integrative or synthesis learning and knowledge-seeking behaviors? Myrick and Tamlyn (2007) dared educators to reflect critically on their teaching and to move to more enlightened approaches that promote student thinking. We are talking about a teaching/learning paradigm shift. That sounds like a big deal, and we'll discuss that shortly, but first let's focus on some easily overlooked but vital "small" things that can help us move to more enlightened teaching/learning.

Make Some Small Changes

Some students, probably more than we think, are affected by seemingly simple comments or actions. Look at **Box 4-3** for a list of such simple comments and nonverbal behaviors that can either promote or squelch CT.

BOX 4-3 | **Comments and Behaviors That Promote or Squelch CT**

Comments and Behaviors That Promote CT	Comments and Behaviors That Squelch CT
• That's an interesting question.	• What a dumb question!
• There's no such thing as a dumb question.	• Don't you know that?
• Do you have a different idea how to do this?	• You should know that!
• Let's explore this.	• We've always done it this way.
• Let's think this through.	• That's the wrong way to do that.
• I'm not sure; can we figure this out?	• That'll never work here.
• Don't believe everything you read or hear.	• Just do it this way.
	• Why do you have to make everything so complicated?
	• That will never fit in our budget.

BOX 4-3	(Continued)

Comments and Behaviors That Promote CT	Comments and Behaviors That Squelch CT
• Show me how you came to that conclusion.	• Just memorize it.
• Can we look at this from a different angle?	• Stop with the questions, already!
• What do you think?	• Because I said so, that's why!
• Walk me through your thinking on this.	• If you're so sure of yourself, you figure it out.
• Tell me about what you learned here.	• Mistakes are not tolerated here.
• Let's see what others have to say.	• Let's get moving; we don't have all day.
• That's one option; let's see what other ways might also work.	• I can't believe you don't know that by now.
• What are some possible outcomes of that approach?	• Come on, use your brain here!
• That was a great example of how you used _____ (insert the CT dimension used, such as inquisitiveness).	• It's too complicated to explain.
	• I can't believe you said/did that!
	• Roll eyes.
	• Smirk.
• That's a good idea; let's expand on it to make it even better.	• Big sighs.
• Use a neutral voice tone.	• Scowl.
• Use an enthusiastic voice tone.	• Foot-tapping or finger-tapping.
	• Other nonverbal demonstrations of anger, frustration, irritation.
• Sit silently and patiently.	• Look at one's watch frequently.

TACTICS 4-1

Promoting CT or Knowledge-Seeking Behavior

Clinicians

Using **Box 4-3**, reflect on your interactions with other staff over the past 2 days. How often have you made comments from the left column of the box, and how often from the right? Be honest now! Think about how you feel when you hear comments from each side of that box.

Educators

Using **Box 4-3**, think about your teaching situation in the past 2 months. How often have you made comments from the left column of the box and how often from the right? Be honest now! Alternatively, ask students to list what they think are the most and least productive teacher comments related to promoting knowledge-seeking behaviors. Use the responses as a self-inventory of the comments you make when teaching.

Discussion

You probably remember some of the CT-promoting and CT-squelching comments directed at you during your education. They stick in your mind, don't they? Especially the squelching ones. It's frightening to acknowledge the potential impact of our small comments, but it's healthy to contemplate how our behavior might help or hinder knowledge-seeking behavior.

Bigger Changes

Now, let's examine the bigger guns of teaching/learning approaches that will transform health professions' education in the 21st century. The philosopher John Dewey wrote *Democracy and Education* in 1916. Because his wisdom has withstood the test of time and because he links thinking and action, Dewey's ideas have particular relevance for teaching and learning in health care. Consider this gem from Dewey that should make you sit up and take note: "Information severed from thoughtful action is dead, a mind-crushing load" (1916/1966, p. 153). Think about that statement the next time you write exam items. Do you want a simple recall of information or a more cognitively sophisticated application item? For those of you who hunger for more of Dewey's thoughts on education and thinking, we've compiled some "Dewey Diamonds" in **Box 4-4**.

Dewey's ideas underpin the problem-based learning movement, which was made popular by McMaster University in Ontario, Canada, and is in common use worldwide today (Rideout, 2001). This student-centered approach to learning

BOX 4-4	**Dewey Diamonds**

(The first bold lines are our translations. Sorry, Dewey.)

Don't be too academic.
"Hence the first approach to any subject in school, if thought is to be aroused and not words acquired, should be as unscholastic as possible." (p. 154)

Both thinking without action and action without thinking get you nowhere.
"Thinking which is not connected with increase of efficiency in action, and with learning more about ourselves and the world in which we live, has something the matter with it just as thought. And skill obtained apart from thinking is not connected with any sense of the purposes for which it is to be used. It consequently leaves a man at the mercy of his routine habits and of the authoritative control of others." (p. 152)

Some people think you can improve thinking separately from what you do.
"Thinking is often regarded both in philosophic theory and in educational practice as something cut off from experience, and capable of being cultivated in isolation." (p. 153)

Teachers, don't make things too hard or too simple.
"A large part of the art of instruction lies in making the difficulty of new problems large enough to challenge thought, and small enough so that, in addition to the confusion naturally attending the novel elements, there shall be luminous familiar spots from which helpful suggestions may spring." (p. 157)

Education is all about thinking.
"[T]he important thing is that thinking is the method of an educative experience. The essentials of method are therefore identical with the essentials of reflection." (p. 163)

Lectures on topics out of context are boring.
"Under the influence of the conception of the separation of mind and material, method tends to be reduced to a cut and dried routine, to following mechanically prescribed steps." (p. 169)

Some teachers think you're a troublemaker if you ask questions.
"Exorbitant desire for uniformity of procedure and for prompt external results are the chief foes which the open-minded attitude meets in school. The teacher who does not permit and encourage diversity of operation in dealing with questions is imposing intellectual blinders upon pupils—restricting their vision to the one path the teacher's mind happens to approve." (p. 175)

It's not all about quick answers.
"The zeal for 'answers' is the explanation of much of the zeal for rigid and mechanical methods." (p. 175)

Some people still want someone to just give them the answers.
"Men still want the crutch of dogma, of beliefs fixed by authority, to relieve them of the trouble of thinking and the responsibility of directing their activity by thought." (p. 339)

Source: Quoted material is from Dewey (1916/1966).

links learning to action in that students are directed by relevant problems or issues rather than a set of topics defined by the teacher. Independent inquiry and reflection are important thinking components of this approach. (Remember, we started this book with a discussion of the value of questions because we believe that questions are the best place to start a thinking journey.)

There are also many references to Dewey in Wiggins and McTighe's *Understanding by Design* (1998). They differentiated real understanding (that which uses learning in new ways) from knowledge that is "superficial, rote, out-of-context and easily tested" (p. 40). We want to promote real understanding, which Wiggins and McTighe viewed as having six facets: "When we truly understand, we can . . . explain . . . interpret . . . apply . . . have perspective . . . empathize . . . [and] have self-knowledge" (p. 44). Have you ever said the best way to learn something is to teach it? Look at those six facets and think about the last time you spent a lot of time and energy preparing a lesson. You probably drew on each of those six facets. A little later in this chapter, we're going to discuss the benefits of picturing yourself teaching something as a way of learning. We'll revisit the six facets then.

Another take on Dewey's ideals is Barr and Tagg's article (1995), which clearly identified the differences between teaching and learning. For example, teaching implies a hierarchy; learning is done in collaboration. Teaching implies covering material; learning implies performance outcomes. Teaching implies that "knowledge exists out there"; learning implies that "knowledge exists in each person's mind and is shaped by individual experience." Teaching implies that "knowledge comes in chunks and bits delivered by instructors"; learning implies that "knowledge is constructed, created, 'gotten' " (p. 17).

In today's healthcare world, where things change almost by the minute, we need to aim for competencies. Performance at competence level necessitates the kind of understanding that allows for transfer of information to fit new situations—what we call *transforming knowledge*. This is what Perry (1970) called "relativism," where knowledge is contextual and relative, and multiple perspectives fit into a big picture. This relativism is in contrast to "dualism," where there are right and wrong answers and the world is seen in absolute categories. In nursing, we are most familiar with the move from dualism to relativism in terms of ways of viewing situations and gaining knowledge from Benner's work (1984). Benner defined these differences as existing between novices and expert nurses. From her work, we have learned to do all we can to move nurses away from novice dualism to the relativistic or contextual thinking of experts.

Old dualistic teaching and learning methods just don't cut it. Clinicians cannot learn about new medications and procedures and expect that information to remain static; it will change, for example, as research reveals better procedures and as medications are shown to be valuable for off-label uses. Clinicians must be able to converse intelligently about new information with the healthcare team and with patients and families.

Educators shouldn't just test students for their recall of textbook information. Who cares what you know today if you won't be able to use that knowledge tomorrow when the context changes? We must help students process information and use it to define their own knowledge. We must move away from shoveling content at students and move toward learning partnerships focused on students discovering things for themselves. And we must develop new habits of the mind to help students do the same. "The development of understanding greatly depends on such attitudes and habits of mind as open-mindedness, self-discipline (autonomy), tolerance for ambiguity, and reflectiveness" (Wiggins & McTighe, 1998, p. 171).

On the academic side of nursing, any suggestion related to changing how content is taught generally sends seasoned faculty running, holding their lecture notes close to their hearts. We are too focused on teaching specific content, fearing that students will not learn content unless it is taught directly. Debates over content often get dichotomized because of the assumption that content and process are parallel and mutually exclusive. This leads to the idea that one must teach either process or content. For those teaching undergraduate students, one of the driving forces behind a rigid focus on content is that students must pass the National Council Licensure Examination. This kind of thinking presupposes that students will not learn content if it is not spoon-fed to them. Does that make any sense? No. We are caught in the providing-information paradigm.

So what needs to be done? Starting with simple steps, we need to redefine the process of acquiring knowledge and understanding (content). A teaching method is not the same as a learning process. Certainly, some teaching methods do seem to promote learning better than others, and we'll discuss some of those shortly. But learning is a whole other process, and it doesn't matter much what we teach and how we do it if no one learns.

We should also clarify what we mean by "content" and "process": Content is information, and process is what we do with that information. There's certainly a necessary marriage of the two in a practice discipline. However, that's too facile; we need to expand on the idea of content or knowledge. We need to distinguish between the acquisition of information and the process of true learning. True learning means internalizing information and transforming it into knowledge until it becomes part of the learner's ideas. Only then can the learner use that knowledge meaningfully (such as for patient care situations). In this context, Dewey's observations are helpful. He said that we don't convey ideas. Ideas form as we do something in our heads with the facts told to us. When facts are shared,

> the communication may stimulate that other person to realize the question for himself and to think out a like idea, or it may smother his intellectual interest and suppress his dawning effort at thought. But what he directly gets cannot be an idea. Only by wrestling with the conditions of the problem at first hand, seeking and finding his own way out, does he think. (Dewey, 1916/1966, pp. 159–160)

If that doesn't stimulate you to plan interactive teaching, nothing will! We'll bet that clinicians are nodding in agreement at this point, though educators may still be a bit skeptical. That's because clinicians are focused on using knowledge, not teaching it. Anyone who uses knowledge knows it's necessary to have it in idea form—what Wiggins and McTighe (1998) called real understanding—that can be used in a variety of ways. Ask clinicians how they learn best, and most will say by practicing or using something. In other words, they are thinking of ideas, not facts. They have done something with what they learned. They have internalized the information so they can use it. Educators need to take a lesson from clinicians and focus on what their students will be doing with the information they are receiving; then educators can adapt their teaching methods to the realities of healthcare practice.

Techniques to Promote Thinking and Knowledge Processing

Thankfully, there are many teaching method resources to promote thinking and the processing of knowledge out there for educators these days. Our favorite is what we call the "CAT" book (*Classroom Assessment Techniques*) by Angelo and Cross (1993). Even though it says "classroom," we think service educators will find it useful, too. Another helpful guide is by Billings and Halstead (2009). We have listed some of the techniques adapted from those sources in **Box 4-5**. Note that these are all interactive approaches.

Many of these teaching techniques can also be used to assess CT competencies. If we view CT as just one of many competencies, then we need to be teaching so that students will be able to demonstrate their CT. Chapter 10 is all about assessing CT, so we'll limit our discussion here to making sure that you link assessment with teaching and learning. **Box 10-2** will give you more ideas for practical teaching methods linked to learning and assessing CT, so for now, consider Chapter 10 an annex to the present chapter.

Teaching as Learning

One of our favorite questions to undergraduate nursing students is this: "How would you explain that to a patient?" Think about that. Inevitably, nurses have to impart most of their knowledge to patients. Remember our discussion of Wiggins and McTighe's (1998) six facets of true understanding—explain, interpret, apply, have perspective, empathize, have self-knowledge. If those ring true in your mind, you will agree that one of the best ways to learn something is to teach it to someone else. And having to teach someone who does not have your working vocabulary will make that an even more valuable learning experience, because now you have to translate the message, too. To do that, you really need to know it.

For our clinician readers, how often do you teach things to patients? Most of you will answer, "continually." Each day, as you learn new things, think about how you would effectively explain these things to a patient. Paolo Freire, the educational philosopher we quoted in Chapter 1, said this beautifully: "Whoever teaches learns in the act of teaching, and whoever learns teaches in the act of learning" (1998, p. 31).

BOX 4-5	Teaching Techniques to Promote Processing and Internalization of Knowledge

*Muddiest Point: After presenting content, have students write on cards the muddiest point and hand in the cards anonymously; the teacher then discusses each of those points.

*One-Sentence Summary: Have students sum up what they just learned in one sentence. Then, in groups, have students explain why they came up with that sentence.

*One-Word Summary: A variation on the one-sentence summary, students choose one word and explain why that word summarizes the idea.

*Concept or Mind Maps: Students map out ideas and the connections among them, questions, answers, and so on, in some way that is meaningful to them.

*Student-Generated Test Questions: Students come up with test questions. These can be collected and used for tests and quizzes.

*Minute Paper: At the end of teaching session, students are asked to answer a question, such as, "What was the most important thing you learned today?" or "What are you most curious to learn more about?" Students are given a minute to write an answer.

*Empty Outline or Empty Mind Map: The teacher gives students a partially completed outline or map; they need to fill in the blanks.

*Memory Matrix: Students set up a grid with some ideas across the top and some down the side; they then fill in the squares to show relationships.

~Algorithms: Break tasks into yes/no steps to solve complex problems.

~Argumentation/Debate: Promotes logical reasoning and open-mindedness as students debate controversial issues. Works well when students have to argue the side opposite to their view.

~Case Studies/Scenarios: Use to teach content; have students share cases with similar or different parts.

~Collaborative Learning: Work groups for assignments or problem solving.

~Newspaper Analysis: Students analyze something written for the lay public, determine/critique sources of information, and discuss relevance to nursing.

~Reflection Projects/Logs: Have students reflect on something, focusing specifically on their thinking.

Source: *Adapted from Angelo & Cross, 1993.
~Adapted from Billings & Halstead, 2009.

Learning in the Workplace

In Chapter 11, we will discuss the realities of practice today and tomorrow, but here we'd like to sow the seeds for the learning environment. Carole Estabrooks (2003), in her discussion of using research in practice, characterized nurses as generating knowledge within their "communities of practice" (p. 60). People don't learn in isolation; they do it with others. Nurses produce knowledge, as well as use it, in their workplaces every day. We don't think Dewey would be surprised to read this, especially if he considered the huge amount of knowledge that nurses must learn and use daily.

This idea of integrating learning and the practicalities of practice is echoed in Carkhuff's (1996) advocacy of reflective learning through the use of work/learning groups in the workplace. This approach is very helpful for service-based educators who want to move from the old goals of adaptive learning that focus on survival and maintenance, to a generative learning model based on creativity and continual learning (Watkins & Marsick, 1993). Carkhuff provided an excellent example of reflective group learning: While checking the competency of nurses to correctly identify and locate equipment on a crash cart, several nurses were unable to meet the criteria. Rather than reteach the crash cart criteria, the staff educator encouraged the group to reflect on and discuss why it was difficult to do this job without error. Together they came up with strategies to increase their competency. The keys to the success of this approach are that the learning was problem based, learner directed, contextual, and reflective.

Reflection in Practice

We'd like to talk more about the value of reflection, not just as a teaching/learning tool, but also as a way to increase clinicians' CT. A word to clinicians: In the last few pages, we've focused on educators, but it would be useful here for you to consider the thinking challenges you deal with daily. You probably do not practice as you once did because of the rapid pace of change in the healthcare arena. "Reflection in practice" is how Schon (1983) referred to this, a wonderful idea that is poignantly relevant today. Schon advocated that practitioners think about what they are doing and thinking while in the midst of action—to be "reflective practitioners" in response to changes in their professions. Although healthcare professionals were one of his intended audiences, he cited many professionals who have experienced a "crisis of confidence" because of "the mismatch of traditional patterns of practice and knowledge [and the] . . . complexity, uncertainty, instability, uniqueness, and value conflict" (p. 18) of the practice arena.

This complexity and uncertainty are especially found in what Schon (1983) called the "swampy lowland where situations are confusing 'messes' incapable of technical solution" (p. 42). Whoa! Does that sound like a typical *when* and *where* for nurses or what, eh? Schon also said that those who choose the swampy lowland "deliberately involve themselves in messy but crucially important problems and, when asked to describe their methods of inquiry, they speak of experience, trial and error, intuition, and muddling through" (p. 43). Can something be done to help clinicians "muddle through" better? Schon's answer is reflection.

How can clinicians use reflection to meet the goals that the IOM has advocated for practice? First and foremost, you must focus on thinking—not as a phenomenon separate from daily work, but as it is joined with action. Now, don't get the idea here that nurses can ever practice without thinking. That is a scary thought. However, reflection in action is thinking about the thinking and the action as one is actively working. That reflection is necessary because of the changing nature of health care. What worked yesterday won't necessarily work today; what we did yesterday is not necessarily what we should be doing today. Thinking and acting are linked out of necessity; we don't have the luxury of sitting back and doing our thinking after the fact, nor would we be comfortable doing that. However, because it is so easy to concentrate on action rather than on the thinking, we need reminders to think.

How Does Reflection in Action Work?

At the risk of being prescriptive, we've come up with a list of questions that clinicians should ask themselves as they reflect (see **Box 4-6**.) As you see, they are essentially based on the CT habits of the mind and skills that we have already discussed. Now, would each clinician reflect on these things in a linear, checklist kind of way? Of course not. But it's helpful to have such a list to help us think about things fully.

BOX 4-6   **Suggestions for Clinicians' Reflection in Action**

Am I . . .

> reasonably sure of my thinking here?
> taking into account the total context of this situation?
> considering more creative, better approaches?
> being too rigid? Too loose?
> asking all the questions I should be asking?
> using any preconceived notions that might be wrong?
> going with my gut reactions or ignoring them?
> closing my mind off to any possibilities?
> sticking with this long enough, or is it time to just make a decision and get on with it?
> breaking this down enough so I'm seeing all the pieces and how they fit together?
> forgetting any important rules here?
> seeing the patterns and details?
> missing anything?
> making conclusions based on solid data?
> able to predict where this is going?
> adapting my knowledge to this situation?

TACTICS 4-2

Reflection in Action

Clinicians

Think about your most recent clinical day. Now think of a specific patient encounter or team meeting. Using the questions in Box 4-6, reflect on these events. Pay attention to how comfortable you are with reflection. Try to picture yourself in the midst of what was happening. Were you reflective at the time? As you recall the situation, do things occur to you now that you didn't consider while the event was happening?

Discussion

If the checklist idea seems a bit scripted to you, think about other ways to promote reflective practice. Perhaps this real-life situation will spark your creativity.

We asked our nurse practitioner colleague Jane Duerr to describe her reflection in action. She talked about *where, when,* and *how* to reflect. (OK, so we prompted her with those words . . . nevertheless, this is what she said.)

> *I try to reflect with another clinician if I can because I think better when I can bounce ideas off someone else. I do that in several ways—both structured and informally. On the structured side, the nurse practitioners at my office get together for breakfast on a regular schedule to talk about practice issues. We make a point of not turning that into a complaining session about things we dislike, but, rather, we focus on things we've seen in practice that we're concerned with, new information we've found and so forth—real collaborative communication. The physicians and nurse practitioners also have a journal club where we reflect on our practice relative to the latest research findings. Less structured reflection occurs in the corridors and lunchroom; sometimes I call one of the docs or nurses to bounce ideas off them in the middle of the day.*
>
> *I also reflect with families and patients. Sometimes sitting down and going over things with them allows me to think aloud; we can think together and often come up with better actions than I would have come up with alone. It's very easy to forget that patients and families are there, too.*
>
> *As to where I reflect, it's everywhere, especially places where I can find some solitude. I go into the lab, find an empty office, I do a lot of reflection in my car on the way home or to and from settings. I often take a longer route home so I can have more thinking time.*

The challenge to clinicians is this: How are you managing reflection in practice? Do you do it enough? Where do you do it? Do you need to reflect on your reflection?

PAUSE
and Ponder

Think Ahead to Change

In this chapter, we've discussed *how* educators and clinicians need to grow to make sure that the competencies of providing patient-centered care, working in interdisciplinary teams, employing evidence-based practice, applying quality improvement, and using informatics become the norm of health care.

This chapter is a bookend on one side of the next chapters, which address the IOM competencies. In Chapter 11, the other bookend, we will revisit some of the ideas introduced here when we consider the day-to-day realities of healthcare practice and education. In this chapter, we described many overt and covert messages about the necessity for change. We'll pick up that theme in Chapter 11, expanding on what thinking is necessary to survive the inevitable complexities of change in healthcare delivery and education.

Reflection Cues

- The *how, when,* and *where* of CT for clinicians and educators are intrinsically interconnected: The *where* is healthcare practice and education; the *when* is today and tomorrow. What remains is to figure out the best *how*.
- The IOM has issued a challenge for health professions "to deliver patient-centered care as members of an interdisciplinary team, emphasizing evidence-based practice, quality improvement approaches, and informatics" and for healthcare educators to produce clinicians who can achieve this task (IOM, 2003, p. 3).
- Errors are inevitable. Blaming individuals is not the way to deal with those errors; errors need to be analyzed to determine ways to prevent them in the future.
- Meeting the IOM's challenge will require major changes in the practice and education of health professionals.
- Education must move away from the status quo of traditional teaching and start focusing on active learning rather than rote memorization.
- Thinking in education and practice requires us to expand our understanding of what Gardner (2006) referred to as the five minds of the future: disciplinary, synthesizing, creating, respectful, and ethical.
- Students must become finders of knowledge, not takers of information.

- Knowledge-seeking behavior can be affected by such simple things as casual comments and nonverbal behaviors directed toward learners.
- A primary goal must be to aim for understanding that allows for transfer of information in a variety of circumstances.
- Dewey's ideas on differences between providing knowledge and forming ideas are relevant to educators today.
- Various teaching techniques lend themselves to promoting knowledge processing.
- Encouraging students and clinicians to imagine themselves teaching patients to think and learn is helpful in developing new skills.
- Clinicians are encouraged to practice what Schon (1983) called *reflection in action* to promote thinking for today's ever-changing practice world.
- Reflecting on the differences between teaching and learning is helpful in gaining a new perspective on *how* to improve thinking.

References

American Association of Colleges of Nursing. (2008, October 20). *The essentials of baccalaureate education for professional nursing practice.* Retrieved October 29, 2008, from http://www.aacn.nche.edu/Education/pdf/BaccEssentials08.pdf

Angelo, T. A., & Cross, K. P. (1993). *Classroom assessment techniques: A handbook for college teachers* (2nd ed.). San Francisco: Jossey-Bass.

Association of American Colleges and Universities and The Carnegie Foundation for the Advancement of Teaching. (2004). *A statement on integrative learning.* Retrieved November 30, 2008, from http://www.carnegiefoundation.org/dynamic/downloads/file_1_185.pdf

Bargagliotti, T., Luttrell, M., & Lenburg, C. (1999, September 30). Reducing threats to the implementation of a competency-based performance assessment system. *Online Journal of Issues in Nursing.* Retrieved February 13, 2009 from http://www.nursingworld.org/search.aspx?SearchMode=1&SearchPhrase=Bargagliotti&SearchWithin=2

Barr, R. B., & Tagg, J. (1995). From teaching to learning: A new paradigm for undergraduate education. *Change, 27*(6), 13–25.

Benner, P. (1984). *From novice to expert: Power and excellence in nursing practice.* Menlo Park, CA: Addison-Wesley.

Billings, D. M., & Halstead, J. A. (2009). *Teaching in nursing: A guide for faculty* (3rd ed.). Philadelphia: Saunders Elsevier.

Binder, F. M. (2000). *So you want to be a college president?* Retrieved June 3, 2004, from http://www.cosmos-club.org/web/journals/2000/binder.html

Carkhuff, M. H. (1996). Reflective learning: Work groups as learning groups. *Journal of Continuing Education in Nursing, 27,* 209–214.

Dewey, J. (1966). *Democracy and education.* New York: Free Press. (Original work published 1916)

Estabrooks, C. A. (2003). Translating research into practice: Implications for organizations and administrators. *Canadian Journal of Nursing Research, 35*(3), 53–68.

Finkelman, A., & Kenner, C. (2007). *Teaching IOM: Implications of the Institute of Medicine reports for nursing education.* Silver Spring, MD: American Nurses Association.

Freire, P. (1998). *Pedagogy of freedom: Ethics, democracy, and civic courage* (P. Clarke, Trans.) Lanham, MD: Rowman and Littlefield.

Gardner, H. (2006). *Five minds for the future*. Boston: Harvard Business School Press.

Giddens, J. F., & Brady, D. P. (2007). Rescuing nursing education from content saturation: The case for a concept-based curriculum. *Journal of Nursing Education, 46*, 65–69.

Hughes, R. G. (Ed.). (2008, April) *Patient safety and quality: An evidence-based handbook for nurses* (Prepared with support from the Robert Wood Johnson Foundation). Rockville, MD: Agency for Healthcare Research and Quality. (AHRQ Publication No. 08-0043)

Institute of Medicine. (2000). *To err is human: Building a safer health system*. Washington, DC: National Academies Press.

Institute of Medicine. (2001). *Crossing the quality chasm: A new health system for the 21st century*. Washington, DC: National Academies Press.

Institute of Medicine. (2003). *Health professions education: A bridge to quality*. Washington, DC: National Academies Press.

Institute of Medicine. (2004a). *Patient safety: Achieving a new standard for care*. Washington, DC: National Academies Press.

Institute of Medicine. (2004b). *Keeping patients safe: Transforming the work environment of nurses*. Washington, DC: National Academies Press.

Myrick, F., & Tamlyn, D. (2007). Teaching can never be innocent: Fostering an enlightening educational experience. *Journal of Nursing Education, 46*, 299–303.

Perry, W. G. (1970). *Forms of intellectual and ethical development in the college years*. New York: Holt, Rinehart and Winston.

Rideout, W. (2001). *Transforming nursing education through problem-based learning*. Sudbury, MA: Jones and Bartlett.

Scheffer, B. K., & Rubenfeld, M. G. (2006). Critical thinking: A tool in search of a job. *Journal of Nursing Education, 45*, 195–196.

Schon, D. A. (1983). *The reflective practitioner: How professionals think in action*. New York: Basic Books.

Tanner, C. A. (2007). Connecting the dots: What's all the buzz about integrative teaching? *Journal of Nursing Education, 46*, 531–532.

Watkins, K. E., & Marsick, V. J. (1993). *Sculpting the learning organization: Lessons in the art and science of systemic change*. San Francisco: Jossey-Bass.

Wiggins, G., & McTighe, J. (1998). *Understanding by design*. Upper Saddle River, NJ: Merrill Prentice Hall.

CHAPTER ———————————— 5

Critical Thinking, Quality Improvement, and Safety

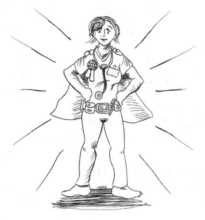

Of the five Institute of Medicine (IOM) competencies discussed in Chapter 4, quality improvement seems to be the one toward which all others are aimed. We have therefore decided to start your thinking journey with this competency. Quality improvement and safety require all healthcare providers, including nurses, to change their thinking as well as their actions. To begin appreciating the impact of critical thinking (CT) or lack of CT on patient quality and safety, read the following patient situation. You should wonder how this could happen in today's state-of-the-art healthcare system.

JW is a 76-year-old 170-pound woman in general good health but has significant immobility and pain secondary to degenerative joint disease in her left knee. She elected to have a knee replacement. Twenty-four hours after surgery to replace her left knee, during a transfer from her hospital bed to a wheelchair, her care providers dropped her to the floor, disrupting the surgical site. After her repair surgery and during her rehabilitation in extended care, she was fitted with a knee support brace in the wrong size. This was discovered after 3 weeks and resulted in another return to surgery to repair the improper and increasingly painful knee alignment. Infection set in after this third surgery, resulting in a long course of antibiotics. After the infections cleared, a fourth surgery fused her left knee, resulting in a permanently straight left leg. JW finally returned home after four surgeries and 5 months of inpatient and extended rehabilitation care. Her mobility is now less than presurgery.

Whether you are a beginning nursing student or have been practicing nursing for years, you can quickly identify the most obvious points at which CT *did not* occur in JW's care. Insufficient thinking contributed to healthcare worker errors (unsafe transferring practice and improper selection of equipment) and system errors (transfer policies and infection control), resulting in severely compromised patient care. Unacceptable outcomes such as those experienced by JW continue to trigger the need for nurses and other providers to engage all 17 dimensions of CT to achieve safe, quality health care.

This chapter examines the thinking that is essential to achieve safe, quality health care. We explore (1) definitions of quality and safety in health care and the stakeholders involved, (2) the scope of the healthcare quality-safety problem, (3) the relationships among quality, safety, and CT within a systems framework of structure, process, and outcomes, (4) the five IOM criteria guiding education and practice toward quality improvement and safe patient care, and (5) nurses as "safety champions" for enhancing quality and safety through thinking. Our goal is to make crystal clear how thinking is the key ingredient in all efforts to achieve safe, quality care for our patients, their families, and their communities.

Defining Quality and Safety in Health Care and Stakeholder Involvement

Definitions

Many groups have defined quality and safety in the last two decades. Such groups include the American Society for Quality, the American Medical Association, and The Joint Commission (Burhans, 2007). The American Nurses Association, the National Quality Forum (NQF), and the Agency for Healthcare Research and Quality (AHRQ) have also weighed in on the issue (Ridley, 2008). The AHRQ (2003) defined safety as "freedom from accidental injury or avoiding injuries or harm to patients from care that is intended to help them" (p. 8).

The IOM (1990) defined quality as "the degree to which health services for individuals and populations increase the likelihood of desired health outcomes and are consistent with current professional knowledge" (p. 4). We believe that they have retained this definition of quality over the years because it recognizes (1) the impact that health care has on quality of life for both patients and communities, (2) the probability of achieving better outcomes, and (3) the reliability of those outcomes stemming from sound information and critical thinking.

Although there are varied definitions within and across disciplines, there are common themes in how we think about quality and safety. Those themes include "deficiency-free excellence; conformity and consistency with standards and current professional knowledge; stakeholder-specific subjectivity; and congruence with the structure-process-outcomes quality triad" (Burhans, 2007, p. 43). Thus, when defining quality and safety, we must think about error-free "top-notch" care, compliance with professional standards and evidence-based practice (EBP), appreciation of multiple points of view, and acknowledgment that thinking must focus on systems (structures, processes, and outcomes) and not simply individuals.

These four themes allow us to dissect the quality improvement issues and the thinking involved in each. The first theme identified by Burhans (2007), deficiency-free excellence, or error-free, top notch care, is the overarching goal for all safety initiatives. However, we need to look at that goal realistically in today's world. The second theme, conformity and consistency with standards and professional knowledge, is addressed in Chapter 8, which covers EBP. The third and fourth themes—stakeholders, and the structure, process, and outcomes of the system—are important areas for CT. We'll start with stakeholders because they are an ever-present influence on quality initiatives.

Stakeholders

Stakeholders are individuals or entities who participate in and/or experience the impact of some activity or event (Alexander, 2007; Burhans, 2007; Lundquist & Axelsson, 2007; Mastal, Joshi, & Schulke, 2007; Melichar, 2007; Needleman, Kurtzman, & Kizer, 2007). We are most concerned about the thinking employed by both individuals and organizations (entities) because thinking is the key if safety and quality care are the desired outcomes.

All stakeholders have a "stake" in the quality of care from the perspectives of cost and benefit/harm. In health care, there are four basic categories of stakeholders: those who pay for care, those who deliver care, those who receive care, and those who monitor the quality of care. The paying stakeholders include the federal and state governments, insurance companies, and recipients of care who pay out-of-pocket costs. Those who deliver care include all healthcare disciplines and providers in health care. Those who receive care include individuals, families, and communities. Recipients of care have been joined by a whole cadre of public and private organizations and agencies whose goal is to improve quality and safety in health care. Examples of those who monitor quality are identified in **Box 5-1**.

Organizations concerned with quality explicitly or implicitly express the need for CT. Consider this example from the AHRQ (1999): "in studying an *intuitively* plausible 'risk factor' for errors, such as 'fatigue,' *analyses* of errors commonly reveal the presence of fatigued providers" (p. 3). (We added the italics to emphasize the thinking language.) Such organizations study and advocate for accurate information, emphasizing the need for collaborative thinking and discussion to find creative solutions. A recently formed organization, Quality and Safety Education for Nurses (QSEN), developed a Web site that invites ongoing critique and input to improve quality and safety strategies (Cronenwett et al., 2007). This group is specifically focused on enhancing prelicensure nursing education. See **Box 5-1** for their Web site.

BOX 5-1	Groups and Organizations That Address Quality in Health Care

Institute of Medicine (IOM):
  http://www.iom.edu
Agency for Healthcare Research and Quality (AHRQ):
  http://www.ahrq.gov
The Joint Commission:
  http://www.jointcommission.org
National Quality Forum (NQF):
  http://www.qualityforum.org
IPRO Quality Improvement Organization:
  http://www.ipro.org
Talking Quality.gov:
  http://www.talkingquality.gov
Quality and Safety Education for Nurses (QSEN):
  http://www.qsen.org

Nurse educators are also a group of stakeholders concerned about delivering quality and safety with patient care. The presidents of both nursing educational professional organizations, the National League for Nursing and the American Association of Colleges of Nursing (AACN), cited the need for changes in the education of prenursing students regarding quality and safety (Bargagliotti & Lancaster, 2007). They described a gap between what nurse educators say they teach about quality and safety, and how nursing graduates apply that teaching in the practice setting. The presidents recommended that faculty embrace "new ways of thinking, interacting and learning" (p. 156) to bridge the gap between education and practice of quality care.

The AACN (2006) also created a Patient Safety Task Force to emphasize the importance of quality and safety in the education and preparation of nurses. It is very important for nursing students and faculty to integrate the knowledge, skills, and attitudes of safe, quality care into all aspects of prelicensure education (Cronenwett et al., 2007)—in other words, integrate quality and safety thinking throughout nursing curricula.

Deficiency-Free Excellence: What Is the Scope of the Quality–Safety Problem?

We probably all agree that much of today's health care would not receive a 10 on a scale of 1–10, with 10 being the best. In contemplating goals for remediation, we first need to reflect on whether reaching 10 is possible. Attempting to achieve perfection in complex systems is not only unrealistic, but also it may actually make matters worse. Attempts at perfection have a tendency to increase the level of system complexity, which in turn potentially leads to more system failures (AHRQ, 1999). "Excellence is not perfection, excellence is striving. Perfection is the enemy of excellence" (E. Tagliareni, personal communication, July 30, 2008).

Given that we cannot score a 10 on healthcare quality and that achieving perfection is unrealistic, let's get a better handle on the scope of the problem in order to employ some thinking to resolve it. We start, of course, with the CT dimensions of *inquisitiveness, information seeking,* and *analysis. Information seeking* enables us to gather useful data about the current state of quality care. *Inquisitiveness* drives us to explore, to find out what is working and what is not, and to wonder why. *Analysis* allows us to examine the parts of the problem in manageable segments so we can thoroughly define and frame the problem before using *logical reasoning* and *transforming knowledge* to find solutions. As you will see, discovering those solutions will require all the CT dimensions from a multitude of stakeholders, but particularly nurses, the "safety champions."

A Bit of History

In the early 1990s, the IOM asked hard questions about healthcare quality and raised awareness of the overuse, misuse, and underuse of healthcare services in the United States. At that point, the IOM recommended switching to computer-based patient records as a way of monitoring healthcare issues (informatics enters the picture; see Chapter 9.) Computerized data provided the means to find out how serious the problem with quality was (IOM, 2004a).

In 2000, the IOM issued *To Err is Human: Building a Safer Health System,* and in 2001, *Crossing the Quality Chasm: A New Health System for the 21st Century.* Both reports revealed growing concerns about quality in health care. The data from the U.S. healthcare system revealed that on a yearly basis:

- 7% of patients suffer a medication error
- Every patient admitted to an intensive care unit suffers an adverse event
- 44,000 to 98,000 deaths [result from errors]
- $50 billion in total costs [result from errors] (Pronovost, 2004)

And to further help put this in perspective, "In the United States, the annual loss of life from medical errors approaches the loss of American combat deaths annually during World War II" (Bargagliotti & Lancaster, 2007, p. 156). These statistics should be a scary call to action.

Quality and Safety "Lingo"

Searching the literature to gain insight and data on safe, quality healthcare provided a plethora of articles that are growing exponentially. There are multiple concepts and terms closely associated with quality and safe care that should be acknowledged in our attempt to be good critical thinkers. **Box 5-2** includes many of the terms and phrases commonly used when discussing quality and safety. Time and space prevent an elaboration on all the lingo, but three of the most prominent phrases deserve special attention: *near miss, adverse event,* and *sentinel event.*

BOX 5-2	The "Lingo" of Quality

Active failures: errors or harm as a result of direct actions or contact with a patient (Mitchell, 2008).

Adverse event: "an event that results in unintended harm to the patient by an act of commission or omission rather than by the underlying disease or condition of the patient" (IOM, 2004a, p. 201).

Continuous Quality Improvement: also referred to as Total Quality Management. Focuses on the healthcare system and its overall structure versus individuals. Keys are measuring performance, making changes, and evaluating the effects of those changes (Newhouse & Poe, 2005).

Culture of Safety: a phrase that describes an organization that acknowledges that (1) most errors are a result of systemic dysfunctional work processes, (2) blaming individuals is counterproductive, and (3) supporting a learning environment for both staff and the organization enhances safety (IOM, 2004b).

Failure to rescue: a situation resulting from delayed detection of changes in a patient's condition *and* slow responses to those changes (IOM, 2004b).

Latent failures: errors or harm as a result of organizational policies, procedures, resources, or allocation of resources (Mitchell, 2008).

Magnet Status: a phrase referring to "Magnet Recognition," which is awarded by the American Nurses Credentialing Center to hospitals that achieve a specific standard of quality nursing care (ANCC, 2008).

Near miss: "acts of omission or commission that could have harmed the patient but did not cause harm as a result of chance, prevention or mitigation" (IOM, 2004a, p. 227).

Nurse dose: a concept with three equal parts: (1) the number or amount of care delivered by nurses (dose), (2) the educational preparation, expertise, and experience (of the nurse), and (3) the receptiveness of the organization and/or the patient (host response) (Brooten & Youngblut, 2006).

Nursing-sensitive care: fifteen national standards for nursing care identified by the NQF and available for use by the public or other stakeholders (National Quality Forum, 2008).

Nursing-sensitive databases: standardized information on nursing quality and patient outcomes (Alexander, 2007).

Organizational system failures: errors or harm as a result of management, organizational culture, processes, communication, or external resources (Mitchell, 2008).

Patient-centered outcome measures: conditions experienced by the recipient of care after the care is provided.

> **BOX 5-2**   **(Continued)**
>
> **Patient Safety Incident (PSI):** measure that facilitates screening for adverse events that can be prevented (AHRQ, 2006).
>
> **Quality assurance:** terminology used to describe projects.
>
> **Quality improvement:** terminology used to describe moving from one level of care to a better level of care.
>
> **Risk management:** label for one department in an organization focused on minimizing both individual and system errors that could result not only in patient harm but also in monetary loss for the institution.
>
> **Sentinel event:** "an unexpected occurrence involving death or serious physical or psychological injury, or the risk thereof. Serious injury specifically includes loss of limb or function. The phrase 'or the risk thereof' includes any process variation for which a recurrence would carry a significant chance of a serious adverse outcome." (The Joint Commission, 2007).
>
> **Six Sigma:** "a system-wide data-driven business strategy [that] focuses on eliminating defects or errors, identifying sources of variation and opportunities for standardization, and applying controls to maintain the improvements" (Newhouse & Poe, 2005, p. 40).
>
> **Surveillance:** a label in the Nursing Interventions Classification system and used to describe the equal role of the ongoing monitoring *and* interpretation of clinical information (Shever et al., 2008).
>
> **Technical failures:** errors or harm due to failure of facilities or resources (Mitchell, 2008).
>
> **Value-added care processes:** indicators that care has improved quality of life.

Near Miss, Adverse Event, and Sentinel Event

Near misses were defined as "acts of omission or commission that could have harmed the patient but did not cause harm as a result of chance, prevention or mitigation" (IOM, 2004a, p. 227). An adverse event was defined as "an event that results in unintended harm to the patient by an act of commission or omission rather than by the underlying disease or condition of the patient" (p. 201). The most adverse event, or the "sentinel" event, was identified by The Joint Commission (2007) as "an unexpected occurrence involving death or serious physical or psychological injury, or the risk thereof. Serious injury specifically includes loss of limb or function. The phrase 'or the risk thereof' includes any process variation for which a recurrence would carry a significant chance of a serious adverse outcome." These terms are discussed in more detail later in this chapter.

The Joint Commission publishes a *Sentinel Event Alert*, which includes a root cause analysis of one problem area at a time. Recent alerts included these: Alert #40: "Behaviors that Undermine a Culture of Safety," July 9, 2008; Alert #39: "Preventing Pediatric Medication Errors," April 11, 2008; and Alert #38: "MRI Safety," February 14, 2008 (The Joint Commission, 2008d). Each alert included root causes and contributing factors. Alert #40 is particularly relevant to this chapter and will be discussed in more detail.

The 2004 IOM report, *Keeping Patients Safe: Transforming the Work Environment of Nurses*, added an additional dimension to the problem with quality in reference to the 44,000–98,000 deaths from errors: "This alarming number, which reflects only deaths occurring in hospital settings, . . . does not reflect the many patients who survive, but sustain serious injuries" (2004b, p. 1). Thus, these data do not address most adverse events, and they do not address any near misses. It is important to recognize that quality and safety issues run the whole gamut of health care and nursing care. Although most of the focus has been on acute care settings, a growing body of literature is addressing quality and safety in long-term care, palliative care, physicians' offices, pharmacies, community clinics, and home care (Davies & Cripacc, 2008; Donaldson & Philip, 2004; Gruneir & Mor, 2008; Lynn et al., 2007; McBride-Henry & Foureur, 2007; Whitson et al., 2008). Concern about quality care is not confined to the acute care setting, and CT cannot be either.

So what is the role of nursing and thinking in all of this? It appears, from a study by Buerhaus et al. (2007), that there are very differing opinions. These researchers surveyed registered nurses (RNs), medical doctors (MDs), chief nursing officers (CNOs), and chief executive officers (CEOs) in health care to get an understanding of the impact of the nursing shortage on hospital patient care. One of their findings was very disturbing. When participants responded to the question, "Do you think the current [nursing] shortage will lead to lower-quality care for patients?" the "yes" responses were as follows (p. 859):

- 69% of the 142 CEOs said yes
- 71% of the 222 CNOs said yes
- 90% of the 657 RNs said yes
- 83% of the 445 MDs said yes

It appears that CNOs and CEOs in this study had significantly different perceptions of the key role that nursing plays in patient safety. *Inquisitiveness* and *perseverance* lead us to some challenging questions: How do these differing opinions make a difference in policies and procedures related to safe, quality patient care? How can nurses use their CT to enlighten policy makers about their role in safe, quality patient care? What impact do these perceptions have on staffing patterns? (What other questions do you have?)

Other studies have strongly acknowledged the significant role of nursing in both the thinking and the doing aspects of quality and patient safety. For example, Mitchell (2008) entitled a chapter section "Nursing as the Key to Improving

Quality Through Patient Safety" (p. 1-3). Numerous other authors support this perspective and the need for some good ol' CT (Kurtzman & Corrigan, 2007; Mastal et al., 2007; Miller & Chaboyer, 2006; Naylor, 2007; Needleman et al., 2007; Ridley, 2008; Schmalenberg & Kramer, 2008), providing more evidence that nurses are safety champions.

Reflection Pause

Now it's time for some *reflection* and *contextual perspective* to look back at the whole picture of the quality problem. A summary of the key points of this section will help us move on to examining the system that needs a good dose of CT to facilitate safe, quality healthcare outcomes:

- Perfection is not a realistic goal; in fact, attempts to achieve perfection probably will make matters worse.
- The volume of errors and deaths is enormous and unacceptable.
- Documented near misses, adverse events, and sentinel events provide concrete evidence of threats to patient safety and quality care.
- Quality and safety concerns and the CT that must accompany those concerns extend beyond acute care in all aspects of health care: long-term care, palliative care, home care, and so on.
- CNOs' and CEOs' perceptions of the role of nursing in patient safety (in one study) do not match with nurses' or physicians' perceptions.

The Relationships Among Quality, Safety, and Critical Thinking Within a Systems Framework of Structure, Process, and Outcomes

Safe, quality health care can result from high-quality thinking and appreciating how systems function. **Figure 5-1** returns to the medallion symbol first used in Chapter 4 to represent the IOM competency of "applying quality improvement." We selected this symbol because it generally represents a mark of excellence or an award for great work.

This more detailed illustration of the medallion acknowledges the overall healthcare system. The center of the medallion represents the healthcare system triad of structure, process, and outcome. Thinking about how these components interact can guide decisions about quality and safety.

Surrounding the three system components is a ring that represents stakeholders' thinking. Beyond that ring are the 17 dimensions of CT used by all the stakeholders, especially the nurse (the safety champion), the interdisciplinary team, and the patient and/or family. The medallion ribbons represent the six IOM Aims for Quality Healthcare: patient centered, effective, safe, timely, efficient, and equitable. For the remainder of this chapter, when we refer to CT, remember that it represents both individual and interdisciplinary thinking. It is this collaborative thinking that ultimately changes the quality of patient care from good to better to best.

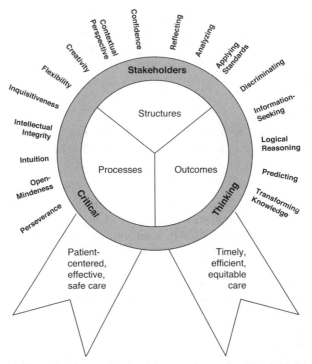

Figure 5-1 Medallion of safe, quality health care through critical thinking.

The Healthcare System and Safe, Quality Care

Attempts at quality improvement in health care have been addressed over the last several decades, beginning in the 1960s with Donabedian's work on quality assurance (Shortell, Bennett, & Byck, 1998). In a nutshell, Donabedian proposed a framework for quality assurance in health care using a systems perspective. Systems have three interacting components—structure, processes, and outcomes. Donabedian was ahead of his time in thinking about systems; unfortunately, the rest of the healthcare industry was not yet into systems thinking, and significant change did not occur. In the last few decades, numerous authors have developed models and tested those models, all based on Donabedian's systems approach to quality assurance (Burhans, 2007; Needleman et al., 2007). According to Leape, Berwick, and Bates (2002), "the clear message of the IOM report, *To Err is Human*, is that safety is primarily a systems problem" (p. 504). Today, as we embrace that awareness and appreciate the complexity of those systems, we move to new levels of thinking.

Healthcare systems have moved well beyond complicated and into the realm of complex. Complex systems are not like machines; they are more like conscious entities (Wheatley, 1994) or living organisms. As such, healthcare systems are constantly adaptive (Plsek, 2003). In other words, people, responsibilities, and workloads do not stay in their nice little boxes on organizational charts. Systems (the inner circle on the medallion in **Figure 5-1**) are dynamic and constantly changing. All aspects of systems (structures, processes, and outcomes) must be actively addressed when looking for solutions to problems of inadequate quality in health care. Chapter 11 will explore in more detail this very important issue of complexity and its impact on change.

Thinking in systems is another level of thinking. Do you remember Einstein's words of wisdom that we quoted in Chapter 1? It's worth repeating here: "The significant problems we face cannot be solved at the same level of thinking we were at when we created them" (Famous Quotes and Famous Sayings Network, n.d.). We will let you imagine the kinds of thinking that "created" the problems of quality in health care, but we are certain it will take a concerted interdisciplinary team effort, using all 17 CT dimensions, to deal with the current level of complexity.

But for now, we need to artificially break down the healthcare system to explore the CT needed to examine the structure, process, and outcomes of healthcare systems as they relate to quality and safety, and thinking. By now, you should be able to say automatically, "Aha, we need some *analyzing*, some *open-mindedness*, and some *reflection* here!" And that's just for starters! Let's use some *analysis* to examine the three major components of a system (structure, process, outcome—the inner circle of our medallion) in health care.

Structure

Structure was a system component addressed in the IOM publication, *To Err Is Human* (2000). Newhouse and Poe (2005) described structure as "having the right things" (p. 61). Structure includes the healthcare system resources and infrastructure such as information, the organization itself, physical aspects, human aspects, and fiscal aspects (Handler, Issel, & Turnock, 2001). When using *reflection* and *inquisitiveness*, think about how the following very simplistic example has an impact on safety related to infection control.

> **Information:** What data are available, and how reliable are they for making decisions about a recent rise in staphylococcal infections?
>
> **Organization:** Who in the organization has authority and responsibility to monitor infection rates? Are there any policies and procedures to guide infection control?
>
> **Physical:** Do the staff have the necessary equipment, such as sterile dressing kits, and antiseptic hand-washing liquid, in convenient locations? Are there sinks in every room?
>
> **Human:** Are there adequate numbers of nurses and ancillary staff to manage the acuity of the patient load with infections? Are the staff adequately prepared for their role in infection control? Are patients and family members, nursing and medical students, and the interdisciplinary members taught how to avoid contamination?
>
> **Fiscal:** Is there money in the budget to install hand-washing sinks in each patient room? Which is more cost-effective, paper gowns or cloth gowns for isolation units? What is the cost of iatrogenic infections if these other factors are not addressed?

What dimensions of thinking help us to understand all these structure resources? An obvious one is *contextual perspective*, or looking at the big picture. It is far too easy to blame someone for a mistake but forget the structural constraints that may have contributed to it. *Discriminating* is vital when you are trying to determine which policies and procedures are working and which aren't. *Logical reasoning* is necessary to ensure that the inferences you draw are based on all the facts.

As broad as the structural components are, they are at least somewhat tangible; they can generally be seen, touched, and even measured in some manner. But the next part of the system, process, is a bit harder to capture, let alone measure.

Process

If structure is "having the right things," then process is what is done with those things. Processes are actions. Processes in health care are not new to nursing students, nurses, or nurse educators. Beginning nursing students consider processes to be the steps or activities taken to achieve a task, such as inserting a urinary catheter. However, when students move from the learning laboratory to the real world of patient care, they soon realize (we hope!) that those "process" steps described in textbooks have limited value without the use of CT. For example, one needs to use *flexibility* and *transforming* knowledge to insert a catheter in a patient with cerebral palsy and severe hip contractures.

Examples of other processes that are used daily and that require constant CT are the nursing process, therapeutic communication, teaching, and working in interdisciplinary teams. More on interdisciplinary team processes comes in Chapter 7, but a related, influential, and somewhat elusive process relevant to this quality discussion is the functioning of the organizational culture. An organization's culture has a powerful influence on quality and safety because it embodies our values, attitudes, and thinking about quality, safety, and care. In short, it affects every process. Later in this chapter, we elaborate on the organizational culture in relation to thinking and errors and, more specifically, "the culture of safety," the goal for our safety champion nurses.

Look back to JW's story at the beginning of this chapter. What are the processes that you can identify? Obviously the nursing process stands out; the parts of that process—assessing, planning, implementing, and evaluating care—may well have been problematic. It is quite possible that JW did not receive proper teaching or that communication went awry. Certainly, there seems to have been a breakdown in the interdisciplinary team interactions. Now, consider how difficult it might be to measure the quality of those processes. In contrast to the tangible qualities of structure, the processes can easily become elusive, taken-on-faith actions.

Outcomes

The third portion of the systems triad (the inner circle of the medallion) is outcomes. Outcomes are results brought on by processes. They are often predetermined as goals toward which providers aim their interventions. Outcomes, specifically patient outcomes, became a major focus over the last decade as health-care providers and quality monitoring organizations began looking at the "value added" aspects/outcomes of health care (Kurtzman & Corrigan, 2007).

It would be hard to imagine anyone in nursing, even a nursing student, who does not recognize the phase *outcome measures*. Typically, outcomes or outcome measures are the part of nursing care plans that we think about ahead of time in order to later determine if our interventions had the planned effect and the patient achieved a goal. That same terminology is used to think about quality. What are we looking for? Alexander (2007) identified three characteristics of outcomes related to quality: (1) measurable, (2) verifiable, and (3) cost-effective. *Measurable* requires something quantitative, such as shorter length of stay, fewer falls, or no postoperative infections; *verifiable* means that more than one person agrees with the outcome; and *cost-effective* refers both to time and money.

Perhaps because outcomes are concrete and measurable, they have become a hot topic. Much has been written about outcomes, and the language to describe them has expanded. There is a wide variety to what is called an "outcome." **Table 5-1** is a sample of the words and phrases associated with safety and quality outcomes in the literature.

After examining Table 5-1, think about what is most obvious about these outcome measures. First of all, several groups and authors have identified similar outcomes measures. But even more significant is the focus on negative outcomes. Although some authors have made a case for identifying positive outcomes (Melichar, 2007; Mitchell, 2008), it appears that this is not the norm. Use some of your *open-mindedness* here and see if you can identify some positive outcome measures for your practice area.

Besides *open-mindedness*, other CT dimensions are important to a consideration of outcomes. *Applying standards* is a necessity. Standards come in many forms—professional, institutional, personal, and ethical, to name a few. Just what should our standards for outcomes be? This is a question on the minds of many nurses and nursing administrators who are *analyzing* outcomes and *applying standards* (Mitty, 2007; Wise, 2007). Although this is hardly a topic that can be dealt with in one paragraph, the need for ethical standards cannot be overemphasized. We encourage those interested to explore documents from the Hastings Center and the report titled "The Ethics of Using QI Methods to Improve Health Care Quality and Safety" from their project (Mitty).

Going back to our example of JW, most of you can probably identify which outcomes were missing. What went wrong? Was it the projected outcome that was amiss, or were the processes and structures the biggest contributing factors to this disaster? We know that reasonable outcomes were not reached. Perhaps you can see that even though outcomes have received lots of attention lately, looking at outcomes alone would not be adequate in figuring out what went wrong in JW's case. We need to remember that outcomes are only one-third of the systems triad. If we want to make a difference in safety and quality, we must engage our thinking to examine all three components—structures, processes, and outcomes—of the whole system (Burhans, 2007).

TABLE 5-1 Selected Samples of Outcome Measures

Outcome Measures of Quality	Citation	Comments
Mortality Morbidity Healthcare costs Nurse satisfaction & burnout Patient satisfaction Organizational performance and clinical information	Brooten & Youngblut, 2006	
Nursing-sensitive measures	Mastal et al., 2007	
Pain management Care coordination Medication management	Melichar, 2007	Need to focus on positive vs. negative measures
27 nursing-sensitive performance measures Failure to rescue Mortality Decubitus ulcers Unspecified infections Cardiopulmonary arrests Several others	Needleman, Kurtzman, & Kizer, 2007 Ridley, 2008	All negative outcomes
Length of stay Incidence of falls	Shever et al., 2008	Focus on "surveillance" from Nursing Interventions Classification
Pressure ulcers Falls	Gruneir & Mor, 2008	Nursing homes

Patient safety indicators
    Provider-level indicators (22)
    Area-level indicators (7)
	AHRQ, 2006	Set of measures that screen for adverse events and are used to focus thinking on reducing injuries with better safety

TABLE 5-1 (Continued)

Outcome Measures of Quality	Citation	Comments
Positive indicators sensitive to nursing input: "Achievement of appropriate self-care, Demonstration of health-promoting behaviors, Health-related quality of life, Perception of being well cared for, and Symptom management to criterion." Negative outcomes resulting from multiple provider input: Mortality Morbidity Adverse events	Mitchell, 2008, p.1	Work is derived from the American Academy of Nursing Expert Panel on Quality Health and the National Quality Forum
Patient-centered outcome measures: Death among surgical inpatients Pressure ulcer prevalence Falls prevalence Falls with injury Restraint prevalence Urinary catheter-associated urinary tract infection Central line catheter-associated blood-stream infection Ventilator-associated pneumonia rate Smoking cessation counseling for acute myocardial infarction, heart failure, and pneumonia Skill mix Nursing care hours per patient day Practice Environment Scale Voluntary turnover	National Quality Forum, 2008	Nursing-Sensitive Care Performance Measures endorsed in January 2004 by the NQF and adopted by The Joint Commission in 2005 (The Joint Commission, 2008e)

Five IOM Criteria Guiding Education and Practice Toward Quality Improvement and Safe Patient Care

Luckily the IOM (2003) established five criteria for the educational changes necessary to improve quality in health care. As you read these five criteria in **Box 5-3**, think about what needs to change in healthcare practice, education, and thinking patterns to move in those directions. Our new level of thinking requires clinicians and educators to engage as many of the 17 CT dimensions as possible and as often as possible.

Although all 17 CT dimensions are necessary to achieve the five IOM criteria, only some will be used in our examples for the sake of time and also to allow you to discover the others on your own. Each criterion and its necessary CT will be discussed separately for the remainder of the chapter.

IOM Criterion #1

#1—Continually understand and measure quality of care in terms of "structure," or the inputs into the system, such as patients, staff, and environments; "process," or the interactions between clinicians and patients; and "outcomes," or evidence about changes in patients' health status in relation to patient and community needs. (IOM, 2003, p. 59)

This criterion addresses the quality improvement concepts of structure, process, and outcomes that we have just discussed. Structure, process, and outcomes are valuable concepts in health care but are more valuable when all three are looked

---

| **BOX 5-3** | **IOM Five Criteria for Achieving Quality** |

1. Continually understand and measure quality of care in terms of structure . . . process. . . and outcomes . . . in relation to patient and community needs.
2. Assess current practices and compare them with relevant better practices elsewhere as a means of identifying opportunities for improvement.
3. Design and test interventions to change the process of care, with the objective of improving quality.
4. Identify errors and hazards in care; understand and implement basic safety design principles. . .
5. Both act as an effective member of an IDT and improve the quality of one's own performance through self-assessment and personal change.

Source: Institute of Medicine, 2003, p. 510.

at as a whole. Remember the saying, "The whole is greater than the sum of its parts"? Basically, this means we have to recognize the whole as its own conscious entity in addition to the contributions of its parts.

To illustrate how these three concepts work together as a system, and the thinking that is involved, complete TACTICS 5-1, which uses Scenario 5-1.

TACTICS 5-1

Thinking for Criterion #1

1. Read Scenario 5-1. Notice that we have inserted some of the CT used by the nurses.
2. Identify any additional CT dimensions we have not cited.
3. Identify the aspects of this situation that represent structure, process, and outcomes.
4. Think about some other possible solutions that the staff did not consider.

Scenario 5-1: Thinking for Criterion #1

*The community health nurses working in the well-baby clinic noticed that fewer and fewer new mothers were bringing in their babies for immunizations over the last 6 months. They were concerned about the potential for increasing incidence of measles during the coming months when measles generally peaks among infants. They wanted to understand both patient and community needs. **(Predicting)***

*They want to find out what is happening that may have precipitated this change in behavior and begin to ask the mothers who come if they have any ideas. They also consult the Centers for Disease Control and Prevention (CDC) Web site to see if this is a national or regional occurrence or unique to their clinic. They consult pediatrician offices as well. **(Information seeking)***

*The mothers who visit the clinic have no idea what the problem could be; they are very pleased with the service they receive. The CDC Web site has no indication that this is a widespread problem; local pediatrician offices have not experienced the problem either. The nurses, however, are not about to give up. They meet with the other clinic staff and try to brainstorm ideas. Are they doing something to discourage the return of certain patients? Are they missing some culturally sensitive information, considering that they serve a population of rural migrant workers? Maybe the parents have been listening to the news reports about mercury in the immunizations causing autism and are afraid of immunizing their children. **(Perseverance, open-mindedness, intellectual integrity)***

The nurses decide to try to contact the new mothers directly to ask them what is happening. Because few have phones, they make several home visits and ask about the missed appointments. They get only vague excuses about not having time or forgetting.

*While driving to a final home visit, the nurse begins to think about one forgotten piece of the whole process of immunizations—access to service. She notices that all the bus stops that used to be in this part of the county are no longer there. When she arrives at the home, she asks the mother about the missed appointments, gets the same vague answer, and then asks about the missing bus stops. (**Contextual perspective**)*

*With some encouragement, the mother admits that she does not have enough money for a taxi to bring her daughter to the clinic for her immunizations. The nurse compares the dates of the decline in immunization appointments with the date that the busses stopped servicing some areas of the county and found a match. She and the rest of the clinic team know that declining immunizations puts the children and the community at risk. They combine their thinking and discuss how to approach this situation using the structure-process-outcomes framework recommended by the IOM. (**Analysis, logical reasoning**)*

Discussion

What other CT dimensions did you identify? What did you see as structure, process, and outcomes? Initially the staff thought that the lack of culturally sensitive interventions for immunizations might be a process problem. It turned out to be a structural problem—transportation. What started as an observation by an inquisitive nurse (declining immunization appointments in a well-baby clinic) became a broader system issue that required CT as the nurses and others examined the structure, process, and outcomes.

The thinking about *structure* included perspectives from the parents of the underimmunized children, from transportation authorities who make bus routes, from city officials who provide tax money to the transportation authority, and from volunteer agencies that provide free transportation. Thinking about *process* included collaboration with all parties to examine causes as well as solutions—for example, considering if the staff were culturally sensitive to this population's needs. Thinking about outcomes ultimately focused on the rates of immunization and led to an increase in the quality of health of the children and the community.

If the staff in the clinic had gone even further in their thinking, they would have reflected on the overall system and how immunization outcomes could be more assured. They might have identified ways to use what they learned in order to deal with other current and future problems. They might have begun to think about how to create a system of mobile satellite clinics that would provide families in outlying areas access to a full range of healthcare services. And they might have thought about how to seek grant money to fund the project.

IOM Criteria #2 and #3

#2—Assess current practices and compare them with relevant better practices elsewhere as a means of identifying opportunities for improvement.

#3—Design and test interventions to change the process of care, with the objective of improving quality. (IOM, 2003, p. 59)

These criteria are being discussed together because they both deal with EBP (refer to Chapter 8 for details on EBP). Criterion #2 implies the use of evidence-based guidelines that would be the "relevant better practices" as comparisons with current practice. Comparisons require information seeking to locate the best practice guidelines and applying standards to select the best fit.

Criterion #3 then pushes for implementation of best practice and testing how the change in practice makes things better (we discuss the CT required for EBP in detail in Chapter 8). As a quick prelude, consider *flexibility, creativity, transforming knowledge*, and *contextual perspective*. *Flexibility* helps clinicians adjust practices as better evidence emerges. *Creativity* is particularly necessary for finding ways to implement evidence-based guidelines. *Transforming knowledge* is used to find evidence and translate it into practice. And *contextual perspective* helps customize best practices to the individual patient.

Criteria #2 and #3 and the incorporation of EBP ultimately lead to safe, effective, and efficient care. The IOM (2000) addressed six attributes for quality health care systems: "(1) safe, (2) effective, (3) patient centered, (4) timely, (5) efficient, and (6) equitable" (pp. 41–42). Of those six, effective and efficient/timely care fit well with criteria #2 and #3 and are discussed next. Patient-centered and equitable care are discussed in Chapter 6. Safe care is discussed with IOM Criterion #4.

Effective Care

Effective care refers to providing the right type and amount of care to specifically address the problem at hand. The right type of care should be what is recommended by solid evidence. We use CT, specifically *logical reasoning*, to accurately match data and conclusions drawn from those data sets with interventions.

Matching the data with conclusions, matching the right provider to patient needs, and matching appropriate tests and procedures to patient conditions are essential aspects of effective care. This can be a delicate balancing act. Providers need to avoid overdoing things, such as ordering unnecessary tests or procedures. Not everyone with neck pain needs an MRI. Antibiotics are not proper treatment for viral infections. Patients with back pain do not necessarily need orthopedic surgery; many will do much better with treatment from a physical therapist who specializes in back pain.

Overuse is wasteful, and underuse can lead to errors and death. For example, for a patient with a brain tumor who complains of headaches and is diagnosed and treated for migraines, care is not effective. The best CT along with the best evidence make the difference between effective-quality and ineffective-quality health care.

Effectiveness has implications for CT in teaching as well, whether it is in the academic classroom or practice setting. Scenario 5-2 illustrates the problems that ensue when quality thinking impacts teaching and quality care.

Scenario 5-2: Earl's Staff Development Teaching Effectiveness

Earl is a staff development instructor for a 30-bed step-down unit in an urban hospital. It is time to do his annual in-service on care of central lines to meet The Joint Commission standards. He has done this several times over the last couple of years and pulls out his file with lecture notes, grabs the video off the shelf, runs to make copies of the quiz he designed when he first prepared the material, and heads off to the conference room.

During his presentation, two nurses seem to be napping, but they scored fine on the quiz, so he decides not to say anything. The one new staff member, Jill, did not score well, however. Earl decides he'd better meet with her and review some of the material. When he talks with Jill, she tells him she learned to do central line dressings differently in school and that's why she answered the way she did. Earl says he will check that out.

Later that week at the weekly staff meeting, the new unit manager shares some data she has been collecting on quality and notices the increasing frequency of infections for patients having central lines on this unit.

Earl looks surprised and says, "I don't know how that can be. I've been doing in-services on central lines consistently for the last few years and everyone attends and passes the post-quiz. I hope we aren't getting another strain of staph on the unit."

TACTICS 5-2

Thinking and Effectiveness

After reading Scenario 5-2, identify the CT skills and habits of the mind that were not used.

Discussion

The obvious missing CT dimensions are these:

- No *information seeking* on Earl's part to update his information. (He clearly did not read Chapter 8 of this book!)
- No *reflection* on Earl's part to consider examining his information, teaching style, or measurement instrument before or after his teaching.

- No evidence of *inquisitiveness* to find out about changes in central line care since he first prepared his teaching material and to ask why Jill has different information.
- No *intellectual integrity* on Earl's part to explore the possibility that he might not be teaching accurate information.

A significant area of improvement would be for Earl to use EBP. Earl could have done a literature review or gone to the Internet (the CDC Web site would have been a good place to start) to look up the latest practice guidelines for central lines. This would have provided him with a better match for the problem—central line care and the proper interventions—thus promoting effective care, as opposed to outdated practice. This behavior requires using at least the listed CT dimensions, plus most other dimensions. Give yourself some stars for additional ones that we did not list, and if you see Earl, tell him about EBP.

Efficient Care

Criteria #2 and #3 also expect efficient care. "Efficiency . . . calls for conducting production activities in as cost-effective and time-efficient a manner as possible" (IOM, 2004b, p. 114). Again, balance is important. Excessive cost-cutting measures without attention to quality frequently lead to decreased staffing, less equipment, and fewer opportunities for catching errors. An example of useful efficiency measures would be to analyze a procedure that has 50 steps, look at all its parts, and see how it could be simplified (by using *logical reasoning*) in order to determine what could be safely eliminated. If that procedure could be reduced to 35 steps without sacrificing safety, then time, money, and energy would be saved. Scenario 5-3 illustrates the problems with efficiency in pain management.

Scenario 5-3 Efficient Pain Control Care

Mr. Cashin, a 63-year-old man with lung cancer metastasized to his thoracic and lumbar spine, was scheduled for his initial assessment prior to receiving radiation. However, his health status was too poor to start the treatment. He was hospitalized with severe back pain. Among his many comorbidities were obesity (5 feet 10 inches and 335 pounds), right- and left-sided heart failure, hypertension, 4+ edema of his lower extremities, and 3+ edema up to the T9 area of his back. He had very limited range of motion. He was very sensitive to narcotics, and in the past, it seemed that half a Vicodin knocked him out. He was prescribed a fentanyl patch. When the nurse practitioner (NP) came to his room to identify the specific point of pain area and prepare him for focused radiation, she found him in pain, with no fentanyl patch. Upon questioning the patient's wife, she discovered that Mrs. Cashin had removed the patch, thinking that it was a band-aid left behind from an earlier procedure. She said her husband kept calling the nurse during the night because he was in so much pain. The patient was unable to identify an area of the back that was causing the pain, stating that it was all over and radiated down his legs. The frustrated NP went to look at his chart and found these entries in the nursing notes: "3 AM: Patient reported pain at level 4 to nursing assistant." "4 AM: When assessed by the nurse, patient reported a pain level of 7/8. Two Vicodin given. Patient continued to use call light every half hour through the night." Wanting to check the specific time of the pain medication administration, the NP looked at the drug-dispensing computer record and found it was 3:40 when the medication was given. When discussing the matter with the nurse, she found the nurse surprised that it had taken 40 minutes for her to give the medication. She reported that the night had been very busy and said, "I'm doing my best; I've been juggling things all night." The NP returned to the radiation oncology department, stating that radiation would be delayed until a full assessment could be completed.

TACTICS 5-3

Thinking and Efficiency for Mr. Cashin

1. After reading Scenario 5-3, how would you describe the efficiency of the night nurse? The NP?
2. Identify what thinking skills and habits of the mind could have been used to make the care more efficient for Mr. Cashin.

Discussion

This situation may be all too familiar to harried nurses trying to do their jobs with too few staff and too many demands. Many of you may immediately become defensive of the harried night nurse because you've been in similar situations. If you could set that defensiveness aside and try to think of efficiency issues, what would you come up with? In terms of efficiency, the delay in pain medication administration created a cascade of events that made both the night nurse and the NP inefficient. Some *contextual perspective* was needed; the nurse needed to realize that the assistant was not equipped to assess pain thoroughly and that, considering the patient's history, she should have assessed pain herself at specific points during the night. If the pain had been controlled, the NP would have been able to accomplish her job of getting the patient ready for radiation. Some *discriminating* by the nurse could have helped her delegate other tasks, not pain assessment, to the nursing assistant. The NP might have been able to be more *discriminating* and assured that the staff knew specifically what the patient needed. *Applying standards* of care would have ensured that the patient's wife was taught about the fentanyl patch. It may be that both the nurse and the NP needed some confidence in their thinking so they could articulate the system problems that led to this patient's pain being ill-controlled.

IOM Criterion #4

#4—Identify errors and hazards in care; understand and implement basic safety design principles, such as standardization and simplification and human factors training. (IOM, 2003, p. 59)

Criterion #4 is aimed at safe care. Safety is the "gold standard" for quality these days. Safety is also something that is very amenable to thinking. *Analysis, logical reasoning, inquisitiveness, predicting,* and *intellectual integrity* are 5 of the 17 CT dimensions necessary to prevent errors and hazards.

Because there is a lot of material in this section, we have provided a road map to help you stay on track. We start with TACTICS 5-4 to examine a safety issue, error identification, in health care. From there, we (1) discuss errors and hazards that hinder safety and how they are categorized, (2) explore how the current organizational culture influences error identification, and (3) identify solutions for better safety.

TACTICS 5-4

CT for Assessing Safety
1. Read Scenario 5-4.
2. Find the dimensions of thinking that are used and those that are missing.
3. Determine what kinds of errors, if any, are present in this situation.

Scenario 5-4 Safety with Medications

Mr. Davis is being discharged today and has a list of medications he needs to take at home. He has been taking Celexa during his hospital stay. His nurse, Betty, who is staffing five patients today because someone called in sick, is in a rush to give blood and doesn't notice the order for Celebrex instead of Celexa. She asks Sara, who just came on, to help out and finish the discharge teaching for Mr. Davis.

Sara is new to this unit; she examines the discharge meds before going in to teach Mr. Davis. She doesn't recognize the name of one drug on the list, Celebrex, but notices from the chart that it looks like what Mr. Davis has been taking. Sara looks for the drug book to check it out but can't find it. She sees

Mr. Davis's doctor rushing off the unit and doesn't want to bother him. She calls the pharmacy, but the line is busy, and just then, Mrs. Davis arrives at the nurses' station.

Mrs. Davis says she has the dog in the car and it's hot outside; she has Mr. Davis all set in the wheelchair and is ready to go. Sara escorts Mr. Davis to the hospital entrance, reminding him to get his prescriptions filled as soon as possible and to call if he has any questions. Mr. Davis goes home with a prescription for Celebrex instead of Celexa.

Discussion

What do you think is the likelihood of this happening? We hope it is not common, but considering the national and international nursing shortage, its potential is rising. Did you find some use of CT dimensions? We came up with these missing CT dimensions. Compare our list with yours, and for all additional dimensions you thought of, give yourself an extra star (or if you're lucky enough to be slim, have chocolate!). If you're not so slim, have the chocolate anyway, but take a break from reading and go for a walk.

Missing thinking:

- Insufficient *discrimination* of the different medications by Betty and Sara.
- Insufficient *applying standards* relative to medication administration by Sara.
- Beginning *perseverance*, but not enough, by Sara in identifying the medication discrepancy.
- No *confidence* in her reasoning, as seen when Sara does not pursue her concerns.

As part of our CT, we would look to the system for ways to protect Mr. Davis and other patients from taking the wrong medication. Many groups, such as The Joint Commission and the U.S. Food and Drug Administration recommend attention to look-alike/sound-alike drugs—that is, medications with similar names, medications with similar packaging, medications that are not commonly used, and commonly used medications that trigger allergic reactions. The U.S. Pharmacopeia has a Drug Error Finder searchable database for drugs that may be mixed up: http://www.usp.org/hqi/similarProducts/drugErrorFinderTool.html. Attention also should be given to drugs that require close monitoring. Mr. Davis would have benefited from his nurses' CT and attention to medications with similar names.

Also, think about who needs to participate in team thinking about how to decrease medication errors. How could those participants create system strategies to alert staff to commonly misread medication names? What should they think about besides assigning blame to individuals? Hold that thought; we'll talk more about a culture of safety shortly.

Hazards and Errors

The first words in IOM Criterion #4 are "Identify errors and hazards in care." We must engage our thinking dimensions to (1) identify and diminish hazards, and (2) minimize errors. Health care is so complex these days that it is foolish to think "things won't go wrong." Once we accept that, we can constructively use *information seeking* and *inquisitiveness* to hunt for hazards and errors and realistically seek to improve safety for patients. Or, as Dr. John Banja, Center for Ethics at Emory University in Atlanta, Georgia, encouraged nurses at the 2008 Michigan nursing summit, "We must accept that the more we are required to make judgments in a complex system, the higher the probability of errors, and the more we need to find ways to close the holes in the Swiss cheese of the healthcare system" (J. Banja, personal communication, July 31, 2008).

Again, we need to examine the concepts. What are hazards? A hazard is an error waiting to happen. Ideally, we will use *predicting* to anticipate hazards and prevent potential errors. And as we examine errors that have occurred with *intellectual integrity* and *logical reasoning*, we can then use *analysis* and *transforming knowledge* to diminish and decrease the probability of future errors.

What is an error? Some prefer the term *complication* because it helps to move away the culture of blaming and redirects us to focus more on thinking about what in the system needs fixing. In general, an "error/complication" can be collecting insufficient data, making the wrong diagnoses, giving the wrong medications, and/or providing the wrong treatments by the wrong providers. All of this and more can result in patient outcomes ranging from discomfort, to increased length of stay, to permanent disability, to death. By initially employing *logical reasoning* and *analysis*, critically thinking nurses are key players in identifying the causes of errors. A lot of *reflection* is also useful for this task.

Reason (2000) used the term *failure* to address underlying causes of errors. He identified two types of failure, or causes of errors: *active failure* (acts of commission or omission that have an immediate effect on a patient), or what we typically consider an error, and *latent failure* (aspects of care that may lie dormant initially but lead to errors). Examples of these latent failures are poor communication among all members of the interdisciplinary team, ineffective management and leadership styles, stressful work environments, short staffing, and poorly designed organizational changes (Currie & Watterson, 2007). Additional latent failures have been identified in long-term care settings. Examples of these include high turnover of staff, adversarial regulatory requirements, and a pervasive system of punishment for errors (Gruneir & Mor, 2008).

Root causes of errors have been addressed by the NQF as (1) latent failures (related to organizational policies, procedures, and resources); (2) active failures (related to actions when directly interacting with patients); (3) organizational system failures (related to management, organizational culture, and communication); and (4) technical failures (related to facilities and external resources) (Mitchell, 2008). Errors have also been identified as adverse events and near misses.

Adverse Events and Near Misses

We defined *adverse events* and *near misses* at the beginning of this chapter, but we'll repeat them here to refresh your memory as we elaborate on the concepts. An adverse event is "an event that results in unintended harm to the patient by an act of commission or omission rather than by the underlying disease or condition of the patient" (IOM, 2004a, p. 201).

These events (errors) are frequently attributed to the poor design, communication patterns, and organization of the healthcare delivery system, not individuals. Such errors generally lead to incident reports and, if the errors lead to death or permanent injury, a sentinel event report. Nurses and others need "not only the knowledge to recognize an error, but also the *confidence* and communication skills to address the issue with appropriate personnel" (Henneman & Gawlinski, 2004, p. 200). That requires both *confidence* (in reasoning) and *intellectual integrity*.

Near misses are defined as "acts of omission or commission that could have harmed the patient but did not cause harm as a result of chance, prevention or mitigation" (IOM, 2004a, p. 227). Near misses occur frequently, as much as 100 times more often than adverse events. Depending on the organizational culture, near-miss data may or may not be reported. *Perseverance* is important in paying attention to patterns and consistently collecting data that are needed to document those patterns and make changes.

Organizational Culture Influences on Thinking and Error Identification

Changing how we think about hazards and errors is a matter of changing our individual thinking. We have to consider the whole of the healthcare system and, in particular, the culture of the organizational system. Organizations are not inanimate objects; they are groups of people who relate, interact, think, and work together for many hours each day. Organizations, therefore, have all the characteristics of any group of people, including a culture. Cultures have values, beliefs, and attitudes that influence behaviors, such as identifying errors.

Look at your organizational culture. What are the values, beliefs, and attitudes that might be promoting errors? When something goes wrong, do people quickly find someone to blame, or does the thinking go further to other possible factors? Does anyone look for a quick fix? All these factors stifle cognitive inquiry and quality in healthcare organizations. Thinking through errors and their prevention requires thinking together with one's team. (That's a cue to appreciate interdisciplinary teams; see Chapter 7.)

Although healthcare cultures vary, historically, all have had two traditional beliefs: (1) avoiding all errors is possible, and (2) finding the one or more persons who are to blame for an error is a goal (IOM, 2004b). We must transform our thinking about the myth that we can avoid all errors because it is counterproductive to developing a new culture of safety. Old beliefs and attitudes about perfection and avoiding errors severely limit our ability to collect accurate data for research and decisions on system changes.

We must also move beyond blaming individuals. According to Benner (2001), a culture of blame and shame actually discourages the reporting of errors for fear of punishment and being singled out for responsibility. Organizational cultures that retain values of blaming and pretending that all errors can be avoided ultimately have a much more difficult job of improving quality (Henneman & Gawlinski, 2004). A more effective approach is to move our thinking to a "culture of safety."

Culture of Safety and Thinking

Healthcare providers must be open and attentive to finding their errors, errors of others, and errors in the system, and not be overtly or covertly punished in the process. If the current culture hinders that openness and attentiveness, the obvious solution is to change the culture. The question is, change it to what, and how?

Benner (2001) had two suggestions for changing the healthcare culture to a focus on safety. One is to accept the fact that "practice is broader and more flexible than the science and technology that support practice" (p. 283). Clinicians who accept that and educators who teach that will be promoting a culture of safety, one that acknowledges the need for *flexibility* and *contextual perspective* in the CT of providers. Benner's second suggestion was to focus on self-improvement, which requires reflection. Both *self-reflection* and *reflection* on the organizational system are essential to changing a culture. We'll discuss this issue of reflection in more detail with Criterion #5.

Affonso and Doran (2002) also addressed solutions for changing the healthcare culture. Their version calls for revolutionary thinking to develop a science of safety by encouraging creative thinking. Their conceptual framework focuses on patient safety through research, education, and practice by creating conditions for critical thinking, ethical practice, and opportunities for learning.

The IOM's (2004b) *Keeping Patients Safe: Transforming the Work Environment of Nurses* confirms the need for more opportunities for thinking to sustain a culture of safety. An entire chapter ("Creating and Sustaining a Culture of Safety") of the report addressed issues of (1) empowering employees with decision-making rights, (2) encouraging staff to question orders with *confidence*, (3) using *creativity* to think of ways to improve procedures, (4) developing staff members' *prediction* abilities to anticipate adverse events, and (5) being able to use *discrimination* abilities to make decisions and select the best practice interventions. The italics are ours (by now you should know why we added them).

CT is also essential for transformational leadership and evidence-based management. The IOM (2004b) emphasized the need for top management to "provide time for thinking, learning and training . . .[;] employees must have sufficient time for reflection and analysis. . . . Only if top management explicitly frees up employee time for this purpose does learning occur with any regularity" (p. 130). With all this focus on thinking, *reflection,* and *analysis*, it makes us wonder if all 17 of our dimensions could be found if we scrutinized that report.

The AHRQ has recently published *Patient Safety and Quality: An Evidence-Based Handbook for Nurses*. In this document, the authors focused an entire chapter (chapter 6) on the paradigm shift needed to "enable nurses to think more critically . . . to ultimately achieve high-quality care in every care setting and for all patients" (Hughes, 2008, p. vi).

Effective communication among nurses, members of the interdisciplinary team, and the patient and family are essential for this cultural paradigm shift (Bartlett, Blais, Tamblyn, Clermont, & MacGibbon, 2008; Currie & Watterson, 2007; Sherwood & Drenkard, 2007; Whitson et al., 2008). For example, improving staff communication was identified as a key goal in the 2009 *Behavioral Health Care National Patient Safety Goals* (The Joint Commission, 2008a). This document is very likely a result of their Seminal Event Alert #40 issue (July 9, 2008), which addressed the "Barriers that Undermine a Culture of Safety" (The Joint Commission, 2008b).

So what is the relationship between communication and thinking, and quality care? That is a subject for another book, but let's focus for a minute on the primary thinking dimension needed here, *confidence*. Remember, *confidence* is focused on your reasoning abilities, not simply being able to do something. Nurses who are *confident* in their reasoning know they have *sought information*; they have used *analysis*, along with *contextual perspective, predicting,* and even some *transforming knowledge*, to draw some inferences with *logical reasoning*. Nurses who have *confidence* in their reasoning are more likely to share their thinking with the interdisciplinary team and *persevere* in being heard by using appropriate communication skills to achieve quality care outcomes.

Processes for Collecting, Monitoring, and Analyzing Errors

Organizations that are conscious entities operate as living organisms that need to be fed (Wheatley, 1994). Information is their food, "informatics" is the grocery store, and CT is the digestive system for the organization, allowing the information to be transformed into usable knowledge. To extend our analogy, we need to look at the "grocery carts," or devices used to collect the information we want transformed.

Some devices used by the experts to collect data include *root cause analysis*, *near-miss analysis*, and *adverse-events analysis* (IOM, 2004a). Once data are collected, CT is used to determine what to monitor and how to analyze the errors that lead to safety gaps.

Root cause analysis is an earlier error identification strategy. This analysis searches for underlying causes and/or system failures that contribute to errors. The major problem with root cause analysis is that it is done after the fact and is considered too subjective. There is little evidence of its value in actually reducing errors (AHRQ, 1999), yet the analysis continues to be used for tracking errors.

Near-miss analysis examines data about situations in which potential errors were caught before they occurred. The IOM identified three goals for near-miss analysis: (1) modeling (gaining qualitative insight into these types of errors), (2) trending (gaining quantitative insight into the patterns of errors), and (3) mindfulness (maintaining a high level of alertness to dangers). Unfortunately, near-miss analysis data are not routinely collected throughout the United States (IOM, 2004a).

The purposes of adverse-event analysis are to define events that need investigating, to design ways to detect the events, and to determine what data should be collected. Adverse-event analyses help identify events labeled as "iatrogenic injuries." The major problem associated with adverse-event analysis is that most events are not reported. The IOM (2004a) recommended three areas for improvement: (1) automated surveillance systems to capture the data, (2) more research to determine the effectiveness of the monitoring, and (3) integration of the data collection systems with patient care standards.

We have designed an adverse-event analysis guideline to emphasize the thinking that is useful in analyzing errors. See **Box 5-4** for the guidelines needed to complete TACTICS 5-5.

TACTICS 5-5

Thinking Through an Adverse Event

Clinicians and Educators

1. Ask nurses or students to record the details of a patient safety incident, paying particular attention to what they were thinking. To maintain anonymity, if that is desired, have those reports typed without names. Even better, have the event voice recorded so verbal nuances can be heard.
2. Give the incident to other nurses to analyze in terms of the CT dimensions.
3. Use the guidelines in **Box 5-4** to help with that analysis. If several nurses analyze the same event, the total scores can be compared.
4. Discuss the how and why of each score.

BOX 5-4	**Guidelines for Analyzing CT in an Event**

Directions: Circle the number that best represents your conclusion.

2 Yes, 1 Maybe, 0 No

1. Was the nurse confident in his/her reasoning?	2 1 0
2. Was the whole situation (relationships, background, environment) taken into consideration?	2 1 0
3. Was there adequate consideration of alternatives, even those that were nontraditional or creative?	2 1 0

(continues)

BOX 5-4	(Continued)			
4. Was the nurse flexible enough?		2	1	0
5. Was the nurse engaged enough to really want to understand fully?		2	1	0
6. Were decisions based on usual practice and/or bias, or was the truth sought even if it went contrary to usual practice?		2	1	0
7. Were there any intuitive signs of this happening?				
8. Were all views considered? (The field was not narrowed too quickly.)		2	1	0
9. Did the nurse keep trying to solve the problem? (Didn't give up too quickly.)		2	1	0
10. Was there evidence of anyone standing back and reflecting on what was happening?		2	1	0
11. Was there evidence of the nurse breaking the situation down to better understand what was happening?		2	1	0
12. Were applicable standards upheld?		2	1	0
13. Were similarities or differences among parts of the issue distinguished carefully?		2	1	0
14. Was all possible information gathered?		2	1	0
15. Was there adequate evidence to support the conclusions drawn?		2	1	0
16. Was there evidence that this incident could have been predicted?		2	1	0
17. Was knowledge applied well in this situation?		2	1	0

Total Score: _____

Interpret Score

0–15: Deficient CT probably contributed to event.

16–25: Insufficient CT possibly contributed to event.

26–30: CT may be insufficient, but consider additional contributing factors.

31–34: CT was good; consider other contributing factors.

Discussion

How did you and/or your colleagues do? Were you consistent in your scoring? In the event recorded, which CT dimensions were strong and which could be enhanced? Consider how you could modify this guideline to fit your practice setting or course content. How can you use this to help emphasize the CT needed to improve safe care?

Safety Goals

Part of IOM Criterion #4 recommended implementing basic safety design principles. The IOM (2004a) began the process by designing safety goals. The Joint Commission established and updated yearly patient safety goals for various healthcare settings, including hospitals (The Joint Commission, 2008c).

These patient safety goals require informatics to collect (*information seeking*), monitor, and interpret the aggregate data (*analysis and logical reasoning*), think about underlying system problems (*reflection* and *inquisitiveness*), and develop strategies to achieve safety goals (*flexibility, creativity, transforming knowledge, intuition, contextual perspective, perseverance,* and so forth). You get the picture?

IOM Criterion #5

#5—Both act as an effective member of the interdisciplinary team and improve the quality of one's own performance through self assessment and personal change. (IOM, 2003, p. 59)

This last criterion addresses CT directly; it refers to self-assessment or *reflection*. As you will recall from Chapter 2, reflection is one of the 10 CT habits of the mind and was defined as "contemplation upon a subject, especially one's assumptions, and thinking for the purposes of deeper understanding and self evaluation" (Scheffer & Rubenfeld, 2000, p. 358).

The standard version of self-assessment (*reflection*) is typically done independently. *Reflection* encourages us to look back at our actions, behaviors, biases, and faulty reasoning. *Reflection* helps us find things we missed, consider things we want to work on differently, see patterns that we did not recognize initially, wonder about solutions we did not consider at the time, and, yes, even celebrate when our thinking was brilliant!

But self-assessment is enhanced when it is validated by thinking and input from other perspectives. Brookfield (1995) identified four lenses, or sources of feedback for reflection: autobiography, theory, students, and colleagues. Each lens is considered to have equal value during reflection. Each lens provides the educator or clinician with another point of view from which he or she can make comparisons and see patterns that confirm or discount what one or more of the other lenses reflect.

Self-Assessment for Educators and Clinicians

Brookfield's (1995) four lenses of reflection can easily be used by educators or clinicians. Scenario 5-5 describes a shortened version of the clinician's use of the four lenses.

Scenario 5-5: Using Four Lenses for Reflection

Carol has been the nurse manager on an inpatient 24-bed psychiatric unit for the last 3 months. She has been trying to implement changes in interdisciplinary teamwork and wonders why the staff show little interest or do not follow through on plans after each staff meeting. She decides to do some reflection to better understand what is happening. Over the course of the next couple of weeks, she uses all four lenses.

Autobiographical Lens: Carol considered herself a facilitative leader and promoter of collaboration. She took a continuing education course in leadership last year and went back to her notes to check off all the things the course recommended. She was doing them. From her perspective, she was doing all the right things.

Patient/Staff Lens: Carol asked some staff what they thought about her leadership. They told her she was doing a great job. It appeared the staff thought she was doing well, but she wondered if they were just being nice. She didn't ask patients.

Theoretical Lens: Carol decided she would get on the Internet. She obtained more updated information on management and leadership. She found others who were having similar problems with getting changes made. Carol found extensive information about management and about interdisciplinary teams. She read the

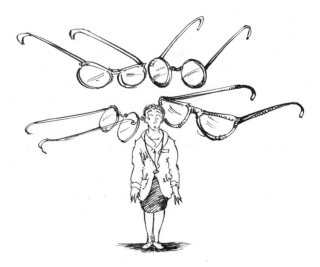

management material, tried to schedule meetings more conveniently, and gave the staff copies of everything she downloaded about interdisciplinary teams.

The results were the same. The staff were not following through.

Colleague's Lens: Carol remembered she had one more lens to use. She asked a colleague to sit in on the next couple of meetings and give her feedback. After the third meeting, the colleague's feedback included, "Have you ever noticed how often you interrupt your staff with your own ideas?" The colleague also suggested how Carol might assign staff to search out reasons why interdisciplinary teamwork such as this would encourage their more active participation. Her colleague reminded her about the "discovery learning" workshop that they attended.

Self-reflection's multiple lenses allow clinicians and educators to examine and think about their practice and teach more effectively and accurately. We must, however, consciously and actively create opportunities to combine our thinking with the thinking of colleagues, patients, and students, and use the best available evidence to achieve the level of self-assessment that will more accurately lead to quality improvement. Again, we believe the IOM would endorse this kind of reflection for clinicians as well as educators.

Summary of the Five IOM Criteria for Quality Improvement

Our journey of thinking through the five IOM criteria for quality improvement has only begun. (And you thought this was the end!) To achieve quality through safe, effective, and efficient care, we need to continually reflect on these criteria and use all dimensions of our CT to make them a reality in practice. Educators must incorporate these criteria into curricula if future practitioners are to be able to effectively apply quality improvement strategies.

We have one last TACTIC to illustrate how CT, the five IOM criteria for achieving quality improvement, and the five IOM competencies all come together.

TACTICS 5-6

Quality Care Through CT

Read the following questions and answer them as you read and reflect on Scenario 5-6.

1. Which of the 17 thinking dimensions were demonstrated in the scenario?
2. How did Jeff achieve the five IOM criteria for quality improvement?
3. Which of the five IOM competencies (patient-centered care, interdisciplinary care, evidence-based practice, informatics, and quality improvement; see **Box 5-3**) were demonstrated in the scenario? And how could you have improved on them?

Scenario 5-6: Quality Care Through Individual and Team Thinking

Jeff is a rural parish nurse. His clinic, 200 miles from the nearest hospital, includes a team of nurses, social workers, an NP, and physical therapists. Contact with the hospital is by phone, e-mail, and fax. Jeff was scheduled to visit Mr. Youngblood, a 30-year-old single farmer, on his first day home from the hospital, where he'd had a bowel resection for diverticulitis. He has a temporary colostomy.

Faxed orders for an initial home visit were for colostomy care. It had been some time since Jeff had done colostomy care, so he got on the Internet to check for EBP guidelines and called the Wound, Ostomy and Continence Nurses Society for their help. Based on the information he found and feedback from the team, he questioned the frequency of the ordered bowel irrigations. He contacted the doctor and explained his concerns, and the order was changed.

The social worker knew Mr. Youngblood and provided information about his healthcare beliefs and how much he valued his privacy. The team would meet again after Jeff's first visit to modify and adjust care planning.

Mr. Youngblood lived about 50 miles from the clinic. He had no phone, but Jeff left a message at the hospital before discharge to tell him the visit would be in the afternoon of his day of discharge.

Based on past experiences with patients in rural areas, Jeff stocked his truck with a variety of items just in case there were some unexpected circumstances. He knew that not all homes had all the amenities needed for standard healthcare procedures. He made sure his cell phone was fully charged even though he would be able to use it only when he was on the tops of the mountain ridges.

When Jeff arrived, he found Mr. Youngblood sitting on his porch. He was sleeping in his rocking chair and needed physical contact to be aroused. With permission, Jeff began his assessment with vital signs. Although Mr. Youngblood was still weak from surgery, the assessment indicated that all systems were within normal limits, with the exception of elimination and possibly his hearing. Assessment of the home environment revealed no indoor plumbing, and water was brought to the house daily from a nearby stream. The home itself was neat and clean, and he had adequate food supplies. Mr. Youngblood still drove. His nearest neighbor was two miles away.

Mr. Youngblood convinced his physician to discharge him early because he believed he would heal more quickly at home, with the fresh air and peace and quiet that did not exist in the hospital. Besides, he did not believe it was good to have young female nurses doing what needed to be done. Mr. Youngblood was also adamant that he couldn't be bothered by doing "all this colostomy stuff more than once a day" because he needed to be in the fields all day long. Jeff did not remind him that work in the fields was probably going to have to wait until his strength returned.

Encouraging Mr. Youngblood to help with the problem solving, they worked out a plan for colostomy care that respected Mr. Youngblood's dignity, personal preferences, and need for quality colostomy care. The plan included Jeff filling empty gallon milk containers with spring water and bringing them to the house to use for irrigation. Because of inadequate lighting in the house, they worked out a plan to do the irrigations and dressing changes by the window that received the best morning light, using an old bucket from the barn for the irrigation waste.

Disposing of the waste in the bucket was a concern. Mr. Youngblood told him not to worry. Jeff had a feeling that Mr. Youngblood, who had been very independent all his life, would try to solve this on his own. Jeff returned to the barn and found an old wagon that still worked. Until his strength returned, Mr. Youngblood agreed to use the bucket in the house, take it outside to the wagon at the end of the porch, and pull it to the outhouse to be dumped. Suspecting that Mr. Youngblood might still try to carry the bucket on his own, Jeff asked him to promise to use the wagon for at least the first few weeks. He reluctantly agreed. An extra couple of gallon water jugs were left by the outhouse for rinsing the bucket.

After returning to the office, Jeff realized that he had misread Mr. Youngblood's antibiotic prescription. He had read "iii" on the Rx as "ii" because of the fuzziness of the fax. He visited the next day to correct his error and notified the physician. Jeff told the team to pay close attention to faxed information in all future orders.

Mr. Youngblood's strength gradually returned; he did use the wagon for a week until he was stronger and able to carry the bucket. He continued to do safe colostomy care with no complications and take the correct dosage of his antibiotic. His second surgery to reconnect his bowel was successful. Jeff continued to visit to monitor progress, working with the healthcare team and following Mr. Youngblood's preferences. Further assessment revealed that Mr. Youngblood was losing his hearing, but he refused suggestions for a hearing test. The team respected his wishes in spite of the increased risk to his safety while living alone.

Discussion

Thinking used:

Transforming knowledge was demonstrated when Jeff had to adapt what he knew were normal procedures for colostomy care in a hospital to a rural environment with fewer resources.

Confidence was demonstrated in challenging the physician's order for frequency of bowel irrigations.

Contextual perspective was demonstrated when Jeff assessed the home environment and Mr. Youngblood's healthcare beliefs and incorporated the input from the social worker.

Creativity was demonstrated when Jeff and Mr. Youngblood came up with several plans for using the available resources to achieve safe care.

Predicting was demonstrated when Jeff thought about the extra supplies he might need in a rural setting.

Intuition was demonstrated when Jeff suspected that Mr. Youngblood would try to be too independent before his strength returned.

Five IOM Criteria for Achieving Quality Improvement:

#1—Jeff considered structure by taking into consideration Mr. Youngblood's preferences and his environment. He paid attention to process in his interactions with Mr. Youngblood and the other healthcare providers. He monitored outcomes in the form of Mr. Youngblood's tolerance for the medications, his ability to stay infection free, and his ability to maintain a quality of life that he preferred.

#2—Jeff assessed current practice and searched for better practice when he used the Internet and conferred with his colleagues for the best approaches.

#3—Jeff very creatively designed and monitored his interventions for effectiveness.

#4—Jeff identified his error and the defect in the fax system. He took steps to avoid this "adverse event" in the future.

#5—Jeff's scenario does not highlight *reflection*, but we will assume he did so when he realized the medication error.

IOM Competencies addressed:

Patient-centered care was demonstrated when Jeff worked to meet Mr. Youngblood's desire to be home during his recovery, and Jeff did not push Mr. Youngblood to follow up on his hearing loss after it was clear that he preferred not to.

Interdisciplinary teamwork was demonstrated when Jeff consulted with the nursing team, the physician, and the social worker, and together they created a plan.

EBP was demonstrated when Jeff searched the Internet for current guidelines for colostomy care.

Informatics utilization was demonstrated when Jeff used the Internet and the fax machine for information.

Applying quality improvement was demonstrated when Jeff provided safe, effective, and efficient care in Mr. Youngblood's home environment. He also applied quality improvement by recognizing a medication error, fixing the error, and addressing the system problem that created it.

Nurses Are "Safety Champions" for Enhancing Quality and Safety Through Thinking

Look back to the first page of this chapter and put your face in the "safety champion" picture! You—the nursing student, the practicing nurse, the nurse educator, the education coordinator—are a safety champion. You are developing, or have, the CT skills to keep patients safe and provide the best quality care possible. The nursing literature is beginning to use the term *champion* in relationship to nursing's role in promoting quality care (Mastal et al., 2007; Miller & Chaboyer, 2006). As Miller and Chaboyer stated, "Nurses cannot afford to remain on the periphery of the patient safety movement but must actively engage with it at personal, institutional and professional levels" (p. 266). You are not alone in this mission, but you will need to continually use your CT to facilitate interdisciplinary thinking and systems thinking in order to make this work. Following are some recommendations to consider along with our thinking:

- Expand research to address issues of quality and safety beyond the acute care setting. Must include home care, long-term care, outpatient settings, palliative care. Better measures to address nursing sensitive outcomes and positive versus negative outcomes.
- Consider whole systems, including structure and process, not just the outcomes.
- Recognize that measuring processes is challenging, but we must find a way.
- Help CEOs and CNOs recognize and appreciate the impact that nurses and the nursing shortage have on quality and safety.

PAUSE _____

and Ponder

Safety Champions of Quality Improvement

Well, here we are at the end of the chapter. Because safe, quality care is the ultimate outcome we seek, it's important to make it the first chapter in our study about the thinking required for the five IOM competencies. If we know what we are aiming for, we are more likely to know when we have achieved it! The current healthcare situation regarding the number of deaths resulting from errors is not tolerable. Engaging thinking to achieve quality and safe patient care is mandatory. What will the future of quality improvement hold? How are you and other providers going to take up the challenge and become the safety champions of quality improvement and safe patient care? You are the providers who will take care of us and our families (and your families) and educate future providers, so we have a vested interest in cultivating all your CT skills and habits of mind to achieve the quality outcomes that we want. We believe that you are up to the challenge of being a "safety champion."

Reflection Cues

- "Quality is the degree to which health services for individuals and populations increase the likelihood of desired health outcomes and are consistent with current professional knowledge" (IOM, 1990, p. 4).
- Errors in health care have led to as many as 98,000 deaths a year.
- Structure, process, and outcomes remain valuable concepts in health care but are more valuable when all three are looked at as a whole.
- Once we accept that errors will occur, we can constructively look for errors and hazards and realistically seek to improve safety for patients.
- *Near misses* and *adverse events* are frequently attributed to the poor design, communication patterns, and organization of the healthcare delivery system, not individuals.
- *Root cause analysis, near-miss analysis,* and *adverse-event analysis* are three strategies for collecting the data necessary to improve systems to decrease errors.
- Refocusing our thinking toward prevention of errors and identifying system problems, as opposed to blaming individuals, is essential.
- Changing the organizational culture to a "culture of safety" requires thinking from individuals, administration, and the interdisciplinary team to change values, attitudes, and beliefs about errors.
- Thinking remains the key to applying quality improvement in health care in order to achieve patient-centered, effective, safe, timely, efficient, and equitable care.
- Matching the data with conclusions, matching the right provider to patient needs, and matching appropriate tests and procedures to patient conditions are essential aspects of effective care.
- Old beliefs and attitudes about perfection and avoiding errors severely limit our ability to collect accurate data for research and for making decisions on system changes.
- Improvements in quality require nurses to be safety champions who (1) use all 17 dimensions of CT in both practice and education, (2) focus on the five IOM Criteria for Achieving Quality, and (3) address the six IOM aims for high-quality healthcare systems.

References

Affonso, D. D., & Doran, D. (2002). Cultivating discoveries in patient safety research: A framework. *International Nursing Perspectives, 2*(1), 33–47.

Agency for Healthcare Research and Quality. (1999). *Making healthcare safer: A critical analysis of patient safety practices.* Rockville, MD: Author.

Agency for Healthcare Research and Quality. (2003). *AHRQ quality indicators.* Retrieved July 25, 2008, from http://www.qualityindicators.ahrq.gov

Agency for Healthcare Research and Quality. (2006). *Patient safety indicators*. Retrieved August 7, 2008, from http://www.qualityindicators.ahrq.gov/downloads/psi/2006-Feb-PatientSafety Indicators.pdf

Alexander, G. R. (2007). Nursing sensitive databases: Their existence, challenges, and importance. *Medical Care Research and Review, 64*(44), 44S–63S. doi:10.1177/1077558707299244

American Association of Colleges of Nursing. (2006). Hallmarks of quality and patient safety: Recommended baccalaureate competencies and curricular guidelines to ensure high quality and safe patient care. *Journal of Professional Nursing, 22*, 329–330.

American Nurses Credentialing Center. (2008). *Goals of the magnet program*. Retrieved July 31, 2008, from http://www.nursecredentialing.org/Magnet/ProgramOverview/GoalsoftheMagnet Program.aspx

Bargagliotti, L. A., & Lancaster, J. (2007). Quality and safety education in nursing: More than new wine in old skins. *Nursing Outlook, 55*, 156–158.

Bartlett, G., Blais, R., Tamblyn, R., Clermont, R. J., & MacGibbon, B. (2008). Impact of patient communication problems on the risk of preventable adverse events in acute care settings. *Canadian Medical Association Journal, 178*, 1555–1562.

Benner, P. (2001). Creating a culture of safety and improvement: A key to reducing medical error. *American Journal of Critical Care, 10*, 281–284.

Brookfield, S. D. (1995). *Becoming a critically reflective teacher*. San Francisco: Jossey-Bass.

Brooten, D., & Youngblut, J. M. (2006). Nurse dose as a concept. *Journal of Nursing Scholarship, 38*, 94–99.

Buerhaus, P. I., Donelan, K., Ulrich, B. T., Norman, L., DesRoches, C., & Dittus, R. (2007). Impact of the nurse shortage on hospital patient care: Comparative perspectives. *Health Affairs, 26*, 853–862. doi:10.1377/hlthaff.26.3.853

Burhans, L. D. (2007). What is quality? Do we agree, and does it matter? *Journal of Healthcare Quality, 29*, 39–54.

Cronenwett, L., Sherwood, G., Barnsteiner, J., Disch, J., Johnson, J., Mitchell, P., et al. (2007). Quality and safety education for nurses. *Nursing Outlook, 55*, 122–131.

Currie, L., & Watterson, L. (2007). Challenges in delivering safe patient care: A commentary on a quality improvement initiative. *Journal of Nursing Management, 15*, 162–168.

Davies, S., & Cripacc, D. G. (2008). Supporting quality improvement in care homes for older people: The contribution of primary care nurses. *Journal of Nursing Management, 16*, 115–120.

Donaldson, L., & Philip, P. (2004). Patient safety—a global priority. *Bulletin of the World Health Organization, 82*, 892–893.

Famous Quotes and Famous Sayings Network. (n.d.) *Famous quotes—Einstein quotes*. Retrieved August 1, 2004, from http://home.att.net/~quotations/einstein.html

Gruneir, A., & Mor, V. (2008). Nursing home safety: Current issues and barriers to improvement. *Annual Review of Public Health, 29*, 369–382.

Handler, A., Issel, M., & Turnock, B. (2001). A conceptual framework to measure performance of the public health system. *American Journal of Public Health, 92*, 1235–1239.

Henneman, E. A., & Gawlinski, A. (2004). A "near-miss" model for describing the nurse's role in the recovery of medical errors. *Journal of Professional Nursing, 20*, 196–201.

Hughes, R. G. (2008, April). *Patient safety and quality: An evidence-based handbook for nurses* (prepared with support from the Robert Wood Johnson Foundation). Rockville, MD: Agency for Healthcare Research and Quality. (AHRQ Publication No. 08-0043)

Institute of Medicine. (1990). *Medicare: A strategy for quality assurance: Executive summary IOM committee to design a strategy for quality review and assurance in Medicare.* Washington, DC: National Academies Press.

Institute of Medicine. (2000). *To err is human: Building a safer health system.* Washington, DC: National Academies Press.

Institute of Medicine. (2001). *Crossing the quality chasm: A new health system for the 21st century.* Washington, DC: National Academies Press.

Institute of Medicine. (2003). *Health professions education: A bridge to quality.* Washington, DC: National Academies Press.

Institute of Medicine. (2004a). *Patient safety: Achieving a new standard for care.* Washington, DC: National Academies Press.

Institute of Medicine. (2004b). *Keeping patients safe: Transforming the work environment of nurses.* Washington, DC: National Academies Press.

The Joint Commission. (2007, July). *Sentinel event policy and procedures.* Retrieved November 2, 2008, from http://www.jointcommission.org/SentinelEvents/PolicyandProcedures/

The Joint Commission. (2008a). 2009 behavioral health care national patient safety goals. *The Joint Commission Accreditation: Behavioral health.* Retrieved July 26, 2008, from http://www.jointcommission.org/PatientSafety/NationalPatientSafetyGoals/09_bhc_npsgs.htm

The Joint Commission. (2008b). Behaviors that undermine a culture of safety. *Joint Commission Sentinel Event Alert, 40.* Retrieved July 26, 2008, from http://www.jointcommission.org/SentinelEvents/SentinelEventAlert/sea_40.htm

The Joint Commission. (2008c). *National patient safety goals.* Retrieved November 2, 2008, from http://www.jointcommission.org/PatientSafety/NationalPatientSafetyGoals/

The Joint Commission. (2008d). *Sentinel event alert.* Retrieved November 2, 2008, from http://www.jointcommission.org/SentinelEvents/SentinelEventAlert/

The Joint Commission. (2008e). *The Joint Commission testing and national implementation of the National Quality Forum endorsed nursing-sensitive care performance measure set: Project summary January 2007-December, 2008.* Retrieved February 12, 2009, from http://www.jointcommission.org/NR/rdonlyres/B14C4B51-10EA-440B-8DCE-C264C78A8D27/0/WebNSCPilotProjectSummary.pdf

Kurtzman, E. T., & Corrigan, J. M. (2007). Measuring the contribution of nursing to quality, patient safety, and health care outcomes. *Policy, Politics, & Nursing Practice, 8*(20), 20–36. doi: 10.1177/1527154407302115

Leape, L. L., Berwick, D. M., & Bates, D. W. (2002). What practices will most improve safety? Evidence-based medicine meets patient safety. *Journal of the American Medical Association, 288*, 501–507.

Lundqvist, M. J., & Axelsson, A. (2007). Nurses' perceptions of quality assurance. *Journal of Nursing Management, 15*, 51–58.

Lynn, J., West, J., Hausmann, S., Gifford, D., Nelson, R., McGann, P., et al. (2007). Collaborative clinical quality improvement for pressure ulcers in nursing homes. *Journal of the American Geriatric Society, 55*, 1663–1669.

Mastal, M. G., Joshi, M., & Schulke, K. (2007). Nursing leadership: Championing quality and patient safety in the boardroom. *Nursing Economics, 25*, 323–330.

McBride-Henry, K., & Foureur, M. (2007). A secondary care nursing perspective on medication administration safety. *Journal of Advanced Nursing, 60*, 58–66.

Melichar, L. (2007). Introduction: Improving health care in America through nursing quality measurement research. *Medical Care Research and Review, 64*(3), 3S–9S. doi:10.1177/1077558707299673

Miller, A., & Chaboyer, W. (2006). Captain and champion: Nurses' role in patient safety. *British Association of Critical Care Nurses, Nursing in Critical Care, 11*, 265–266.

Mitchell, P. H. (2008). Chapter 1. Defining patient safety and quality care. In R. G. Hughes, (Ed.), *Patient safety and quality: An evidence-based handbook for nurses* (Volume 1, pp. 1-1-1-5, Publication No. 08-0043). Rockville, MD: AHRQ.

Mitty, E. (2007). Hastings Center special report: The ethics of using QI methods to improve health care quality and safety. *Journal of Nursing Care Quality, 22*, 97–101.

National Quality Forum. (2008). *Nursing care quality at NQF.* Retrieved November 7, 2008, from http://www.qualityforum.org/nursing/

Naylor, M. D. (2007). Advancing the science in the measurement of health care quality influenced by nurses. *Medical Care Research and Review, 64*(144), 144S–169S. doi: 10.1177/1077558707299257

Needleman, J., Kurtzman, E. T., & Kizer, K. W. (2007). Performance measurement of nursing care: State of the science and the current consensus. *Medical Care Research and Review, 64*(10), 10S–43S. doi:10.1177/1077558707299260

Newhouse, R., & Poe, S. (Eds.). (2005). *Measuring patient safety.* Sudbury, MA: Jones and Bartlett.

Plsek, P. (2003, January). *Complexity and the adoptions of innovation in healthcare.* Paper presented at the National Institute for Healthcare Management Foundation and National Committee for Quality Healthcare conference, Accelerating Quality Improvement in Healthcare Strategies to Speed the Diffusion of Evidence-Based Innovations, Washington, DC.

Pronovost. P. J. (2004, March). *Healthcare safety and quality revolution.* Presentation at the American Association of Colleges of Nursing spring annual meeting, Washington, DC.

Reason, J. (2000). Human error: Models and management. *British Medical Journal, 320*, 768–770.

Ridley, R. T. (2008). The relationship between nurse education level and patient safety: An integrative review. *Journal of Nursing Education, 47*, 149–156.

Scheffer, B. K., & Rubenfeld, M. G. (2000). A consensus statement on critical thinking in nursing. *Journal of Nursing Education, 39*, 352–359.

Schmalenberg, C., & Kramer, M. (2008). Essentials of a productive nurse work environment. *Nursing Research, 57*, 2–13.

Sherwood, G., & Drenkard, K. (2007). Quality and safety curricula in nursing education: Matching practice realities. *Nursing Outlook, 55*, 151–155.

Shever, L. L., Titler, M. G., Kerr, P., Qin, R., Taikyoung, K., & Picone, D. M. (2008). The effect of high nursing surveillance on hospital cost. *Journal of Nursing Scholarship, 40*, 161–169.

Shortell, S. M., Bennett, C. L., & Byck, G. R. (1998). Assessing the impact of continuous quality improvement on clinical practice: What it will take to accelerate progress. *The Milbank Quarterly, 76*, 755–757.

Wheatley, M. J. (1994). *Leadership and the new science: Learning about organization from an orderly universe.* San Francisco: Berrett-Koehler.

Whitson, H. E., Hastings, S. N., Lekan, D. A., Sloane, R., White, H. K., & McConnell, E. S. (2008). A quality improvement program to enhance after-hours telephone communication between nurses and physicians in a long-term care facility. *Journal of the American Geriatric Society, 56*, 1080–1086.

Wise, L. C. (2007). Ethical issues surrounding quality improvement activities. *Journal of Nursing Administration, 37*, 272–278.

CHAPTER ——————————— 6

Critical Thinking and Patient-Centered Care

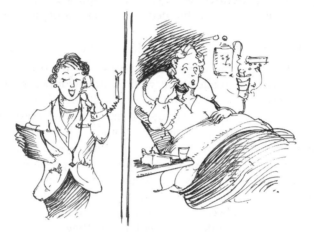

'OH... MS. McGREGOR LOOKS GOOD. HER BLOOD PRESSURE IS DOWN AND SHE'LL BE DISCHARGED IN A DAY OR TWO!'

Perhaps you heard the joke that went around before strict patient privacy laws were instituted? It goes something like this: One night the nurse on the 600 unit gets a phone call from somebody asking about Mary McGregor. The nurse grabs the chart and says, "Oh, Ms. McGregor looks good. Her blood pressure is down and she'll be discharged in a day or two!" The caller replies with obvious glee, "Oh, thank you." The nurse asks, "Are you a relative?" to which the caller replies, "No, I'm Mary McGregor and I haven't been able to get anyone to tell me anything about how I'm doing." Funny as it is, if the Institute of Medicine (IOM) gets its way, no one will be able to relate to that joke because it will be so preposterous.

Providing patient-centered care has been defined by IOM (2003) as being able to

identify, respect, and care about patients' differences, values, preferences, and expressed needs; relieve pain and suffering; coordinate continuous care; listen to, clearly inform, communicate with, and educate patients; *share decision making* [italics added] and management; and continuously advocate disease prevention, wellness, and promotion of healthy lifestyles, including a focus on population health. (p. 4)

The italicized words highlight how nurses' critical thinking (CT) interfaces with patients' CT. In this chapter, we focus on the thinking involved in patient-centered care. But first, let's consider circumstances that probably instigated our joke. And we'll look at the state of provider–patient relationships and why this IOM competency is so important. (It is important, you know, not just for being "nice," but to improve patient satisfaction and outcomes.) For providers who have not yet made this paradigm shift, patient-centered care will require a drastic modification in their thinking about the relationship between patients and providers.

Changing Patient–Provider Relationships

Let's take a look at that traditional patient–provider relationship. As a patient, what decisions have you made about your health issues? Have you ever had a health provider dismiss you when you offered what you thought was a reasonable solution to your health problem? Worse yet, have you had a provider remind you that he or she knows better and that you should do what you're told? How did you feel? Angry? Stupid? Inept? Devalued? All of the above? This scenario exemplifies the all-powerful and disrespectful healthcare provider. And, until confronted about their behavior, most healthcare providers who behave this way are usually oblivious to other options for provider–patient relationships.

When the IOM vision becomes a reality, healthcare professionals and patients will work in partnerships. In this new relationship, they will respect each other for having different, but valuable, knowledge. In the IOM version of patient-centered care, patients will no longer tolerate the traditional relationship. They will expect care tailored to their individual needs. Providers, in turn, will expect patients to do sophisticated research on the Internet, think through their health situations, and come up with conclusions and questions that they will expect to have considered. Gone will be the days when health providers are viewed as all-knowing.

Patient-centered care is not just an IOM concept, nor is it a new one. Some of you, especially those practicing in mental health, will remember the tenets of Hildegard Peplau (the mother of psychiatric nursing) regarding the collaborative relationship required between patient and nurse to achieve what we now call "patient-centered care" (Peplau, 1952). Under a variety of other terms, such as "client-centered" (Brown, McWilliam, & Ward-Griffin, 2006; de Witte, Schoot, & Proot, 2006), "partnerships" (Enehaug, 2000; Lee, 2007), "informative relations" (Benbassat, Pilpel, & Tidhar, 1998), "relationship-centered care" (Nolan, Davies, Brown, Keady, & Nolan, 2004), "patient-focused care" (McCauley & Irwin, 2006; Medina, 2006), and "person-centered care" (Crandall, White, Schuldheis, & Talerico, 2007; Landers & McCarthy, 2007; McCormack, 2004; McCormack & McCance, 2006), this movement has been studied from moral/ethical perspectives (Hewitt-Taylor, 2003), with a "consumer specialist" focus (Calabretta, 2002), and as a service partnership (Buch & Edgren, 2001). McCauley and Irwin called it "care we would want for our own family members" (p. 1573). In spite of the differences in nomenclature and focus, the underlying messages are quite similar. In

BOX 6-1	Examples of Descriptors of Patient-Centered Care

- Balance of power between provider and patient
- Empowered patients
- Focus on interpersonal relationships
- Shared decision making
- Understanding others' perspectives
- Collaboration and partnership
- Common goals
- Patient autonomy promoted
- Mutual respect for each other's expertise
- Negotiation
- Acknowledgment of provider as not having all the knowledge
- Discussions of uncertainty OK
- Patient responsibility for health behaviors
- Open communication and information exchange
- Consumer control over information
- Connectedness
- Truthfulness and honesty
- Culture of caring
- Mutuality
- Customized, individualized care

Sources: Buch & Edgren, 2001; Calabretta, 2002; Carter et al., 2008; Crandall et al., 2007; Enehaug, 2000; Hewitt-Taylor, 2003; McCormack, 2004; Nolan et al., 2004; O'Donovan, 2007; Sidani, 2008; Slater, 2006.

Box 6-1, we've compiled some examples of patient-centered care descriptors we've found. Although there are many more phrases, these should give you a snapshot of what patient-centered care looks like.

Where does your experience fit in terms of the descriptors shown in the box? Are you more familiar with the old-fashioned paternalistic provider relationships, or are these examples part of your experience? If it's the latter, you recognize the wisdom of the IOM's vision. We hope that by now, patient-centered care is becoming more common; unfortunately, Redman (2008) might be right—patient-centered care is still "an aspiration, not a reality" (p. 5). One thing we know for sure is this: This alternative to traditional approaches will affect and be affected by the thinking of both providers and patients.

Patient-Centered Care and CT

Patient-centered care acknowledges and celebrates patients as critical thinkers. This may be a shift in perception for many. Nurses and other providers need to consider not just their CT, but how their thinking interfaces with patients' CT. Because most patients have one or more family members and significant others who actively participate in their healthcare decision making, the actual group of affected thinkers can get fairly large. In Chapter 7 we will discuss interdisciplinary teams, and there you will see that nurses, patients, and significant others are all part of the sizable thinking/decision-making team. In the IOM's ideal healthcare delivery world, everyone's thinking would "merge" to find resolutions to the issues at hand. **Figure 6-1** depicts this model of thinking through a patient's healthcare issue.

Those thinking "clouds" should merge naturally, but in fact, this doesn't happen automatically. We have a long history of viewing health providers as experts to whom patients must defer; the expert model gives power to the provider, with an implication of compliance for the patient (Brown et al., 2006). Many older patients, especially, have that deferential attitude. However, that patient–provider relationship is changing rapidly. Patients of all generations can access vast amounts of health information today. With implementation of patient-centered care, providers will be more likely to acknowledge and value patients' knowledge and collaborate with them in addressing health issues. However, providers cannot yet assume that patients have the necessary level of knowledge even though so much information is out there.

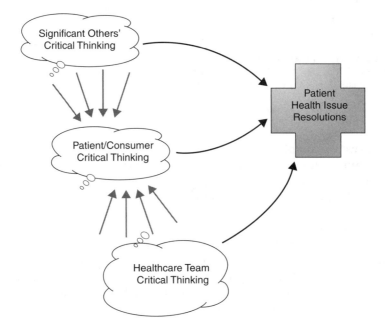

FIGURE 6-1 Critical thinking for patient-centered care.

Health literacy is becoming an important topic as we move toward patient-centered care (Clancy, 2008). Patient thinking has been studied by several authors. Anderson (2007) found that couples' decision making for genetic issues could be enumerated into nine types of thinking: analytical, ethical, moral, reflective, practical, hypothetical, judgmental, scary, and second sight. Because people use other patients' experiences as an important part of their decision making relative to newly acquired conditions, one Web site (http://www.dipex.org) has been set up specifically to report controlled and analyzed narratives of people who have various health conditions (Ziebland & Herxheimer, 2008). Consumer health informatics is a burgeoning field, but it is not without its drawbacks—not the least of which is the often undependable quality of the knowledge now available (Eysenbach & Jadad, 2001). Therefore, providers will need to assess patients' knowledge much more critically in the future (Coulter, Entwistle, & Gilbert, 1999). (We will examine this problem in Chapter 9 in our discussion of healthcare informatics.)

Our challenge for now is threefold. We must (1) assess the patient's readiness, willingness, and ability to participate in the healthcare thinking process, (2) facilitate patients' actual process of thinking about their own health care, and (3) merge our thinking and the patient's thinking to create a mutually satisfying and functional process that leads to quality outcomes. According to the IOM (2001), "in many cases, the best window on the safety and quality of care is through the eyes of the patient" (p. 45).

Assessing Patient Readiness, Willingness, and Ability to Participate in CT and Patient-Centered Care

Perhaps 50 years from now, all patients will be accustomed to ready access to information (and the standards to judge its quality) and self-diagnostic kits. But we're not there yet. Some patients might be uncomfortable with what they see as the extra burden of being full participants in healthcare decision making; others might be dissatisfied that they are not included in the thinking process. For now, we need some way to estimate how engaged a patient is, or wants to be, and to track potential growth in that engagement. For that, we can look at CT habits of the mind.

Keeping in mind that habits of the mind are dynamic states and reflect one's penchant for CT, we could use a checklist to rate patients' thinking tendencies. Assessing habits of the mind is different from assessing the patient's actual skills at thinking (which we will address later); habits of the mind focus more on readiness and willingness. Before rating a patient's thinking tendencies, however, engage a bit of *contextual perspective* in your thinking. Look at yourself (*reflection*) and consider how your habits of the mind will correlate with the patient's habits. Remember, partnership in care decisions is at the core of patient-centered care, not simply out of respect, which is important, but to achieve quality outcomes.

Now, move to the patient's context. First, the basics: Can the patient speak and understand English? (Nailon, 2007). What is the status of the patient's senses; can he or she see and hear adequately to be a partner in decision making? Second, consider the magnitude of the physical and emotional stress experienced in the current health situation. Pain and anxiety can powerfully override natural thinking habits of the mind. Third, there may be cognitive deficits that are due to developmental factors, neurological disease, and conditions such as dementia and delirium. Although not considered cognitive deficits per se, the patient's educational level may affect thinking. In these cases, don't forget the patients' significant others as thinking team members; complete the checklist with them in mind. Fourth, cultural or generational issues might cause a patient to think it disrespectful to openly participate in health-issue thinking. (We discussed some of these ideas in Chapter 3.) In these cases, it is our responsibility to let those people know that it is not only OK but desirable to think along with us.

Once you have considered the contextual issues, look at the checklist in **Box 6-2** and think about how you might use such a checklist in your practice. Even if you don't specifically rate patients' thinking habits of the mind, asking yourself these questions about each patient will help you focus on the patient as a thinking person and not some blank slate on which you and the team "do" things.

| **BOX 6-2** | **CT Habits of the Mind Patient-Rating Checklist** |

Insert your patient's name in the blank for each item. Rate each habit of the mind as 1 (no), 2 (maybe), or 3 (yes) and mark this on the line. Remember that circumstances can change these scores, so use this information to assess where your patient is today. If your patient scores between 10 and 15, he or she is probably less likely to be an active team thinker; between 16 and 21, he or she is probably a moderately active team thinker; between 22 and 30, he or she is a very active team thinker.

____ *Confidence:* Does _____ seem sure of himself/herself in thinking through this situation?

____ *Contextual perspective:* Is _____ thinking of the whole picture?

____ *Creativity:* Is _____ likely to adapt to the situation with plans not immediately obvious to us?

____ *Flexibility:* Is _____ able to adapt his/her thinking to this health situation?

____ *Inquisitiveness:* Will _____ seek out information on his/her own?

____ *Intellectual integrity:* Will _____ consider the truth about this situation even if it goes against his/her hopes and wishes?

____ *Intuition:* Is _____ likely to respond at a "gut level"?

____ *Open-mindedness:* Will _____ choose the best path toward health even if it means changing his/her behavior?

____ *Perseverance:* Will _____ hang in there and work this through?

____ *Reflection:* Is _____ someone who stops to think back on things?

_____**Total Score**

TACTICS 6-1

Reflect on Your Patients' Habits of the Mind

Clinicians and Educators

Think back to a patient encounter you (or, for educators, your student) had recently. Use the checklist in Box 6-2 to rate that patient. Then think: How did it feel to rate the patient? Can you see how such a rating might be valuable? How did it help you consider your patient in a different light?

Discussion

If you have patients who rate very low on this scale, what were possible reasons? To what can you attribute higher scores? How did you use contextual perspective to find these contributing factors? Are any of those factors changeable and, if so, how?

Facilitating Patients' Critical Thinking Skills

Once we have a feel for patients' CT tendencies, we can better gauge how much encouragement, if any, they need to exercise their thinking skills alongside ours. In other words, for patients and significant others, we need to determine what's in those thinking "clouds" shown in Figure 6-1 on page 136. To help you focus on their thinking, let's look at each of the seven CT skills, explore how patients use those skills, and consider what we can do to promote them. We have addressed the skills in alphabetical order, but this does not imply any ranking of their importance.

Analyzing

Separating or breaking a whole into parts to discover their nature, function, and relationships. Can you imagine patients breaking down options for their care, such as for treatment of diabetes? Of course you can. Studying the pros and cons of insulin therapy and oral hypoglycemics is an analytical process. Helping patients *analyze* the complexities of a diabetic diet helps them follow recommendations. It's not enough to hand dietary guidelines to patients; they need to break that down into something that translates into their breakfast, lunch, dinner, snacks, grocery lists, restaurant options, vacation diets, sick days, and so on. Coulter et al. (1999), using focus groups, found that patients were dissatisfied with the information they got from healthcare providers. They wanted a full range of treatment options and to learn the pros and cons of each. They wanted materials to help them feel knowledgeable enough to participate equally in decision making. They didn't want simplistic conclusions; they wanted empowerment through knowledge. If providers and patients together analyze situations—break things down to essential information—they will better understand which options are appropriate and make more informed decisions. Patients then will be more likely to adhere to treatments such as dietary changes because those treatments will be tailored to their lifestyle.

Applying Standards

Judging according to established personal, professional, or social rules or criteria. This is an interesting cognitive skill. It is closely aligned with what one values. In a recent class exercise, we asked registered nurse (RN)/bachelor of science in nursing (BSN) students to share personal standards they applied in their practices. Here are some of their answers: "I always check to see if my patients need pain medication right at the end of my shift, and I remind them that staff will be in transition for the next hour. I don't want them sitting there waiting for pain medication." "I always talk about what I'm doing while I'm doing tasks in patients' rooms." "I try to teach something every time I'm in the room." "I always ask patients, 'How can I help you today?'" Aren't those wonderful standards?

Now, let's think about patients' standards. How often do we ask patients what they expect of us? What is their definition of standard of care, and might their definitions be in conflict with ours? Healthcare providers are apt to forget that patients don't know the usual routines that are taken for granted in health care. Patients might expect every nurse to ask about pain medication at the end of the shift, as the nurse just mentioned did. If the nurse on the next shift doesn't, patients are apt to think that she isn't doing her job.

Think about the patient who is constantly pressing his call light for seemingly trivial reasons. Might that patient think this is the expected standard of nursing care on an evening shift on a medical floor? People often think of nurses as being like waiters—you just call them when you want something. Rather than getting frustrated with patients like this, we can try to educate them about the norms and standards of care and ask them what they expect as routines.

A common example of conflicting standards is the patient who is angry at having to wait in the office for 45 minutes for his or her physician or nurse practitioner (NP). These patients obviously have an expectation that a 3 p.m. appointment means that they'll be seen within 5 minutes or so—as they do at the hairdresser, for example. Sometimes a straightforward explanation of what life is like in a medical office—people have unexpected needs that disrupt schedules—is enough to help a patient develop a more realistic standard and expectation of care. Patients and providers must have a full knowledge of how the system works for a true partnership to exist (Enehaug, 2000).

Another consideration concerning *applying standards* is linked to patient access to information. Patients not only read about healthcare issues in magazines, but also, for example, can go online and retrieve the same guidelines for diabetes management that their health provider is using. In line with this diabetes management example, the National Institutes of Health Web site Making Systems Changes for Better Diabetes Care (http://betterdiabetescare.nih.gov) cited several dimensions of patient-centered care, including respect; information and communication; and coordination and integration of care (National Diabetes

Education Program, n.d.). This site promotes a true partnership between patients with diabetes and their providers. Patients who use the thinking skill of *applying standards* will keep us on our toes. If we focus only on our application of standards without considering the patients' application of those same standards, we will create conflict, waste time, and diminish patient-centered care.

One final word and a bit of caution when *applying standards*: Standards change, such as acceptable measures for blood pressure and blood glucose. Some standards are also culturally biased. For example, most height and weight charts for children are normalized for Caucasians. An Asian-Pacific colleague has to keep that in mind when her pediatrician's records show her son as consistently in the lower percentile for height. The lesson there is that we need CT even with standards in order to customize patient-centered care.

Discriminating

Recognizing differences and similarities among things or situations and distinguishing carefully as to category or rank. We might not think of this as a cognitive skill that we readily identify from patients' perspectives. After all, we see distinguishing the finer points in healthcare situations as requiring our expert eyes, ears, and intuition. However, when we consider patients' abilities to make fine distinctions about their bodies, we can appreciate their ability to discriminate.

Pain assessment, for example, requires patient *discrimination*. Consider the question, "On a scale of 0 to 10, with 10 being your worst pain, what number do you rank your pain at now?" The answer requires mighty powers of *discrimination*, with potentially dire consequences (often unrealized by patients). Nurses decide between Tylenol and Vicodin based on those numbers! Should we pay more attention to how well patients are able to *discriminate* when we ask that question? And we must not let our own biases invade. Imagine the scenario going through this nurse's mind as she asks a patient to rate pain: "This patient ranks her pain at a 3 on the 1–10 scale. She is a woman, so the worst pain she's had is probably childbirth. I had a baby so I have a good idea of what her 3 would be. OK, so she's in reasonable pain." But, what if this woman suffers from migraine or cluster headaches? She may be using that pain as her standard.

The point is, the number is minimally relevant unless we can relate it to a baseline. The number allows for accurate *discrimination* only when the patient shares what the pain compares with. We must ask about that comparison to find out how the patient is making the distinction between, say, a 5 and a 3. Patient-centered care depends on understanding the patient's unique perspective, thinking, and *discriminating* skills.

Calabretta (2002) went so far as to call patients "consumer specialists" because of this acute self-discriminating ability relative to their health. "Because patients can afford to focus narrowly on their own concerns, learning only about their condition, they have the possibility of ultimately becoming 'consumer specialists.' In addition, all patients have the inherent knowledge of their own symptoms and the experience of living with a disease that physicians lack" (p. 33).

Information Seeking

Searching for evidence, facts, or knowledge by identifying relevant sources and gathering objective, subjective, historical, and current data from those sources. In today's world of easy access to information, patients can and will access information with or without our help. They can, for example, go to the American Diabetes Association Web site, pull up the section for healthcare professionals, and read the recommendations for care. Increasingly, we find patients doing just that. They read self-help books and magazine articles and view TV shows, all of which provide information. Whereas some patients are able to do extensive research on their health issues on their own, others could and might do so if healthcare providers guided them by identifying resources such as Web sites, patient-information libraries, and self-help books.

Providers must coach patients to be seekers of information. We must help them evaluate which sources of information are legitimate. We are well past the days when our role in patients' information-seeking is simply to hand them brochures. We now need to be partners in seeking information. We must listen to and value what our patients find and respond not in a dismissive manner but collegially in deciding together the value of that information. Sharing and valuing each other's information promote patient-centered care.

As we have mentioned earlier and will discuss in Chapters 8 and 9, the issue of judging information, especially that found on the Internet, is still problematic. Some organizations are working diligently to improve this situation and develop instruments to judge the quality of Web site information. (We list some in Chapter 9.) Unfortunately, we have a long way to go before these instruments are consistently validated. Gagliardi and Jadad (2002) found 51 new Web site rating instruments; only 5 had information allowing them to be evaluated, and none of those had been validated. They questioned the value of these incompletely developed instruments, asking, "Is it desirable or necessary to assess the quality of health information on the internet? If so, is it an achievable goal given that quality is a construct for which we have no gold standard?" (p. 571). Until these questions are answered, we must use our CT and help patients use their CT to choose the best sources of information and evaluate the quality of that information. The folks at Vanderbilt University have an interesting system to help patients get the best information. Their medical center and Eskind Biomedical Library have developed the Patient Informatics Consult Service, which gives patients "information prescriptions" that they can take to librarians who then collect the information and create a report that is delivered to the clinician and patient (Williams, Gish, Giuse, Sathe, & Carrell, 2001). Now that's CT creativity at work!

Logical Reasoning

Drawing inferences or conclusions that are supported in or justified by evidence. This cognitive skill is used by everyone to some degree. Most patients today will not accept pat answers that aren't supported by the evidence of their symptoms. They will, and should, question these answers. On the other hand, we can also point out to patients that there is much we still don't know—that we don't have evidence for some things. "Healthcare professionals should acknowledge that they do not possess complete and irrefutable knowledge . . . [and] enter into discussions with patients in which uncertainties and conflicting views can be explored openly" (Hewitt-Taylor, 2003, p. 1327). Working together with patients and using available information, however incomplete it might be, we can help patients draw conclusions that are easier to accept because they can see the logic behind them.

Consider this case study: Mrs. Jones is 75. She has a diagnosis of diverticulosis and colonic stricture; she has been suffering from diarrhea since finishing one course of antibiotics for a recent urinary tract infection. Based on her physical exam findings, she was placed on metronidazole to cover both clostridium difficile colitis and diverticulitis. When she sees her NP on a follow-up visit, she states that she has stopped taking the metronidazole because it made her nauseated and she didn't like the taste it left in her mouth. When the NP said she needed a referral to a gastroenterologist and an abdominal scan, Mrs. Jones replied, "I don't like that doctor and I'm not having another scan." Continuing to ask for something to help stop the diarrhea but refusing all suggestions, the patient was a challenge to the NP, who was struggling alone with the logical reasoning. Totally frustrated, the NP finally laid all the facts in front of the patient, including ways to disguise the taste of the pill, and said, "Here are the only conclusions I can make with these facts. Do you see a different conclusion here?" The patient replied, "Oh, I thought there were other things I could do, but I see that these are my choices."

Initially, this passive patient wanted the nurse to draw all the conclusions and make the decisions. Ultimately, however, when presented with the facts and given the option to draw her own conclusion, the patient engaged her logical reasoning and drew inferences based on the available evidence. (By the way, the patient reported that metronidazole and peanut butter taste great!) This situation is not unusual. Patients who see health providers as all-knowing don't engage in the decision making, but wait passively until a conclusion is passed down. Patients often can state what they don't want without knowing all the possible choices. When faced with making decisions themselves or in partnership with providers, they can see the logic used by the provider and add their own *logical reasoning*.

Predicting

Envisioning a plan and its consequences. Patients may be better at the cognitive skill of predicting than healthcare providers are; they can see how their lives will change by the health issue at hand. A good question to help patients use this skill, for example, is, "Knowing that diabetes is a progressive condition (meaning that you will likely need more medications over time), how do you see yourself dealing with this over the next few years?" This question helps patients think about the future and increases the chances that they will recognize the consequences of their decisions. It is important for providers to help patients see alternative "right" answers. There may be good, better, and best options, or even three "betters" and two "bests."

Helping patients with *predictive* thinking is valuable because patients know themselves and the circumstances of their daily lives best. *Predicting* is especially important when patients are first faced with a chronic illness that will change their lifestyle. The process of *predicting* helps them internalize their new health situation and accept their realities. *Predicting* consequences may not come naturally to some and can be based on culture as well as be dependent on cognitive and developmental skills. Our job as providers is to facilitate opportunities for patients to use this skill to promote patient-centered care.

Predictive thinking, so important in dealing with chronic illness, is a driving force behind the shift away from provider-centered care, a paradigm for acute illness management (National Diabetes Education Program, n.d.). In the case of an acute illness, the provider takes more control, but with chronic illness management, once the patient is out the hospital or office door, he or she is the one in control. Predictive thinking about what's outside that door must be the result of a partnership between patients and providers.

Transforming Knowledge

Patients probably have to transform knowledge (*change or convert the condition, nature, form, or function of concepts among contexts*) more than their providers do. Patients with this skill use information to take control of new health situations. Consider patient education: You know that you need to impart medical knowledge in a way that patients can understand. Among the most successful *knowledge transformation* examples are consumer self-help groups, which allow patients with similar conditions to talk to each other, teach each other, and translate medical lingo into something they can learn from.

It behooves healthcare providers to think about how they can learn from consumer groups. Some primary care settings have done this by having group appointments for patients with similar conditions, such as diabetes or pregnancy. The provider saves time by not having to repeat things, and patients benefit by receiving information from both the provider and others in similar situations. Group interactions are great facilitators for transforming knowledge. Transforming the provider's knowledge into the patient's reality, and vice versa, provides increased opportunities for patient-centered care.

How to Merge Our Thinking with Patient Thinking

With this perspective of how patients can and do use their thinking skills, what can educators and clinicians do to make this collaborative thinking the norm? Kleiman (2007) would say that we need to revitalize "the humanistic imperative in nursing practice" (p. 209). Eldh, Ekman, and Ehnfors (2006), while studying patients' participation in health care, found that two conditions were necessary for true participation—recognition of each patient's unique knowledge, and respect for the patient. Even though it seems a ludicrous statement, it is easy to forget the patient, a human being deserving of our respect and honesty, as we go along our way as healthcare providers.

The first job, then, is to remember the patient and acknowledge his or her "natural standpoint" (Anderson, 2007, p. 15). The second is to validate, validate, validate our conclusions with the patient. The third job is to coax and coach patient thinking.

Remember the Patient

In our nursing classes, when we get to the part about drawing conclusions—such as nursing diagnoses—we often ask our students, "Now that you've concluded that there is a problem needing nursing care, what will your next step be?" The typical response (based on the students' familiarity with the assessing, planning, implementing, and evaluating phases of the nursing process) is, "Start planning." The answer we are looking for, however, is "Validate that conclusion with the patient." In all our years of teaching, neither of us has ever gotten that response without prompting. And that's even with teaching patient-centered care from the get-go. Why is it so easy to "forget the patient" when we keep saying that we value patient-centered care?

Here's an example. A student caring for a patient whose wife had died 4 months earlier made a nursing diagnosis of dysfunctional grieving based on evidence that the patient could not speak of his wife without crying. That student, with the teacher's prompting, sought the patient's validation of that conclusion by asking, "Mr. Jones, based on my assessment, I'm thinking that my nursing diagnosis is dysfunctional grieving. What do you think?" Mr. Jones was quick to put the student in her place. "I am grieving, but there's nothing dysfunctional about crying over my wonderful wife who left me only 4 months ago!" In response, this student, with the help of Mr. Jones, changed her diagnosis to "incomplete grieving," even though the NANDA (Herdman, 2009) classification had no such label (and still doesn't—it has "grieving," "complicated grieving" and "risk for complicated grieving" only). There wasn't a problem—just a conclusion, based on facts, made jointly with the patient. In this example, the patient's *logical reasoning* was better than the student's. She was more focused initially on following context-free rules—a common occurrence with novice-level thinking. But she was able, with the patient's partnership, to demonstrate *logical reasoning* and *transforming knowledge*.

Validate, Validate, Validate

The process of validation cannot be overemphasized. Think about your practice; how often do you solicit patients' validation to see if your thinking is on track? How often do you validate with yourself that you are valuing the patient's part in the thinking process? See **Box 6-3** for examples of remarks that support both kinds of validation.

BOX 6-3	**Validation Remarks to Promote Patient Participation in Decisions**

- Here's what I think; do you agree?
- What would you say is going on here?
- How is all of this affecting you?
- Does it seem that way to you? It does to me, but I want your opinion.
- Let's think about this together for a minute.
- Only you know your daily living situation.
- Can we find a way through this together?
- Let me explain my thinking to you.
- What do you think?
- How does this feel?
- Do you agree with this?
- This is what I'm thinking; what do you think?
- I'm interested in your take on all of this.
- If you could change this, what would be different?
- If you had a magic wand, what would you have it do?

TACTICS 6-2

Reflect on Your Validation Remarks

Clinicians

Carry a copy of the validation remarks in Box 6-3 in your pocket for a couple of days as you work with patients. Periodically, pull it out and check off which comments you've made. At the end of each day, look at how many comments you've made.

Educators

Distribute a copy of Box 6-3 to your students and ask them to track how many times they make such remarks over the course of a day or two when working with patients. You might also think about how many of these comments you use with students to validate your thinking with them.

Discussion

These remarks may seem simple, but many important things we do as nurses are simple. Remember the old adage, "For want of a nail the shoe is lost, for want of a shoe the horse is lost, for want of a horse the rider is lost." There's a lot of truth to that; don't forget the simple things; they have huge consequences. Simple can be powerful.

Buch and Edgren (2001) suggested that patients be interviewed soon after admission to the hospital to "explore expectations, needs and demands" (p. 69). Doing that would set the stage for thinking partnerships at the outset of the patient–provider encounter. The patient would expect to be a partner in decision making, either as a direct participant or by validating conclusions.

Coaxing and Coaching Patient Thinking

Most patients respect healthcare providers; they don't want to step on their toes or take up their time. They are also reluctant to push for collaborative thinking if their providers don't indicate that this is desirable. Using the validation remarks listed in Box 6-3 might help providers encourage patient participation, but there's more to it than that. We must do more than just verbally validate our thinking with them; we have to personify openness to their thinking and show them that we value them as people, not only as patients. That's a tough one to put in a box— it's linked to our personal interaction styles and requires subtle nonverbal communication. We asked some nurses how they show patients that they are open to "sitting down and thinking" together. **Box 6-4** lists ideas that those nurses shared. Add your unique ideas to this list.

BOX 6-4	**Strategies to Help Healthcare Providers Encourage Patient Participation in the Thinking Process**

- Stay in the room; don't talk to them from the doorway.
- Pay attention to your body language and to theirs.
- Sit down so you're at eye level with them.
- Use open questions and comments, such as, "Tell me about . . ." instead of closed questions, which imply that you expect a short answer.
- Touch them, but be respectful of their space and cultural norms.
- Use collaborative thinking language such as, "We should think this through," "Let's look at some possible conclusions," and "Can we analyze this together?"
- Use phrases that let them know that their situation is not so unusual that they can't discuss it; for example, "Some people feel anxious when . . ."
- Address them respectfully; find out if they prefer Mr. or Mrs. or Professor, Reverend, and so on.
- Don't look at your watch, no matter how busy you are.
- Be direct and honest; for example, tell them when the schedule is backed up and why.
- If you feel like avoiding a patient, reflect on why you feel that way.

Are There Negatives to Patient-Centered Care?

Clearly, we value patient-centered care, but are there negatives to this? Certainly. Two of the biggest are time and power. It takes more time to practice true patient-centered care—or so it would seem on the face of it. As providers, we have to give up power and share it with patients, and, if we consider that honestly, that makes us feel vulnerable. It's hard to admit that we don't have all the control or all the answers.

Time

Let's look at time. Say you have a passive patient who doesn't push to get involved in decisions. What do you do? You probably answer, "Get the patient involved, of course." Now, picture yourself on a particularly busy medical unit and ask yourself what you'd do. If you're like most, you'd be happy that the patient is not slowing you down, asking questions, or expressing opinions on how things should be done. This is our reality; we're busy people, and practicing patient-centered care can be very time-consuming. That's probably the real reason why it's not the norm.

We ask you to reconsider this assumption. Does patient-centered care really take more time in the long run, or does it seem that way in the short run? How much time do we spend doing things that we decide are best for the patients, only to find that those patients have no investment in our ideas because they weren't involved in the decisions? How many extra trips down the hall do we have to make because our patients feel isolated and at the mercy of all those providers who are making decisions for them? What is the price of making our patients feel powerless?

Power

Now, let's look at power—ours and patients'. According to the IOM (2003), "the patient is the source of control" (p. 47), and providers must "allow patients to have unfettered access to the information contained in their medical records" (p. 52). Are you old enough to remember the days when it was unheard of to show a patient his chart? Do you work in a setting where patients who ask to look at their charts are still put off? "You'll need to wait until the doctor can sit down with you." When we were students, we were usually taught phrases to use when patients asked us what their blood pressure was: "It's just fine, don't worry about it; it's a little high, but it's fine." What nonsense such approaches seem now, with the new focus on patient-centered care! Some of you might be saying, "Gee, that's still done on our unit!" We hope not, but we wouldn't be surprised.

Don't you wonder why we kept patients' health information secret from them? We think some of it had to do with a misplaced sense of power and a desire to protect patients and ourselves. Perhaps it was predicated on a fear of litigation, which is certainly a consideration in the United States. Traditionally, we believed we were burden-carriers for patients. We are the experts and we do things for them (Brown et al., 2006). We know what's best for them. At the same time, we keep their identities as people separated from our identities; otherwise, we might spend too much time worrying about what it would be like to be in their situation. We want to distance ourselves from the horror of being sick. You can probably think of other reasons to keep your distance, too.

Oops, it's time for therapy again. Maybe it's time that educators help students deal with their mortality as a way to promote patient-centered care. That's not such a far-fetched idea. If we can help providers, right at the start of their education, see how similar they are to patients instead of making them feel superior to and separate from patients, then we will minimize the power issues that interfere with patient-centered care.

We need to accept that we are not there to protect patients from the truth and that health care is a collaborative process. Providers are supposed to help patients think through health issues with open eyes. Hickson et al. (2002) studied patient complaints and malpractice risk; their results were consistent with earlier similar studies. "Patients who saw physicians with the highest numbers of lawsuits were more likely to complain that their physicians would not listen or return telephone calls, were rude, and did not show respect" (p. 2955). Although fear of litigation should not be a primary force driving patient-centered care, it can serve as a reminder that we want to avoid adversarial relationships and that we want patients in the loop in the decision-making process. In the long run, withholding information is not protection—it's simply not good practice.

Before we leave the topic of power issues, you might want to look at your environment. Tellis-Nayak (2007) concluded that a person-centered workplace would turn workers into person-centered caregivers. Can we provide patient-centered care if we don't care about the people we work with?

A discussion of caring about the people we work with probably requires a whole chapter, if not a book or two. But, for a capsular version, think about the big picture for a minute—the whole system and all the stakeholders we have been pondering in this book. Nurses are a major part of that system, as are patients and families, but so are nursing assistants (NAs), technicians, physical therapists, unit clerks, physicians, pharmacists, and so on, and so on. Now, think about all the things that contribute to the functioning of those stakeholders in the system. The bottom line of a working system depends on caring about and trusting the people you work with. Although caring about people is considered a natural characteristic of nurses, unfortunately, it doesn't always carry over to those we work with. The old, very sad adage that "we eat our young" is still in play in some settings. It is time to ban that phenomenon and move to a new paradigm of caring for new nurses, old nurses, and all other healthcare providers. The more we care about each other, the more we work together. The more we work together, the better the care we provide. We'll discuss the "thinking together" part of that working together in Chapter 7, but now it's time for a marvelous example of how the nurses in one large healthcare organization are clearly capturing the essence of patient-centered care:

A Patient-Centered Care Story

from Diane DiFiore, RN, MSA, Director, Nurse Recruitment & Retention, and
Sandra Schmitt, RN, BSN, Manager, Nursing Development Specialist
Oakwood Healthcare System, Michigan

Nurses at Oakwood Healthcare System in Michigan are finding the change to patient-centered care an eye-opening one. Listen to this story:

> *One nurse asked a very ill elderly woman if she wanted to get up. The patient replied, "I'm done." The nurse took that to mean she didn't want to get up, but the answer seemed strange. When she went back later and asked again, the patient replied with the same answer, "I'm done." The nurse then asked the patient to explain her answer, and the patient said, "I'm ready to have hospice care now; I'm done with life."*

Really listening to the patient in this situation made a big difference in how she was cared for. Several things occurred to make that happen. Two nurse leaders who were intimately involved in this transitional endeavor talked to us.

> *We had no patient care delivery model, so Oakwood made a conscious decision to adopt relationship-oriented care (ROC). This model is broader than just patient-centered care; it focuses on all relationships—those among staff as well as those among clients and staff. It's important that staff consider their relationships too. We want their work environment to be best practice as well.*
>
> *ROC is our version of Ruth Hansten's model, Relationship and Results-Oriented Healthcare (Hansten, 2005). Her model is evidence based and emphasizes measurement of outcomes and the use of critical thinking. Choosing this model was a top-down and bottom-up decision as well as process. Once we decided this was what we wanted, we met with Ruth Hansten and did a 2-day training with 20 nurses who would be our Level 1 Specialists; they completed the certification portfolio over 5–6 months. Each week, there was an assignment to complete; there was always a self-reflection piece in each assignment. Critical thinking and clinical judgment were key elements of the project.*
>
> *The Level 1 Specialists developed the framework and the presentations for the system rollout. We went out to the four hospitals and did in-service training with all shifts—nurses and ancillary staff; over 3,000 employees were involved, and we held about 300 classes. One critical thinking dimension emphasized during the training was reflection. Opportunities for reflection brought out lots of good ideas and opportunities to engage in serious thinking about patient care issues.*
>
> *Nurses were excited about the project because it got them back to the bedside. A lot of this approach is not new, but ROC brought it to the foreground. After the training, the first performance improvement change we made was to replace taped*

shift reports with bedside reporting. A unit reporting tool was designed—one for the RN and one for the NA. The first phase of ROC implementation consisted of three steps: bedside reporting, use of the unit report tool, and staff introduction (making sure we introduce ourselves properly to patients). When we started this, nurses said they'd do this if it would save time. It used to take about 30 minutes to listen to taped report. When bedside reporting was started, it took 25 minutes; the nurses did not think saving only 5 minutes was a marked improvement. What was happening was that when they went to the patient bedside, patients would ask for help with various tasks—going to the bathroom, getting a drink, etc. To resolve this, the off-going and oncoming NAs, whose shifts overlap by a half hour, went ahead of the nurses in addressing basic patient care needs. This saved the nurses a lot of time. Now report took 15 minutes, so we saved 15 minutes on both sides of the shift. Patient satisfaction went up to 99% (from less than 50% before), so bedside reporting was really effective.

Even more important than satisfaction is that bedside reporting improves safety. If you have to stand at the bedside and hand over your shift to the next nurse, you are not apt to leave an IV that is almost dry.

The second phase of ROC implementation was an RN/patient-focused interview for every shift, RN–NA report, and RN–NA checkpoints and feedback. In the interview, we ask the patient what he or she would like to accomplish during that particular shift. This plan is shared in report by the RN with the NA. Together they establish times for checkpoints and feedback (even/odd hours) to update each other on work completed. We introduced "care boards," which is like a white board that includes the plan for the day, phone numbers, patient and family communication, and physician communication.

There's an interesting story about the interview and care board. When a nurse asked one patient, Aloysius, what name he wanted to be called, he thought for awhile and then said, "Al." His daughter looked up and said, "Dad, since when have you wanted to be called Al?" He replied, "All my life but nobody ever asked." We always say we're listening to patients, but I'm not sure we really have been doing that. They know and appreciate when we're listening; it builds trust.

The ROC report tools and mechanisms, such as bedside reporting and hourly rounds, help nurses organize their thinking. Nurses at Oakwood now find they are more systematic; they used to be focused on their task perspective—"This is what I need to do." Now they are thinking about the patient as a person—"What does the patient want/need?"

Nurses have been inundated with new technology and tasks. The healthcare focus is becoming more specialized all the time. It's easy to forget the patient. Here's an example: A patient was recently extubated. In the past, I would have anticipated what the patient needed—a drink, mouth care, etc., but when we asked the patient, she said, "I want my hair washed; it's been 4 days and I feel grungy." That may seem like a simple thing, but it's not. We are now putting the patient's needs first.

PAUSE _____

and Ponder

Where Is the Balance?

What else can educators and clinicians do? We will leave this question for you to ponder. Keep in mind that there are no easy answers to these complex issues. We'll bet that every reader can think of a patient who was so controlling that the only solution seemed to be to say, "Could you just listen to me and do as I ask?" Such negative situations always seem to stand out more than the positive ones. We've also had many patients who reached wonderful "a-ha" points after collaborative problem solving. There will, of course, always be extremes that challenge our commitment to patient-centered care.

One useful guideline to remember is balance. Ideal patient-centered care is a balance of patient thinking and provider thinking within the realities of each situation. Many factors—knowledge, access to knowledge, overt and covert permission to think, cultural beliefs about roles, habits of the mind and thinking skills, power and control—affect thinking and patient-centered care. Our job is to keep thinking in spite of time constraints, taking advantage of our CT and that of our patients.

Reflection Cues

- Patient-centered care, as envisioned by the IOM, must include a focus on patient and provider thinking.
- Traditional patient–provider relationships were hierarchical, with the provider doing the thinking for the patient.
- Patient-centered care must start with a collaborative nurse–patient relationship.
- Patients, significant others, and the team of healthcare providers must work to merge their thinking toward one end—a safe, high-quality healthcare issue outcome.
- Challenges for providers who want to think with patients are threefold. We must assess the patient's readiness, willingness, and ability to participate in the healthcare thinking process; help patients with the actual process of thinking about their own health care; and merge our thinking and the patient's thinking to create a mutually satisfying and functional process.
- Assessing readiness, willingness, and ability to participate in collaborative thinking can be done by considering patients' CT habits of the mind and taking into account contextual factors that might affect those habits of the mind.
- Helping patients with their thinking processes can be done by focusing on each of seven CT cognitive skills.

- Patients can be encouraged to *analyze,* breaking issues down into manageable parts.
- Providers can determine patients' expectations of standards of care and share with patients their *application of standards.*
- Patients are often able to *discriminate* the nuances of their responses as well as, or better than, providers.
- Sharing *logical reasoning* processes with patients can help them see how we come to conclusions, enabling them to draw their own conclusions.
- *Predictive* thinking helps patients see the reality ahead and may help them through a grief process brought on by a change in health.
- *Transforming knowledge* is crucial to effective patient teaching; consumer groups often do very well at transforming medical knowledge into a usable form for consumers.
- Merging provider and patient thinking means remembering to engage patients' thinking and validating conclusions with them.
- Negative aspects of patient-centered care can be seen as time and power issues.
- Although patient-centered care may seem time consuming, in the long run, it may save time.
- Giving up the power of the traditional hierarchical provider–patient relationship can make us feel vulnerable.
- Power issues between providers and patients may be addressed by having providers consider their own mortality.
- Two nurses describe their success with relationship-centered care: It can be done.
- The best patient-centered care occurs when providers also care about each other and work together.

References

Anderson, G. (2007). Patient decision-making for clinical genetics. *Nursing Inquiry, 14*(1), 13–22.

Benbassat, J., Pilpel, D., & Tidhar, M. (1998). Patients' preferences for participation in clinical decision making: A review of published surveys. *Behavioral Medicine, 24*(2), 81–88.

Brown, D., McWilliam, C., & Ward-Griffin, C. (2006). Client-centered empowering partnering in nursing. *Journal of Advanced Nursing, 53,* 160–168.

Buch, T., & Edgren, L. (2001). Patients as partners in intensive care units: A conceptual analysis of the literature. *Nursing in Critical Care, 6,* 64–70.

Calabretta, N. (2002). Consumer-driven, patient-centered health care in the age of electronic information. *Journal of the Medical Library Association, 90,* 32–37.

Carter, L. C., Nelson, J. L., Sievers, B. A., Dukek, S. L., Pipe, T. B., & Holland, D. E. (2008). Exploring a culture of caring. *Nursing Administration Quarterly, 32*(1), 57–63.

Clancy, C. (2008, May) *What is your health literacy score? Navigating the health care system: Advice columns from Dr. Carolyn Clancy.* Rockville, MD: Agency for Healthcare Research and Quality. Retrieved July 17, 2008, from http://www.ahrq.gov/consumer/cc/cc052008.htm

Coulter, A., Entwistle, V., & Gilbert, D. (1999). Sharing decisions with patients: Is the information good enough? *British Medical Journal, 318*, 318–322.

Crandall, L. G., White, D. L., Schuldheis, S., & Talerico, K. A. (2007). Initiating person-centered care practices in long-term care facilities. *Journal of Gerontological Nursing, 33*(11), 47–56.

de Witte, L., Schoot, T., & Proot, I. (2006). Development of the client-centered care questionnaire. *Journal of Advanced Nursing, 56*(1), 62–68. doi:10.1111/j.1365-2648.2006.03980.x

Eldh, A. C., Ekman, I., & Ehnfors, M. (2006). Conditions for patient participation and non-participation in health care. *Nursing Ethics, 13*(5), 503–514.doi:10.1191/0969733006nej898oa

Enehaug, I. H. (2000). Patient participation requires a change of attitude in health care. *International Journal of Health Care Quality Assurance, 13*, 178–181.

Eysenbach, G., & Jadad, A. R. (2001). Evidence-based patient choice and consumer health informatics in the internet age. *Journal of Medical Internet Research, 3*(2), e19. Retrieved May 14, 2009, from http://www.jmir.org/2001/2/e19/HTML

Gagliardi, A., & Jadad, A. R. (2002). Examination of instruments used to rate quality of health information on the internet: Chronicle of a voyage with an unclear destination. *British Medical Journal, 324*, 560–573.

Hansten, R. (2005). Relationship and results-oriented healthcare. *Journal of Nursing Administration, 35*, 522–524.

Herdman, T. H. (Ed.). (2009). *NANDA international nursing diagnoses definitions and classification 2009–2011*. West Sussex, England: Wiley-Blackwell.

Hewitt-Taylor, J. (2003). Issues involved in promoting patient autonomy in health care. *British Journal of Nursing, 12*, 1323–1330.

Hickson, G. B., Federspiel, C. F., Pichert, J. W., Miller, C. S., Gauld-Jaeger, J., & Bost, P. (2002). Patient complaints and malpractice risk. *Journal of the American Medical Association, 287*, 2951–2957.

Institute of Medicine. (2001). *Crossing the quality chasm: A new health system for the 21st century*. Washington, DC: National Academies Press.

Institute of Medicine. (2003). *Health professions education: A bridge to quality*. Washington, DC: National Academies Press.

Kleiman, S. (2007). Revitalizing the humanistic imperative in nursing education. *Nursing Education Perspectives, 28*, 209–213.

Landers, M. G., & McCarthy, G. M. (2007). Person-centered nursing practice with older people in Ireland. *Nursing Science Quarterly, 20*(1), 78–84. doi:10.1177/0894318406296811

Lee, P. (2007). What does partnership in care mean for children's nurses? *Journal of Clinical Nursing, 16*, 518–526. doi:10.1111/j.1365-2702.2006.01591.x

McCauley, K., & Irwin, R. S. (2006). Changing the work environment in ICUs to achieve patient-focused care: The time has come. *Chest, 130*, 1571–1578. doi:10.1378/chest.130.5.1571

McCormack, B. (2004). Person-centeredness in gerontological nursing: An overview of the literature. *Journal of Clinical Nursing, 13*(3a), 31–38. Retrieved from CINAHL Database with Full Text database. (Document ID: 2004093693)

McCormack, B., & McCance, T. V. (2006). Development of a framework for person-centered nursing. *Journal of Advanced Nursing, 56*(5), 472–479. doi:10.1111/j.1365-2648.2006.04042.x

Medina, J. (2006). A natural synergy in creating a patient-focused care environment: The critical care family assistance program and critical care nursing. *Chest, 128*, 99–102. doi:10.1378/chest.128.3_suppl.99S

Nailon, R. E. (2007). The assessment and documentation of language and communication needs in healthcare systems: Current practices and future directions for coordinating safe, patient-centered care. *Nursing Outlook, 55*(6), 311–317. doi:10.1016/j.outlook.2007.04.005

National Diabetes Education Program. (n.d.) *What we want to achieve through systems changes*. Retrieved August 3, 2008, from the Making Systems Changes for Better Diabetes Care Web site: http://betterdiabetescare.nih.gov/WHATpatientcenteredcare.htm

Nolan, M. R., Davies, S., Brown, J., Keady, J., & Nolan, J. (2004). Beyond "person-centered" care: A new vision for gerontological nursing. *Journal of Clinical Nursing, 13*(3a), 45–53. Retrieved from CINAHL Database with Full Text database. (Document ID: 2004093694).

O'Donovan, A. (2007). Patient-centered care in acute psychiatric admission units: reality or rhetoric? *Journal of Psychiatric and Mental Health Nursing, 14,* 542–548.

Peplau, H. E. (1952). *Interpersonal relations in nursing: A conceptual frame of reference for psychodynamic nursing.* New York: Putnam.

Redman, R. W. (2008). Whither patient-centered care? *Research and Theory for Nursing Practice: An International Journal, 22*(1), 5–6. doi:10.1891/0889-7182.22.1.5

Sidani, S. (2008). Effects of patient-centered care on patient outcomes: An evaluation. *Research and Theory for Nursing Practice: An International Journal, 22*(1), 24–37. doi:10.1891/0889-7182.22.1.24

Slater, L. (2006). Person-centeredness: A concept analysis. *Contemporary Nurse, 23,* 135–144.

Tellis-Nayak, V. (2007). A person-centered workplace: The foundation for person-centered caregiving in long-term care. *Journal of the American Medical Directors Association, 8,* 46–54. doi:10.1016/j.jamda.2006.09.009

Williams, M. D., Gish, K. W., Giuse, N. B., Sathe, N. A., & Carrell, D. L. (2001). The patient informatics consult service (PICS): An approach for a patient-centered service. *Bulletin of the Medical Library Association, 89,* 185–193.

Ziebland, S., & Herxheimer, A. (2008). How patients' experiences contribute to decision making: Illustrations from DIPEx (personal experiences of health and illness). *Journal of Nursing Management, 16,* 433–439. doi:10.1111/j.1365-2834.2008.00863.x

Critical Thinking and Interdisciplinary Teams

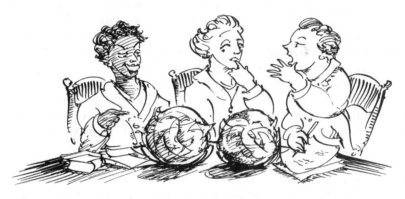

'I DON'T THINK THAT'S WHAT THEY MEANT'

"Two Heads Are Better Than One."

It's hard to imagine anyone who has not heard this saying. The basic idea is that the combined thinking of two individuals produces better outcomes than trying to solve a problem from only one perspective. Now, we know you are thinking, "Yeah, well, lots of times if I want to get it done properly, I just have to do it myself!" You are right; there are those times, but the key is to be able to use your critical thinking (CT) to discriminate between the best times for individual thinking and the best times to use interdisciplinary team (IDT) thinking to produce the best outcomes.

Participants in the Institute of Medicine (IOM) study (2003) strongly believed that combining "heads" was essential to improving health care and therefore included "work in interdisciplinary teams" as one of their five competency recommendations for practice and education. They envisioned IDTs as having the ability to "cooperate, collaborate, communicate, and integrate care in teams to ensure that care is continuous and reliable" (p. 45). These teams are composed of members from different professions who are able to "integrate their observations, bodies of expertise, and spheres of decision making" (p. 54). This team approach is particularly important today. "Interdisciplinary teams are critical in dealing with the increasing complexity of care, coordinating and responding to multiple patient needs, keeping pace with the demands of new technology, responding to the demands of payers, and delivering care across settings" (p. 54).

The IOM did not address CT directly. But let's use some *logical reasoning* here. How can individuals, let alone IDT members, address all the factors in the last IOM quote without solid CT skills? Look at the language used by the IOM: "dealing with," "coordinating," "responding," "integrate their observations," "expertise," "decision making." CT is the engine that drives those activities. All 17 dimensions are required, but consider just a few examples. *Open-mindedness* and *flexibility* are needed to consider alternative approaches and suggestions from other disciplines. *Logical reasoning* and *perseverance* are needed to consider solutions beyond those that first come to mind. *Confidence* helps members know that the IDT solutions are well reasoned based on the expertise of all team members.

We suspect that the IOM was simply assuming we could see the underlying CT. But such assumptions contribute to why details of thinking are frequently overlooked in complex processes such as IDT work. When we make these basic assumptions and do not emphasize the underlying CT, we make IDT work harder to learn and harder to teach others.

Recently, however, authors have acknowledged the need for thinking in IDT activities (Apker, Propp, Ford, & Hofmeister, 2006; Erickson, Ditomassi, & Jones, 2008; Falise, 2007; Rossen, Bartlett, & Herrick, 2008). Some have even used the terms *inquiry* and *information seeking* as operational concepts important for IDT work (O'Daniel & Rosenstein, 2008). But more focus on thinking is needed to facilitate healthcare practice and education moving toward effective IDT work.

This chapter begins with an explanation of IDT work, a brief history of IDT in both practice and education, and a clarification of the different terminology used to describe IDT work. This background helps us understand the complexity of the thinking embedded in IDT work. We then explore the uniqueness of IDT thinking and the growing examples of IDT work and thinking in health care. In the last two sections, we focus your thinking on these questions: What interferes with IDT thinking, and what cultivates it?

What Is Interdisciplinary Team Work?

Before examining the thinking necessary for teamwork, let's identify what IDT work is. Basically IDT work occurs when folks from different backgrounds or disciplines (two or more "heads" ☺) work together to accomplish a task. Employing an interdisciplinary approach to work and recognizing the value of team thinking began long ago. Civilization as we know it would not have survived without the collaborative thinking of folks with different skills needed to save the clan from saber-toothed tiger attacks, to harvest crops, to build factories, and to fly into space. We have vivid examples of teamwork today in the Amish culture, for example, where large tasks such as barn-raising are only accomplished by teams. Other recent examples are the IDTs of health professionals, first responders, contractors, volunteers, and others who come together to help in times of major disasters, such as the tsunami in Southeast Asia, the hurricane in New Orleans, and the earthquakes in Pakistan and China.

There are many levels of working together. Shortly we will discuss the different levels of working together in the healthcare arena. A look at history's influence will help us see today in context.

IDT Work in Healthcare Practice Settings

IDTs in healthcare practice have a somewhat shorter history than IDTs in other settings. Baldwin (1996), in an article describing the history of IDT in practice, traced some of the earliest healthcare teams to mission hospitals in India prior to the 1900s. These teams were composed of physicians, nurses, and "auxiliaries." London's Pioneer Health Centre focused on collaborative healthcare teams and a "positive health" model in the 1920s. The London Centre inspired similar projects in South Africa and Israel with the development of primary health teams in community-based health programs. The Montefiore Hospital in New York City began using healthcare teams of physicians, social workers, and nurses in 1948. It too focused on health and illness prevention models more than medical models of care.

Baldwin (1996) also described seven phases of IDT work in the United States. Phase I began in the 1940s with federal funding and included primary care health team development through IDT education and training. Phases II and III occurred in the 1960s and 1970s, concurrent with the community mental health movement and the start of groups such as the Institute for Health Team Development. By the end of the 1970s, federal funding for IDT projects declined significantly. Phases IV and V, beginning in the early 1980s, included the Veterans Administration work on IDT training in geriatrics and a national focus on rural populations. Phase VI saw a change in funding sources, from public to private, including the Robert Wood Johnson Foundation and the Kellogg Foundation. Phase VII began in the mid-1990s with a renewed interest in the potential for IDTs to enhance healthcare quality.

In each phase, the IDTs are composed of many health professionals (nurses, physicians, social workers (SWs), physical therapists (PTs), occupational therapists (OTs), pharmacists, recreational therapists, dentists, optometrists, osteopathic physicians, and psychologists, to name the predominant professions). Baldwin (1996) alluded to thinking as a key component of success when he said, "Interdisciplinary healthcare teams are not an end in themselves, but a means for more effective communication and cooperation" (p. 183). Communication and cooperation are effective only with CT to back them up. Later in this chapter, we will elaborate on communication issues as the foundation for effective IDT functioning.

IDT Work in Healthcare Educational Settings

IDT work in healthcare education also has a short history. Healthcare education, from the beginning of the 20th century, essentially occurred in isolated "silos." Each discipline did its own thing! A change in that approach began in the 1930s, when Dewey challenged the learning paradigm of rote memorization. But it wasn't until the 1970s, 1980s, and 1990s that organizations such as the federal- and state-funded Area Health Education Centers began to stress the need for multidisciplinary and interdisciplinary clinical education to better meet the needs of care consumers. The early 1970s also heralded reports on healthcare education. For example, the 1972 Carnegie Commission studied higher education, proposing "a lessening emphasis on professional boundaries, a holistic approach, and a call for 'curricular bridges' across disciplines" (Kuehn, 1998, p. 424). As early as 1972, the IOM recommended that all teaching hospitals, faculty involved in healthcare education, and public and private funding agencies focus on interdisciplinary education, delivery systems, and funding support.

The IOM recommendations were supported in a position statement from the National League for Nursing in 1973, which proposed that nursing faculty and nursing students share experiences across disciplines. Although practitioners in gerontology and mental health embraced the concept, less attention was paid in the mainstream of healthcare education (Kuehn, 1998).

As health care became increasingly complex, examining the whole system and not just the parts became paramount in the 1990s (Erickson et al., 2008; Falise, 2007; Kuehn, 1998; Mitchell, 2005; Redman, 2006; Rossen et al., 2008). Agencies of the federal government in the United States as well as private foundations (Pew Research Center, Robert Wood Johnson) began funding research to help educational institutions develop models for interdisciplinary education.

Acknowledging the growing complexity of the healthcare system has facilitated both practitioners and educators in appreciating the new kinds of thinking required to deliver quality patient care in any setting. Dealing with complexity can seem overwhelming, so let's use some *analyzing* here and break things down into manageable pieces. For starters, let's examine the different terms used to describe "working together."

Clarification of IDT Terminology

The literature frequently chooses an adjective preceding the word *team* that describes the composition of a group whose purpose is to reach some goal. The most common adjectives include *unidisciplinary, intradisciplinary, multidisciplinary, interdisciplinary, interprofessional,* and even *transprofessional*. Refer to **Table 7-1** for some descriptions and examples of these terms.

In 2000, the IOM convened a panel of 17 experts representing 11 disciplines involved in health care to review over 750 citations using the terminology, *interdisciplinary health care*. The term *interprofessional* was recommended by the National Academies of Practice (Simpson et al., 2001) and is seen more commonly in the literature today, but the majority of the literature continues to use the term *interdisciplinary* (Erickson et al., 2008; Falise, 2007; Reeves & Freeth, 2006; Rossen et al., 2008).

The goal of the National Academies of Practice (Simpson et al., 2001) was "to promote the implementation of cost-effective interprofessional health practice

TABLE 7-1 Descriptions of Healthcare Teams

Term/Label to Describe a Team	Description of the Team	Example of the Team
Unidisciplinary	Members of the same discipline and same area of work working together. Leadership is typically the unit manager.	Nurses on the cardiac rehabilitation unit meet to modify unit protocols for medication administration.
Intradisciplinary	Members of the same discipline but with different specialties working together. Leadership is typically one of the managers.	Nurses from the emergency department (ED), the trauma/burn unit, and infection control work together to design a plan for continuity of care.
Multidisciplinary	Members of different disciplines share information about their specialty and its impact on patient care. Leadership and membership are generally fixed.	Information from the physical therapist, occupational therapist, respiratory therapist, nurse, physician, and dietitian is shared to create a discharge plan.
Interdisciplinary or Interprofessional	Members of different disciplines collaborate to achieve interdependence and group accountability. Leadership and membership can vary depending on which area of expertise is most prevalent.	The school nurse, the teachers, the parents, the student, and the school psychologist focus on joint problem identification and joint problem solving. The school nurse initiates the team, but the student becomes the leader over time, with all members assuming responsibility for outcomes.
Transdisciplinary	Significant discipline boundary blurring because members highly value one another's knowledge and skills. Strong acknowledgment of complementary expertise. Leadership may vary. This level of complexity is most common in effective research teams.	Nurses, nurse researchers, social workers, oncologists, hospice workers, and oncology patients meet regularly to create a new model for end-of-life care. They work and think as a dynamic entity beyond each individual.

Sources: Adapted from Austin, Park, & Goble, 2008; Dyer, 2003; Lessard, Morin, & Sylvain, 2008; Mitchell, 2005.

that leads to better healthcare outcomes" (p. 6). They focused on three recommendations for achieving the goal: (1) disseminating information on successful models of IDT practice, (2) increasing opportunities for healthcare professionals to make referrals to one another and practice collaboratively, and (3) advocating for changes in legal and reimbursement policies to support IDT practice.

Based on these recommendations, it may be difficult to make clean distinctions among these teams in the real world of health care, where there are no neat boxes as in book chapters. In practice, there are hybrids of these teams. The predominant form of teamwork and thinking found in health care today matches the "multidisciplinary" description as demonstrated in TACTICS 7-1 and Scenario 7-1 in the next section.

Teamwork and Team Thinking in Healthcare Practice

We will elaborate on the thinking aspects of IDT thinking in practice and education later in the chapter, but before we tell you our ideas, we'd like you to reflect on IDT thinking. Perhaps you've seen the application of team thinking in practice similar to that in the first TACTICS for this chapter.

TACTICS 7-1

Practice-Setting Team Meeting and Thinking

1. Read Scenario 7-1.
2. Find the thinking that occurred.
3. Identify the thinking done by the individuals by comparing the scenario descriptions with the CT vocabulary on your "17 dimensions" card.
4. Compare the events with the characteristics of the different kinds of teams in Table 7-1.
5. Make a list of what you would do to make the team more interdisciplinary and, to yourself or with a colleague, explain the CT needed to do it more effectively.
6. Think about the kind of thinking that may have occurred beyond individual thinking. This last task is challenging at this point in the chapter because we have not yet begun a discussion of team thinking, but all good thinkers enjoy a challenge, so see how you do.

Scenario 7-1: Practice-Setting Team Meeting and Thinking

CD is a 75-year-old married male admitted to a subacute unit for rehabilitation following a mild right-sided ischemic stroke, attributed to atrial fibrillation, that has affected his left side. He agreed to a short stay to improve his strength and functional abilities. Medications were adjusted prior to discharge from the hospital. Now, a week later, he is participating in the care conference, which includes his PT, OT, speech and language pathologist (SLP), primary nurse (RN), registered dietitian (RD), physician (MD), SW, and charge nurse. Fortunately, his regular doctor and nurse practitioner (NP) are on staff and round at this facility regularly. No other family members are present. He says, "I want to go home tomorrow. I am really feeling good and I don't see any sense in wasting everyone's time."

Going home has been a recurrent theme since he arrived. The SW has done his evaluation and learned that CD is the primary caregiver to his wife, who has dementia. She is being cared for by their son, who flew in when CD was hospitalized. The SW reports that CD is a retired engineer with good insurance benefits.

PT, OT, and SLP all report that CD has made great progress this past week. He is ambulating 50 feet with contact guard. He is "a bit" impulsive in his movements and decision making; he needs frequent cues to attend to tasks at hand. He makes his needs known. They believe he could benefit from at least 2 more weeks of therapy, twice daily, for safety and strength reasons. SLP says that his swallowing problems are also improving, and he has advanced to a Dysphagia II diet. He continues to take his meals in his room to avoid distraction, maintaining aspiration precautions. He eats impulsively, gulping and not chewing his food completely. The RD tells the group that CD's weight has been stable, and his nutritional needs are being met based on a completed calorie count.

The RN identified the following problems: impaired physical mobility, toileting self-care deficit (requires post-void residual bladder scanning and clean intermittent catheterizations), unilateral neglect, impaired skin integrity (Stage 3 pressure ulcer on coccyx), and knowledge deficit regarding medical condition. High risk for falls was identified on admission; she notes that he fell last night while confused. The NP saw him; no injuries were found, but he is still quite confused this morning. Because he had an indwelling catheter while hospitalized and is still not emptying his bladder, she is checking for a urinary tract infection. The nurse is also worried because his Coumadin (warfarin) dose is still not stable, and his recent international normalized ratio (INR) was 4.0. The NP ordered this to be checked STAT today because of the fall. If he needs an antibiotic, this may affect his INR further. If his confusion worsens, he will have to go back to the hospital to be evaluated for a "bleed."

Discussion

The scenario is abbreviated, but you get the idea. On a scale of a good-better-best ranking in terms of team CT and the "two heads are better than one" approach, how would you rate it?

This typical team meeting in the clinical arena gives everyone some input and provides opportunities for bringing up problems and concerns, but that is about the extent of its function. Most team meetings in practice best match the characteristics of a multidisciplinary team, or what Bensimon and Neumann (1993) would classify as a "utilitarian team," whose activities consist of "deliver[ing] information, coordinat[ing] and plan[ning], mak[ing] decisions" (p. 34).

We are sure you came up with a long list to make the team interaction a better fit with the interdisciplinary descriptions in Table 7-1. For starters, those changes might include (1) openly discussing with CD his desire to go home and the implications for his safety and that of his wife if he plans to continue caring for her, (2) discussing options with CD for community resources available for his wife's care, and (3) helping CD see the patterns of impulsive behavior and implications for his safety. All issues discussed in the meeting are important to patient care, but the team did not move beyond simply sharing information into true collaborative thinking.

Teamwork and Team Thinking in Healthcare Education

One might assume that academic nurse educators engage in teamwork and team thinking as a natural part of their scholarly endeavors. Unfortunately, nurses in academe appear to be even less skilled at IDT thinking than nurses in practice. In reality, educators have very little opportunity to collaborate across disciplines. The traditional reward systems in higher education favor independent, not interdependent, thinking. That tradition is changing as institutions of higher learning begin to recognize the value of interdisciplinary work. That change is being facilitated by external funding sources (federal and private) that are prioritizing funding to interdisciplinary projects.

Here is an opportunity to examine an educator's team meeting and see how thinking occurs. Again, this is just an example to help your thinking expand, knowing that we have lots more to discuss about thinking in teams later in the chapter.

TACTICS 7-2

Educator Team Meeting and Thinking

1. Read Scenario 7-2 and reflect on the following:
   a. The thinking being demonstrated by the individuals.
   b. The process of thinking as a team.
   c. The outcome of the thinking for achieving one of their goals—increasing nursing student understanding of IDT work.
2. Compare this team's characteristics to those in Table 7-1.
3. Make a list of what you would do differently, and, to yourself or a colleague, explain why. Again, use the thinking vocabulary of the 17 dimensions to reflect or share your thinking with a peer.

Scenario 7-2: Educator Team Meeting and Thinking

Janet is the lead nursing faculty member in the community health nursing courses. Bob and TaNisha are the other tenured nursing faculty. There are three part-time nursing faculty who teach in the clinical sections of the course. Janet, Bob, and TaNisha each teach a third of the classroom portion of the course. Janet calls a meeting with Bob and TaNisha to review the syllabus for the following year and asks for input.

Bob reminds the others that the paper assignment needs changing; it requires too much grading, and he isn't sure that students even read all of his extensive feedback on each paper.

TaNisha wants to change the textbook and has a recommendation. TaNisha also shares a need to change how they teach primary, secondary, and tertiary prevention, based on the feedback in student evaluations and the low scores on test items in that area.

Janet brings up the need to deal with the new program objective related to increasing students' abilities to work in IDTs. She reminds the others of the faculty decision to incorporate that aspect of the IOM recommendations.

Bob suggests a plan to have guest speakers from occupational therapy, physical therapy, and social work make presentations to the class and explain the role of each in patient care.

TaNisha says, "I don't know how we will ever fit that in; we have so much critical information to teach already, I can't give up any of my time. Maybe you or Bob can."

In the end they decide to:

1. *Change the paper assignment to include a peer-reviewed first draft component.*
2. *Change to a newer textbook.*
3. *Add some additional readings on IDT work to each topic in the course.*

Discussion

What thinking occurred? With regard to individual thinking, we can make a case for *reflection* when Bob and TaNisha looked back at the past year and identified assignments and textbooks that needed modifications. TaNisha also used *logical reasoning* when she inferred that a different teaching approach was needed to present primary, secondary, and tertiary prevention concepts, based on low student evaluations of that assignment and low test scores in that content area.

But where is the evidence of team thinking? How did the three think differently as a team than as individuals sharing information? Was team thinking necessary, or was this group interaction enough?

This scenario does not even approach the multidisciplinary level of work, let alone IDT thinking, because there are no other disciplines represented. The team in Scenario 7-2 consists of only the three educators who teach the classroom content. It does not include the part-time nursing faculty who work with students in the clinical setting to apply classroom concepts. Their insights could have significantly affected the team thinking. Students or even alumni could have added valuable insights as well.

Even with these additional members, however, the thinking would still be limited to nurses. Including faculty from the other disciplines, such as occupational or physical therapy and/or social work, would have increased the probability of an interdisciplinary thinking perspective for both ideas and solutions.

Having examined the terminology of team thinking and looked at some examples of team activities in practice and education, let's now look at who thinks IDTs are important. IDTs have been getting a great deal of support over the last decade because, as Baldwin cited (1996), they can improve quality health care.

What Is Interdisciplinary Team Thinking?

The literature on IDT work in health care is growing but still offers little to describe the CT needed either individually or jointly by IDT members. To better understand team thinking, we must first examine the literature from other disciplines. Studies of organizations and leadership in business and industry, education, and adult learning provided useful guidance for arriving at descriptions of IDT thinking that we can apply to healthcare settings with some TACTICS. Then we need to look at the growing body of healthcare literature that (1) acknowledges the complexity of thinking in interdisciplinary healthcare teams and (2) begins to provide examples of how IDT work is making a difference.

IDT Thinking Outside Healthcare Settings

It is important at this juncture to make a distinction between team thinking and "groupthink." According to Bensimon and Neumann (1993), *groupthink* was a negative term that described what happens when groups mistakenly assume that harmony is the way to achieve group goals. Originating in the early 1970s, *groupthink* described a phenomenon of "assumed consensus" that discouraged group members from voicing their concerns, doubts, or points of view, or sharing data that did not fit with the predominant conclusions. Groupthink does not describe thinking as a team; instead, groupthink describes a quick method to reach a conclusion, frequently directed by an individual with power. Groupthink is a very different phenomenon from IDT thinking.

Are there ways for team members to pool their thinking without settling for groupthink? The answer is yes, and one solution is "systems thinking." Senge (1990) explained how to use systems thinking to create team-oriented learning organizations in business. As shown in **Box 7-1**, systems thinking goes beyond the thinking of the individual and helps counter some of the linear thinking habits that adults have developed over the years. Systems thinking is ideally suited for IDT work.

Senge believed that the key to systems thinking was dialogue among members of the team as they "enter into a genuine 'thinking together'" (p. 10). Genuine thinking together requires that thinkers suspend assumptions (*open-mindedness* and *flexibility* are helpful here) and allow for "free flowing of meaning through the group, allowing the group to discover insights not attainable individually" (p. 10). The IOM (2003), used the language of system-mindedness to capture this same idea—cooperation and thinking together.

BOX 7-1	Senge's View: Systems Thinking Is . . .

- A discipline of seeing wholes, seeing interrelationships rather than things, seeing patterns of change versus static snapshots.
- Recognizing that members are part of that pattern, not separate from the patterns.
- Seeing relationships versus linear cause-and-effect chains of actions.
- The ability to avoid merely shifting problems around and making today's solutions tomorrow's problems.
- Recognizing that our basic skills in systems thinking are underdeveloped or repressed by formal education in linear thinking. Reality is made up of circles, but we tend to see only straight lines that limit our systems thinking.
- A process that requires more dialogue than discussion, interactions of the mind as opposed to simply sharing information.

Source: Senge, 1990.

Ubbes, Black, and Ausherman (1999) wrote that systems thinking is a tool for thinkers to modify their "value dualisms" of linear thinking (yes/no, black/white, body/mind) to more real-world dimensions of yes/no/maybe, black/white/gray, mind/body/spirit. They described systems thinking as the means to see multiple perspectives and broaden understanding by recognizing relationships between and among pieces of data. (Contextual perspective and transforming knowledge dimensions should come into play.)

Bensimon and Neumann (1993) have used the term *team thinking* in their writings about collective thinking. **Figure 7-1**, based on their findings, is an illustration of the continuum of team types and the different thinking at the ends of that continuum. The ideal is on the far right and may not be realistic for

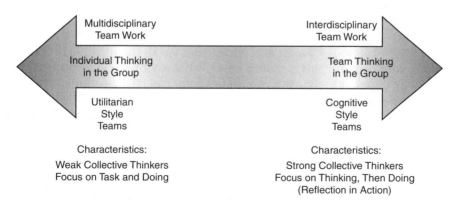

FIGURE 7-1 Continuum of thinking in teams.

all organizations in health care or education, but it gives us something to strive for. Remember, in reality, clinicians and educators often need to adapt ideas and create hybrid teams to work in their worlds (*creativity* needs to emerge!). Use this illustration to visualize some of the gradations of IDT thinking before reading about them in more detail.

Bensimon and Neumann (1993) conducted a comprehensive qualitative research study to identify the thinking necessary for teams to function effectively in higher education settings. They studied leadership teams in 15 universities in the United States over a 3-year period, making two visits to each university during that time. They identified several patterns of thinking skills necessary for effective team functioning and described "thinking as a conglomerate verb, referring to a wide variety of mental processes (for example, defining, analyzing, synthesizing)" (p. 59).

Bensimon and Neumann (1993) used the terminology of *team thinking* to represent "the art of thinking together" (p. 55), a condition necessary to move from "utilitarian"-style teams to "cognitive"-style teams. Utilitarian-style teams simply achieve tasks, and their members are generally weak at collective thinking. Cognitive-style thinking teams achieve more than task completion. These authors believed that accomplishing a task was only the tip of the iceberg of real teamwork. The inner workings of real teams, not visible in task outcomes, include "team members' thinking, talking, wondering, asking, speculating, arguing, correcting, trying, rethinking, creating, trying again" (p. 55). (Looks like they were recommending that all members use at least *inquisitiveness, information seeking, analyzing, logical reasoning*, and *transforming knowledge* as a group!)

According to Bensimon and Neumann (1993), real teams functioning at the cognitive level recognize their purpose as "sense making." In a real team,

> its members are collectively involved in perceiving, analyzing, learning, and thinking . . .[;] the team is a brain-like social structure that enlarges the intelligence span of individual team members . . . [and] allows the group to behave as a creative system . . . a) viewing problems from multiple perspectives, b) questioning, challenging, and arguing, and c) acting as a monitor and feedback system. (p. 41)

From their research, Bensimon and Neumann (1993) identified eight member thinking roles when teams function effectively. Any of the eight roles can be assumed by different individuals over time and/or can change during the course of the discussions, but the more thinking roles that are present, the better the team thinks. **Box 7-2** includes their eight roles with brief descriptions. Attention to these roles helps team members become aware of group thinking processes— what is helping and what is hindering achievement of IDT goals.

Brookfield and Preskill (1999) offered another perspective on team thinking. They referred to "'group talk' as a blending of conversation, discussion and dialogue . . . to create new meanings, [incorporating] reciprocity . . . , exchange and inquiry,

BOX 7-2	**Eight Team Thinking Roles Identified by Bensimon and Neumann**

1. The definer (voices and creates the team's reality)
2. The analyst (assesses all the parts of the issue)
3. The interpreter (provides insight on how outcomes might be perceived)
4. The critic (redefines, reanalyzes, and reinterprets)
5. The synthesizer (elicits all thinking perspectives and helps provide linkages for solutions)
6. The disparity monitor (assesses how outcomes are perceived)
7. The task monitor (removes obstacles to team thinking and facilitates the teamwork)
8. The emotional monitor (addresses the human, personal, and emotional aspects of team thinking during the thinking process)

Source: Bensimon & Neumann, 1993.

cooperation and collaboration" (p. 6). They described thinking habits of collaboration that include critical analysis and reflective speculation. Bensimon and Neumann (1993) and Brookfield and Preskill recommended group self-assessment and reflection to monitor thinking and its outcomes.

Applying IDT Thinking to Nursing Situations

Let's see how this group assessment might work. We have created a Team Thinking Inventory (**Box 7-3**) based on the works of Bensimon and Neumann (1993), Brookfield and Preskill (1999), and Senge (1990) to help clinicians and educators discriminate how team thinking is different from individual thinking. TACTICS 7-3 helps us assess team thinking and use the CT dimension of *discriminating* to sort out the differences and similarities.

TACTICS 7-3

Team Thinking Assessment

This activity can be performed by both clinicians and educators.

1. Select a team of which you are a member.
2. Think about the function of that team, its purpose, the way it operates, and the ways in which its members participate. Compare the functioning to Figure 7-1 and see where on the Utilitarian–Cognitive Continuum your team fits.

3. Using the Team Thinking Inventory (Box 7-3), assess that team.
4. Compare the behaviors demonstrated by team members with the eight team thinking roles in Box 7-2.
5. Using your critical thinking skill of *discriminating*, identify differences and similarities between individual thinking and team thinking.

BOX 7-3	Team Thinking Inventory

1. What strategies are used to help team members think about the big picture as well as the parts?

2. What strategies are used to help team members see the situation from different perspectives?

3. What strategies are used to help team members see their biases and assumptions?

4. What strategies help team members think about patterns and interrelationships of issues and parts of problems?

5. What strategies are used to help team members think beyond cause and effect consequences?

6. Does the thinking that occurs in the team resemble simple sharing of information or discussion/dialogue? Why? How can you move in the direction of discussion/dialogue?

7. What is done to encourage team members to share their thinking or feel comfortable enough to talk about it?

8. How is conflict managed in the team to promote thinking instead of discouraging it?

9. What other sources of gratification are available for team members to socialize, obtain recognition, and interact, besides interdisciplinary team work?

10. How were the interdisciplinary team members prepared for their thinking roles?

11. How does the team deal with ambiguity? How long can they tolerate not having a solution?

12. How does the team examine its own thinking processes (e.g., *how* it works, not *what* it is doing and *who* is doing it)?

Sources: Adapted from Bensimon & Neumann, 1993; Brookfield & Preskill, 1999; Senge, 1990.

Discussion

What did you discover? Does your team function at the Utilitarian or the Cognitive end of the continuum, or somewhere in between? How did the team thinking manifest itself on the Team Thinking Inventory? Which of the eight thinking roles were present, and which were not? What can you and the others on the team do to modify your team thinking? When you used *discriminating*, were you able to see some similarities and the differences between individual thinking and team thinking? These are tough questions, and the answers probably require more than just your CT. It may be time to share this activity with the team and initiate some team thinking to answer these questions.

Now let's eavesdrop on another team meeting in health care that demonstrates a minimal degree of team/systems thinking. Scenario 7-3 represents an inpatient psychiatric unit IDT meeting.

TACTICS 7-4

Finding the IDT Thinking

Read the very condensed dialogue of Scenario 7-3.

Identify aspects that do or do not fit with team/systems thinking.

Scenario 7-3: *Intake Note:*

Mary James is a 34-year-old Caucasian married female with two children aged 3 and 1. She was admitted yesterday in the early afternoon to the inpatient psychiatric unit with suicidal ideation, and the following DSM-IV-TR Axis I diagnosis was made: Major depressive disorder: recurrent with generalized weakness.

Psychiatric History: One episode of postpartum depression after second child born. Wellbutrin was effective after trying several different antidepressants but was discontinued by the patient after 6 months.

Intake Nursing Assessment: Pt has lost 10# over the last 3 months, little appetite. Denies ETOH intake, denies smoking, drinks about 8–10 cups of coffee a day. Complains of problems sleeping, averaging 2–3 hours per night for the last three months. Very tired and having difficulty keeping up with child care; husband has had to take off work to help out during the day. Husband appears very supportive but concerned about the reoccurrence of depression. All other assessment data WNL.

Beginning dialogue occurring during the first IDT meeting after Mrs. James's admission.

Social worker:	*"Mr. James, we are meeting as a team to plan for your wife's care and encourage you to be an active participant until your wife is able to join us. Welcome to the team."*
Mr. James:	*"Thanks. I don't know what I can do, but I'll do what I can."*
Nurse:	*"We include patients and/or family members on the team to help make sure we don't miss important pieces of information unique to their situation. It makes for safer, quicker, and better care. We also want you to help with making decisions."*
Psychiatrist:	*"I assume we have all read Mrs. James's history. According to Mr. James and his wife, they believe this recent episode of depression and suicidal ideation began building after Joy, their second child, was born. Outpatient treatment and restarting bupropion have not been successful. I'm thinking we need to try one of the newer SSRIs. I want to wean her off bupropion for a couple of days and then try escitalopram to see if we can't attack different neurotransmitters sites."*
Physical therapist:	*"Mr. James, did you understand all that?"*
Mr. James:	*"Not exactly."*
Psychiatrist:	*"Sorry about that. Let me translate that doctor jargon. Your wife is experiencing a clinical depression. All of the symptoms you described about her not eating, having trouble sleeping, thinking about hurting herself, etc., all fit with that diagnosis. Basically the chemicals in her brain that affect how she feels are not working properly and that brings on these symptoms. These chemical imbalances can be triggered by pregnancy and childbirth. The medication your wife was taking, Wellbutrin, is one way to treat depression. When one way doesn't work, we need to try something else. Luckily, there are several to choose from, and I would like to try one called Lexapro. It is in a different classification of antidepressants, meaning it works on different parts of the brain and therefore may work better. Does that help?"*
Mr. James:	*"Yes."*
Physical therapist:	*"I've done a preliminary eval. and think we can start some strengthening activities slowly. Mrs. James has really lost a lot of muscle mass; besides, the activity will stimulate some endorphins and help with the depression as well."*
Mr. James:	*"But what about her headache? It was getting worse all yesterday and no better when I had to leave at 4:00 to get the kids from the neighbors. [Starts to get tears in his eyes.]*

	I'm afraid she might have a brain tumor because the medicine you ordered yesterday didn't help at all."
Psychiatrist:	"Let's not jump to conclusions about tumors, but what's going on with the headache?" [looking to the nurse]
Nurse:	"I think we figured out what the headaches are about. Last night, the student nurse working with your wife did an excellent assessment, and we realized that her caffeine intake had significantly changed since admission. Because there was no reason to restrict caffeine, we made sure she had a couple cups of coffee before and during dinner. She told the night nurse the headache was almost gone."
Mr. James:	"She does drink lots of coffee. She says it helps her get through the day."
Psychiatrist:	"Caffeine shouldn't be a problem; she can have her coffee, so lets move on to the depression issues."
Nutritionist:	"Before we skip over caffeine and nutrition too quickly, let's talk about how it can contribute to the depression. I haven't had an opportunity to meet with Mrs. James yet, but from what I've heard, it sounds like her nutritional intake or lack of nutrients along with lack of activity [looking at physical therapist] might be contributing as well. I would also like to share some of the new research on Omega 3 Fatty Acids and treating depression. . . . "
Social Worker:	"I think we should also explore Mr. James's comment about a brain tumor to see what is behind that concern, and then, Dr. Jones, could you explain to him what you would do to rule out that possibility?"

This dialogue continued, focusing on treating the depression and the suicidal ideation; ongoing contracting for safety; combinations of medication, activity, and nutritional changes; and exploring existing and new ways of coping for the family, including resources to help Mr. James with child care during his wife's hospitalization and support groups for the parents after discharge. Each professional then shared what he or she would specifically focus on for discharge planning as well as the day's care.

Discussion

Wasn't finding the team thinking a very challenging task? It is really hard to clearly identify actual thinking by an individual or a group. You probably used some of the same comparisons you chose for TACTICS 7-1 to help find the thinking. Although the thinking in this team was moving in the right direction and there was somewhat more discussion, it still has a long way to go to achieve true interdisciplinary collaboration.

Examples of IDT in Healthcare Settings

Effective teams in health care are increasing. One example is the Program for All-Inclusive Care for the Elderly (PACE), a team model for managed long-term care (Mui, 2001). This model was designed to provide the frail elderly with options for living in communities instead of nursing homes. The goals of the program were to maximize the residents' autonomy while providing quality at lower costs.

Based on a British day-hospital concept, the first PACE program was developed in San Francisco in 1971. As of 2001, there were 70 organizations in 30 states operating at different stages of the PACE model, serving over 9,000 frail elderly. Their IDT members include SWs, nurses, physicians, PTs, OTs, recreational therapists, home health aides, pharmacists, psychologists, psychiatrists, dentists, durable medical equipment suppliers, hospice staff, housing personnel, and chaplains.

It has taken more than 25 years to move from conception to supportive legislation and nationwide implementation of the PACE model, but it is working. A key factor in its success was identified as team members who are "competent and strong in their individual disciplines and have the skills and attitudes to work collaboratively to achieve broader objectives" (Mui, 2001, p. 64). Mui cited the team members' courage to embrace the change from traditional forms of care to this collaborative approach.

A large research study by Wheelan, Burchill, and Tilin (2003) examined the impact of IDTs on patient outcomes in 17 intensive care units (ICUs) in nine hospitals in the eastern United States. Two instruments were used—APACHE III to predict risk of dying, and the Group Development Questionnaire to assess staff perceptions of their team functioning. At the end of a 5-day period, patient mortality was lower on the units where the personnel scored higher on the Group Development Questionnaire. In other words, there was statistically significant evidence to support that units whose staff believed they had effective teamwork in place had lower patient mortality rates.

There are many examples in current literature of how IDT and thinking are being used successfully, from improving patient outcomes to job satisfaction. **Table 7-2** highlights some of the current IDT work in a variety of settings and with a variety of healthcare conditions. There appears to be growing evidence that IDT work and thinking provide for enhanced patient compliance and satisfaction, reduced costs, decreased hospitalizations, lowered infant and geriatric mortality rates, reduced lengths of stay, and improved staff morale.

Kurtzman and Corrigan (2007) have emphasized the need to look beyond the acute care setting for IDT work and thinking. They cited the creation of the Interdisciplinary Nursing Quality Research Initiative to help us better engage the thinking of all the disciplines to achieve the levels of patient care we want in multiple settings.

Time for another TACTIC. Let's explore how our individual thinking dimensions also work with IDT thinking.

TABLE 7-2 Selected Examples of IDT Successes

Focus of Interdisciplinary Activities	Where Studied	Authors
Glucose control in ICU	Austria	Holzinger et al., 2008
Bladder retraining program	New Zealand	Karon, 2005
Nurse–physician collaboration on medical-surgical units	California and Arizona	Nelson, King, & Brodine, 2008
Hospice care	Missouri and Texas	Oliver, Wittenberg-Lyles, & Day, 2006
Self-medication success with stroke patients	Connecticut	Purdy, 2007
Assessment of the elderly	England	Ross, O'Tuathail, & Stubberfield, 2005
End-of-life education	Michigan	Schim & Raspa, 2007
Rheumatic diseases	Finland	Suominen, Savikko, Kukkurainen, Kuokkanen, & Doran, 2006
Cognitive behavioral psychotherapy	England	Townend, 2005
Diabetic workshop	Texas	Valdez, Boswell, & Vickers, 2007
Fibromyalgia	Minnesota	Luedtke et al., 2005
Homelessness	Utah	Gundlapalli et al., 2005
Gerontology	New Hampshire	Ferris, 2008

TACTICS 7-5

Matching Some CT Dimensions with IDT Thinking

1. Pull out that handy tear-out card with the 17 CT dimensions in order to reflect on the definitions of the dimensions listed in **Table 7-3**.
2. Read Scenario 7-4.
3. Study the grid that follows the scenario (Table 7-3), and compare and contrast the differences between the thinking examples provided as they relate to the scenario.
4. Fill in the empty squares.
5. Share your ideas with colleagues at work or in class and discuss your different approaches to thinking.
6. What are your conclusions about the similarities and differences in individual thinking and IDT thinking?

Scenario 7-4

JW is a 48-year-old Hispanic male with a diagnosis of asthma and chronic low back pain. He is currently homeless. He has just been admitted to the inpatient unit from the ED to get his asthma under control. This is his third hospitalization within the last 6 months. During his stay, he receives care from an IDT consisting of an SW, a nurse, a pulmonologist, a nutritionist, and a PT.

TABLE 7-3 Comparing Individual and IDT Thinking

CT Dimension	Individual Thinking	IDT Thinking
Flexibility	Physical therapist thinks about ways to customize PT activities for JW to minimize complications with his asthma.	The team thinks about ways to customize all of JW's care to fit his needs regarding recidivism, housing, finances, nutrition, activity, pain management, respiratory health, medication, and health teaching.
Open-mindedness	Nutritionist acknowledges that JW's food preferences are not always the healthiest but that he has the right to choose.	The IDT acknowledges their temptation to judge JW for frequent visits to the ED and for not getting his prescriptions filled for his asthma medication.
Applying Standards		
Transforming Knowledge		

Discussion

What did you discover? Use of the thinking dimensions by groups is not so different from their use by individuals, is it? What is different is using the thinking dimension on a larger scale and with more input. It is also helpful to use the dimensions very overtly. Comments such as, "Let's use our *flexibility* thinking for a minute here and see if we can't. . . ." or "If we all put on our thinking caps and use some *inquisitiveness,* what are some of the things we need to know but don't know?" or "If we try what _____ recommends, what can we *predict* as possible outcomes?" or "What part of the big picture *(contextual perspective)* are we missing?" or "We really need to break this down and look at the parts *(analyzing)* before we try to draw any conclusions *(logical reasoning)* about how to fix things."

For more practice, try adding other dimensions and different scenarios to discriminate the subtle and overt differences between thinking from an IDT perspective and an individual perspective.

The next sections address some of the barriers to, as well as what helps, IDT thinking. The better we understand the factors that influence IDT thinking, the better we are able to use our individual thinking to modify and enhance it.

What Interferes with IDT Thinking?

The literature cites numerous factors that interfere with IDT thinking. We have classified these barriers to IDT thinking by the following categories: (1) time, resources, and support; (2) professional preparation; and (3) personality, including communication skills and behavioral patterns. Communication and behavior are paramount because IDT work and thinking are totally dependent on our ability (or inability) to interact with one another.

Time, Resources, and Support

The lack of time constantly plagues healthcare providers. With all the work that needs to be done, it is difficult to convince people that more time needs to be found for meetings within the discipline, let alone interdisciplinary ones. It is even harder to convince folks if their only experience with meetings is wasting time. What's that old saying? A meeting is where you keep minutes but lose hours.☺ Creative solutions for IDT thinking without meetings are proposed later in the chapter. We bet that piqued your interest!

Lack of resources and support can also restrict movement toward IDT work and thinking (O'Daniel & Rosenstein, 2008). A few examples of resources and support include:

1. Physical space for IDTs to meet, where staff can talk and think together with limited distractions

2. Functioning computers and Internet access so that physicians, nurses, SWs, PTs, and so on, can continually update their knowledge about their discipline and how others are using IDT work to improve patient outcomes

3. Leadership, policies, and procedures that acknowledge the value of IDT work and thinking, and empower IDT members to work together

Professional Preparation

Most professional disciplines pride themselves on their discipline autonomy. Nurses have been working very hard since the 1950s to establish their profession as unique and separate from medicine. They have achieved that goal through the development of a solid knowledge base, discipline-specific research, a code of ethics, and standards of care. However, in the process, they may have also promoted clinicians who avoid collaborative thinking for fear of being traitors to the nursing profession. Nursing, like other disciplines, is a bit ethnocentric—or should we say, discipline-centric? We have been educated in our own domains with our own paradigms for thinking and problem solving separately instead of together. The literature refers to this as working in disciplinary silos (Herbert et al., 2007; Kuehn, 1998; Verma, Paterson, & Medves, 2006). It is time to apply new professional standards—interdisciplinary work standards—that include strategies for IDT thinking.

Thinking and working together is not easy; it requires preparation for teamwork both in the educational arena and in the practice arena. Lack of preparation for teamwork significantly hinders team members from thinking together, let alone working together. Although teamwork has been given lip service over the last few decades, unidisciplinary teams are still the most common. For the most part, nurses talk with nurses, doctors talk with doctors, nurse educators talk with nurse educators, and so on. This isolation limits thinking to the paradigms of the discipline.

Because of the nature of their work, SWs, case managers, discharge planners, and community health nurses are probably the groups most skilled at engaging more than one discipline in team thinking and activities. Their jobs require extensive collaboration in order to connect clients with necessary resources. Doing that job effectively demands communication and thinking collaboration with other disciplines.

Personality

Ego, Ego, Ego. President Harry S. Truman once commented, "It is amazing what you can accomplish if you do not care who gets the credit" ("The Quotations Page," n.d.). If team members need to feel important, believe they have the best ideas, or have difficulty accepting good ideas from other members, team thinking suffers. If team members use the team's thinking time to meet their personal needs for socialization, team thinking suffers. IDT thinking requires the *intellectual integrity* to go beyond one's beliefs and assumptions and seek a better truth.

Low tolerance for ambiguity hinders folks from taking the extra time to go beyond acceptable to better or best solutions. Lack of *open-mindedness, flexibility*, and *contextual perspective* contributes to low tolerance for ambiguity. If team members are uncomfortable because there are no obvious answers to problems, they are more likely to rush to quick solutions. Quick solutions may ease the anxiety of the team, but they are not always the best choices.

Comfort level in working together is another personal factor to consider. How comfortable are you with team membership? For example, what about when patients are present? Will the presence of patients prevent you from saying what you really think for fear of hurting their feelings, creating unnecessary worries, or challenging data? How much you value *contextual perspective* may influence your comfort with the patient being part of the context.

And perhaps one of the most essential personality factors is emotional intelligence (EI). Goleman (1995) asserted that EI is critical to success in any area of life. EI is particularly critical in developing the collaboration needed for effective IDT thinking (McCallin & Bamford, 2007; McQueen, 2004). In a nutshell, EI is a constellation of personality characteristics that requires several thinking dimensions. Individuals with high levels of EI are better team thinkers because team thinking is complex. The more complex a situation is, the more knowledge and thinking need to converge, moving from one point of view to a synthesis (Kuehn, 1998). Sure sounds like *transforming knowledge* to us!

McCallin and Bamford (2007) referred to the thinking skill needed for the complexity of IDT work as pluralistic dialogue. Pluralistic dialogue allows IDT members to use *reflection, open-mindedness, contextual perspective, transforming knowledge*, and *confidence* to break through stereotypes, come to grips with different ways of approaching problems, synthesizing, and exploring alternative solutions, and be assured that their reasoning is sound. Without EI, effective team thinking is difficult, if not impossible.

Communication Skills

The medium for IDT collaborative thinking is language. Discipline-specific language and jargon are cited repeatedly as limiting factors for working in IDTs (Case, 1998; O'Daniel & Rosenstein, 2008; Schofield & Amodeo, 1999). Converting to the language of thinking may become the unifying factor for IDT communication and collaboration.

When individuals in the same or different disciplines communicate, conflict is inevitable. One's inability to handle conflict can hinder CT and IDT work. Conflict creates anxiety, which prevents higher order thinking (Hart, 1983). The secret is not to try to eliminate conflict (which, by the way, is impossible), but to use conflict to improve the effectiveness of teams (Northouse & Northouse, 1985; O'Daniel & Rosenstein, 2008; Sessa, 1998). Strategies for improving your ability to use conflict constructively depend on *confidence* in your reasoning, *flexibility*, and *intellectual integrity*.

An analysis of the current interaction style in healthcare practice and education indicates a developmental delay. Many providers' interaction styles might best be described as parallel play or, at best, multidisciplinary. Parallel play refers to the interaction style used by 2- and 3-year-old toddlers as they begin their socialization process beyond self. Toddlers using parallel play are aware of others; they enjoy being in the vicinity of others, but basically they do their own thing, not having figured out how to play together. Does this sound like the way we operate sometimes in health care? Moving beyond parallel play to collaborative interactions will likely require *perseverance* to learn better ways to work and think as teams instead of in silos.

The current literature on IDT work and IDT thinking repeatedly emphasizes that communication skill has the most important impact on whether outcomes of IDT work are positive or negative (Charlton, Dearing, Berry, & Johnson, 2008; O'Daniel & Rosenstein, 2008; Reader, Flin, Mearns, & Cuthbertson, 2007; Seago, 2008; Williams, Vares, & Brumbaugh, 2006).

Behavioral Patterns

Our behavior patterns can reflect our thinking. For example, some of us behave by removing ourselves to a quiet place to think. Others behave by pausing to think before offering ideas. And many behave as active listeners, respectfully absorbing the information that others are sharing before responding.

Our behavior toward others is a primary measure of how well we have been socialized as thinking human beings in a civilized society. Disruptive, counter-productive behavior patterns that have been around for years in health care and elsewhere are finally being identified as totally unacceptable. These patterns are particularly problematic because they literally make IDT thinking and IDT work impossible.

These patterns have been referred to as disruptive or bad behavior ("Bad Behavior No Longer Acceptable," 2008; O'Daniel & Rosenstein, 2008), lateral violence (Martin, Stanley, Dulaney, & Pehrson, 2008; Sincox & Fitzpatrick, 2008), and incivility (Clark, 2008a, 2008b). Whether it is covert (passive aggressiveness, ignoring, rudeness) or overt (yelling, belittling, bullying, physical violence), this behavior represents flagrant disrespect for colleagues. Disruptive behavior/lateral violence/incivility in health care can occur between any individuals—nurses and nurses, physicians and nurses, administrators and healthcare workers, nursing faculty and nursing students, and so on. The Center for American Nurses (2008) prepared a position paper calling for zero-tolerance policies related to disruptive behavior/lateral violence. IDT thinking can work only with a foundation of respect and trust for one another. Confronting negative behaviors and modeling positive behaviors are essential for quality patient outcomes.

What Cultivates IDT Thinking?

Brookfield and Preskill (1999) made a strong case for how discussion enhances learning through the cultivation of critical reflection and thinking. They offered strategies promoting CT through discussion with exercises called Critical Incident Questionnaires (p. 49), Telling Tales from the Trenches (p. 77), and Circle of Voices (p. 80), to name just a few.

Thinking in an effective team environment does not happen automatically; it takes time, effort, and a commitment to think beyond your discipline's knowledge bases, aspirations, and values (McCormack, 2001; Salmon & Jones, 2001). It also takes a shift in organizational culture to mutually respect working partnerships (Coombs, 2001). Bottom line: Cultivating IDT thinking is hard work. We do not have any magic bullets, but we have some helpful suggestions.

For starters, not all IDT thinking requires meetings. The IOM talks about IDT work, not IDT meetings. This is an important distinction and helps us to think outside that ol' box! This awareness can lead to all kinds of creativity and flexibility to change the IDT work environment mindset for clinicians and educators.

Clinicians

The IOM (2003) summarized eight conditions necessary for effective IDT work in the practice setting. Although they do not specifically mention thinking, we believe that if you examine **Box 7-4**, you will decide that it is impossible to achieve anything on the list without thinking. These too can all occur in providers' daily interactions in addition to meetings.

Case (1998) identified several similar factors that need to be in place for teamwork to occur in the practice setting: (1) a common language, (2) a common knowledge base, (3) shared core values, (4) understanding the roles of the team members, (5) respect for team members, and (6) mutual sharing among the members. Case encouraged staff development specialists to pay attention to these factors when they promote IDT work. Note that Case did not say "meetings." All of her recommendations can occur in corridor discussions as long as privacy is not violated, of course.

BOX 7-4	**IOM Conditions for Effective IDT Work**

- Learn about other team members' expertise, background, knowledge, and values.
- Learn individual roles and processes required to work collaboratively.
- Demonstrate basic group skills, including communication, negotiation, delegation, time management, and assessment of group dynamics.
- Ensure that accurate and timely information reaches those who need it at the appropriate times.
- Customize care and manage smooth transitions across settings and over time, even when the team members are in entirely different physical locations.
- Coordinate and integrate care processes to ensure excellence, continuity, and reliability of the care provided.
- Resolve conflicts with other members of the team.
- Communicate with other members of the team in a shared language, even when the members are in entirely different physical locations.

Source: Institute of Medicine, 2003, p. 56.

An excellent example of nonmeeting IDT thinking is offered by Halm, Goering, and Smith (2003), with the use of interdisciplinary rounds (IDR). These are enhanced discharge planning rounds in which each discipline reviews the patient record, identifies problems from the discipline's perspective, shares information with the team, collaborates on approaches, identifies barriers to the approaches, and identifies individual and team learning needs. The goals for IDR were timely and safe discharges, improved documentation of collaborative care, and increased awareness of each discipline's skills and resources.

They implemented IDR in a large midwestern hospital on medicine, orthopedics, neurology, rehabilitation, surgery, cardiology, oncology, behavioral health, and birthing center units. The plan was to use IDR as a means of engaging all disciplines in discharge planning. Participating clinical nurse specialists used the Internet to collaborate with other institutions using similar processes. Sharing of ideas and constant modifications took place as new information became available. At the end of 6 months, outcomes of the IDR included "greater participation by all the disciplines in achieving patient and family outcomes, increased early recognition of patients at risk, and improved communication among members of the healthcare team" (Halm et al., 2003, p. 133).

Seago (2008) reviewed 36 studies focused on professional communication. She found empirical evidence of the strong relationship between effective communication and positive patient outcomes. O'Daniel and Rosenstein (2008) synthesized findings focused on teamwork and team thinking. They identified 13 components of successful teamwork and focused very clearly on issues of open communication, a respectful atmosphere, and processes for acknowledging and dealing with conflict, among others. One effective strategy they cited was "SBAR" (situation-background-assessment-recommendations) as a guide for nurse/physician reporting. Developed at Kaiser Permanente and becoming increasingly popular, this simple approach not only facilitates communication but also "helps develop desired critical-thinking skills" (O'Daniel & Rosenstein, p. 2-277). You can see how thinking would be enhanced by the reminders. Consider how some of the CT dimensions come through:

Situation—What is going on with the patient? What *information seeking* have I done? How has my *discriminating* helped me clarify signs and symptoms?

Background—What is the clinical background or *contextual perspective*?

Assessment—What do I think the problem is? What are the results of my *analysis* and *logical reasoning*?

Recommendation—What would I do to correct it? What would I *predict*?

Educators

The IOM conditions for effective IDT in Box 7-4 and the issues identified by O'Daniel and Rosenstein (2008) are also valuable for thinking about implementing IDT work in the educational setting. Implementation in the academic arena, however, has some additional challenges because IDT activities are not generally rewarded in that arena. Value in education has traditionally been given to independent work. These traditions must be changed to prepare educators and students of all the professions for IDT practice in the real world.

Rice (2000) recommended a dual socialization process in academic education. For example, nursing students would not only learn their profession but also have courses and clinical experiences together with students from other disciplines; as a result of thinking and working together as groups, they would learn to share and respect each other from the start. Rice based her recommendation on her experience as an SW and her extensive literature review of 302 articles.

Some professional education programs are taking IDT concepts to heart. Two deans in Colorado, one from a medical school and one from a nursing school, worked together to change scheduling so that students in those programs could take courses together (P. Pronovost, MD, PhD, personal communication, March 28, 2004).

We have firsthand knowledge of one IDT course that has been very successful. Faculty from the School of Nursing, the School of Social Work, and the School of Associated Health Professions at Eastern Michigan University worked collaboratively to develop and teach a course called "Aging to Infancy: A Retrospective Approach to Life." The disciplines involved were nursing, social work, occupational therapy, and dietetics. All four faculty participated before, during, and after the class periods to coordinate their teaching, discuss issues arising in class, and assess students' learning. A major goal of this course was to demonstrate to students how the disciplines collaborate in both thinking and doing to address healthcare issues across age groups. Course enrollment increased from 25 students the first year to over 100 students 2 years later.

Educational collaboration across disciplines is being encouraged at policy-making levels. In its *Excellence Initiatives* document (2004), the National League for Nursing addressed the importance of nursing curricula's inclusion of multidisciplinary approaches to care. The National League for Nursing Accrediting Commission (2008) also included in their accreditation standards (Standard 4-Curriculum) the need for curricula to address interdisciplinary collaboration. The American Association of Colleges of Nursing (2008) and their corresponding accreditation body, the Commission on Collegiate Nursing Education (2008), also acknowledged the necessity of interdisciplinary and collaborative work.

Since this text was first published, numerous articles and texts have emerged that address the need for educational models to promote interdisciplinary thinking. Rodehorst, Wilhelm, and Jensen (2005) proposed the use of simulations for interdisciplinary courses to illustrate differences in norms, values, cultures, and professional orientations to patient care. In their text for nurse educators, Bradshaw and Lowenstein (2007) offered several learning activities to stimulate interdisciplinary thinking: Interdisciplinary Case Study Analysis (p. 51), Developing Collaborative Creativity Skills (p. 76), and An Interprofessional Problem-Based Learning Course on Rehabilitation Issues in HIV (p. 137), to name just a few.

Verma et al. (2006) identified core competencies for curricula and ideas for assessing interdisciplinary learning outcomes, elaborating on the stages of learning how to work and think collaboratively. Reeves and Freeth (2006) discussed the development of a model of interprofessional education in community mental health in England. Golanowski, Beaudry, Kurz, Laffey, and Hook (2007) offered a model for interdisciplinary decision making. Dellasega, Milone-Nuzzo, Curci, Ballard, and Kirch (2007) described a discipline-neutral model, in which all professionals are on equal ground. This model was used in a humanities course to explore interdisciplinary thinking and problem solving. Weaver (2008) proposed a model for examining the antecedents, processes, and outcomes that need to be addressed for successful IDT. All aspects of this model require what Weaver described as "integration of thought" and "synergy" (p. 112).

Perseverance Is Needed

Whether in practice or education, initial efforts to enhance IDT work will take time, energy, and CT. It may seem overwhelming; you will want to fall back on, "It's easier to do it myself." At first we will likely continue using hybrid versions of IDT. But once IDT thinking is integrated into daily activities that go beyond having more meetings, the time factor will become less of an issue.

Before finishing this chapter, let's return to the "two heads are better than one" idea and expand on it. Consider this. Compare the positive outcomes of IDT thinking to a molecule of sugar!

Think back to your organic chemistry course. For some, this may be a bit painful, but bear with us a minute. Remember how the elements of carbon, hydrogen, and oxygen combine to make sugar? Each of the elements has unique properties and is distinct. But when certain conditions exist, those elements work together to create sugar, a whole new entity (**Figure 7-2**).

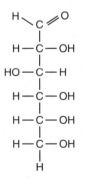

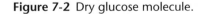

Figure 7-2 Dry glucose molecule.

Sugar is a totally different substance from any of its three elements—carbon, hydrogen, and oxygen. Sugar is something new (and much tastier than any of the three elements by themselves) that results from the combined efforts of energy, the right amounts of elements, and the right conditions. But even as sugar, the elements of carbon, hydrogen, and oxygen maintain their basic molecular integrity.

IDT work and IDT thinking work in similar (sweet?) ways. Healthcare providers (the elements) collaborate using energy to combine their thinking and disciplinary knowledge (the necessary conditions) to create quality patient outcomes (sugar). And, as with the sugar molecule, all the healthcare providers (elements) maintain their unique identity, disciplinary knowledge, and thinking skills.

Now, if you are really into organic chemistry, you know there are lots of different types of sugar and starches that result from combining these elements in different amounts. IDT work and thinking have the same kinds of results, if not more. Imagine the quality patient outcomes possibilities that IDT thinking could create.

PAUSE

and Ponder

Future Implications of IDT Thinking

According to growing evidence, moving toward IDT thinking is no longer a choice; it is a necessity. IDT thinking is the catalyst for moving us from disciplinary silos to collaborative outcomes. Our job is to better understand IDT work and IDT thinking. We must value IDT thinking, overcome the barriers to it, nurture the factors that cultivate it, respect each other's thinking, teach it, and model it as we strive for quality patient outcomes. You and your peers will be the new generation of leaders in practice and education to achieve that goal. Today's clinicians may have to learn IDT thinking on the job, but it is hoped that tomorrow's clinicians will have learned IDT thinking in school.

Reflection Cues

- IDTs are essential for dealing with the increasing complexity of health care.
- Most team meetings in practice best match the characteristics of a multidisciplinary team or a "utilitarian team" whose activities consist of delivering information, coordinating and planning, and making decisions.
- IDTs focus on collaborative problem identification and problem solving.
- IDTs occur less frequently in academic settings than in practice settings.
- Research studies indicate that IDTs enhance patient compliance, produce greater patient satisfaction, reduce costs, decrease hospitalizations, lower infant and geriatric mortality rates, reduce lengths of stay, and improve staff morale.

- Multiple factors—time, resources, support, professional preparation, personality, communication skills, and behavior patterns—can interfere with team thinking.
- Discipline autonomy tends to promote working and thinking in silos.
- Lack of preparation and training to work in IDTs is a major impediment to IDT work.
- Thinking in IDTs is more than simply adding ideas together; IDT thinking blends ideas and creates new ones that individuals would not have considered independently.
- Attention to Bensimon and Neumann's (1993) eight thinking roles of teams is helpful in assessing IDT work.
- Not all IDT thinking requires meetings; IDR are one alternative.
- New educational models and research are demonstrating effective IDT strategies and outcomes.
- IDT work takes time and energy, effective leadership, and critical thinking to be successful.

References

American Association of Colleges of Nursing. (2008, October 20). *The essentials of baccalaureate education for professional nursing practice.* Retrieved October 29, 2008, from http://www.aacn.nche.edu/education/pdf/BaccEssentials08.pdf

Apker, J., Propp, K. M., Ford, W. S. Z., & Hofmeister, N. (2006). Collaboration, credibility, compassion, and coordination: Professional nurse communication skill sets in health care team interactions. *Journal of Professional Nursing, 22*(3), 180–189. doi:10.1016/j.profnurs.2006.03.002

Austin, W., Park, C., & Goble, E. (2008). From interdisciplinary to transdisciplinary research: A case study. *Qualitative Health Research, 18*(4), 557–564. doi:10.1177/1049732307308514

Bad behavior no longer acceptable. (2008). *Michigan Nurse, 81*(5), 13–14.

Baldwin, D. C., Jr. (1996). Some historical notes on interdisciplinary and interprofessional education and practice in healthcare in the USA. *Journal of Interprofessional Care, 10,* 173–187.

Bensimon, E. M., & Neumann, A. (1993). *Redesigning collegiate leadership: Teams and teamwork in higher education.* Baltimore: Johns Hopkins University Press.

Bradshaw, M. J., & Lowenstein, A. J. (2007). *Innovative teaching strategies in nursing and related health professions* (4th ed.). Sudbury, MA: Jones and Bartlett.

Brookfield, S. D., & Preskill, S. (1999). *Discussion as a way of teaching: Tools and techniques for democratic classrooms.* San Francisco: Jossey-Bass.

Case, B. (1998). Competency development: Critical thinking, clinical judgment, and technical ability. In K. J. Kelly-Thomas (Ed.), *Clinical and nursing staff development: Current competency, future focus* (2nd ed., pp. 240–281). Philadelphia: Lippincott.

Center for American Nurses. (2008). *The Center for American Nurses calls for an end to lateral violence and bullying in nursing work environments.* Retrieved October 19, 2008, from http://www.centerforamericannurses.org

Charlton, C. R., Dearing, K. S., Berry, J. A., & Johnson, M. J. (2008). Nurse practitioners' communication styles and their impact on patient outcomes: An integrated literature review. *Journal of the American Academy of Nurse Practitioners, 20*, 382–388. doi:10.1111/j.1745-7599.2008.00336

Clark, C. M. (2008a). Student voices on faculty incivility in nursing education: A conceptual model. *Nursing Education Perspectives, 29*, 284–289.

Clark, C. M. (2008b). Faculty and student assessment of and experience with incivility in nursing education. *Journal of Nursing Education, 47*, 458–465.

Commission on Collegiate Nursing Education. (2008). *CCNE standards for accreditation of baccalaureate and graduate degree nursing programs.* Retrieved November 18, 2008, from http://www.aacn.nche.edu/accreditation/

Coombs, M. (2001). Towards collaborative and collegial caring: A comparative study. *Nursing in Critical Care, 6*, 23–27.

Dellasega, C., Milone-Nuzzo, P., Curci, K. M., Ballard, J. O., & Kirch, D. G. (2007). The humanities interface of nursing and medicine. *Journal of Professional Nursing, 23*, 174–179.

Dyer, J. A. (2003). Multidisciplinary, interdisciplinary, and transdisciplinary educational models and nursing education. *Nursing Education Perspectives, 24*, 186–188.

Erickson, J. I., Ditomassi, M. O., & Jones, D. A. (2008). Interdisciplinary Institute for Patient Care: Advancing clinical excellence. *Journal of Nursing Administration, 38*, 308–314.

Falise, J. P. (2007). True collaboration: Interdisciplinary rounds in nonteaching hospitals—It can be done! *AACN Advanced Critical Care, 18*, 346–351.

Ferris, M. (2008). Where are the geriatric nurses? Multidisciplinary forums need your expertise. *Journal of Gerontological Nursing, 34*(2), 3–4.

Golanowski, M., Beaudry, D., Kurz, L., Laffey, W. J., & Hook, M. L. (2007). Interdisciplinary shared decision-making: Taking shared governance to the next level. *Nursing Administration Quarterly, 31*, 341–353.

Goleman, D. (1995). *Emotional intelligence: Why it can matter more than IQ.* New York: Bantam Books.

Gundlapalli, H., Hanks, M., Stevens, S. M., Geroso, A. M., Viavant, C. R., McCall, Y., et al. (2005). It takes a village: A multidisciplinary model for the acute illness aftercare of individuals experiencing homelessness. *Journal of Health Care for the Poor and Underserved, 16*, 257–272.

Halm, M. A., Goering, M., & Smith, M. (2003). Interdisciplinary rounds: Impact on patients, families, and staff. *Clinical Nurse Specialist, 17*, 133–142.

Hart, L. A. (1983). *Human brain and human learning.* New York: Longman.

Herbert, C. P., Bainbridge, L., Bickford, J., Baptiste, S., Brajtman, S., Dryden, T., et al. (2007). Factors that influence engagement in collaborative practice: How 8 health professionals became advocates. *Canadian Family Physician, 53*, 1318–1325.

Holzinger, U., Feldbacher, M., Bachlechner, A., Kitzerger, R., Fuhrmann, V., & Madl, C. (2008). Improvement of glucose control in the intensive care unit: An interdisciplinary collaboration study. *American Journal of Critical Care, 17*, 150–158.

Institute of Medicine. (2003). *Health professions education: A bridge to quality.* Washington, DC: National Academies Press.

Karon, S. (2005). A team approach to bladder retraining: A pilot study. *Urologic Nursing, 25*, 269–276.

Kuehn, A. F. (1998). Collaborative health professional education: An interdisciplinary mandate for the third millennium. In T. J. Sullivan (Ed.), *Collaboration: A health care imperative* (pp. 419–465). New York: McGraw-Hill.

Kurtzman, E. T., & Corrigan, J. M. (2007). Measuring the contribution of nursing to quality, patient safety, and health care outcomes. *Policy, Politics, & Nursing Practice, 8*(1), 20–36. doi:10.1177/1527154407302115

Lessard, L., Morin, D., & Sylvain, H. (2008). Understanding teams and teamwork. *The Canadian Nurse, 104*(3), 12–13.

Luedtke, C. A., Thompson, J. M., Postier, J. A., Neubauer, B. L., Drach, S., & Newell, L. (2005). A description of a brief multidisciplinary treatment program for fibromyalgia. *Pain Management Nursing, 6*(2), 76–80.

Martin, M. M., Stanley, K. M., Dulaney, P., & Pehrson, K. M. (2008). The role of the psychiatric consultation liaison nurse in evidence-based approaches to lateral violence in nursing. *Perspectives in Psychiatric Care, 44*(1), 58–60.

McCallin, A., & Bamford, A. (2007). Interdisciplinary teamwork: Is the influence of emotional intelligence fully appreciated? *Journal of Nursing Management, 15,* 386–391.

McCormack, B. (2001). Clinical effectiveness and clinical teams: Effective practice with older people. *Nursing Older People, 13*(5), 14–17.

McQueen, A. C. H. (2004). Emotional intelligence in nursing work. *Journal of Advanced Nursing, 47,* 101–108.

Mitchell, P. H. (2005). What's in a name? Multidisciplinary, interdisciplinary, and transdisciplinary. *Journal of Professional Nursing, 21,* 332–334.

Mui, A. C. (2001). The Program of All-Inclusive Care for the Elderly (PACE): An innovative long-term care model in the United States. *Journal of Aging and Social Policy, 13*(2/3), 53–67.

National League for Nursing. (2004). *Excellence initiatives.* Retrieved September 18, 2008, from http://www.nln.org/excellence/hallmarks_indicators.htm

National League for Nursing Accrediting Commission. (2008). *NLNAC Standards and criteria baccalaureate.* Retrieved November 14, 2008, from http://www.nlnac.org/manuals/SC2008_BACCALAUREATE.pdf

Nelson, G. A., King, M. L., & Brodine, S. (2008). Nurse-physician collaboration on medical-surgical units. *MEDSURG Nursing, 17*(1), 35–40.

Northouse, P. G., & Northouse, L. L. (1985). *Health communication: A handbook for health professionals.* Englewood Cliffs, NJ: Prentice Hall.

O'Daniel, M., & Rosenstein, A. (2008). Professional communication and team collaboration. In R. G. Hughes (Ed.), *Patient safety and quality: An evidence-based handbook for nurses* (Vol. 2, pp. 2-271–2-284). Rockville, MD: Agency for Healthcare Research and Quality. (AHRQ Publication No. 08-0043)

Oliver, D. P., Wittenberg-Lyles, E. M., & Day, M. (2006). Variances in perceptions of interdisciplinary collaboration by hospice staff. *Journal of Palliative Care, 22,* 275–280.

Purdy, M. (2007). Increasing stroke patients' success in self-medication programs using an interdisciplinary cognitive rehabilitation approach. *Rehabilitation Nursing, 32,* 210–213, 219.

The quotations page. (n.d.). Retrieved August 11, 2004, from http://www.quotationspage.com/quotes.php3?author+Harry+S+Truman

Reader, T. W., Flin, R., Mearns, K., & Cuthbertson, B. H. (2007). Interdisciplinary communication in the intensive care unit. *British Journal of Anaesthesia, 98*(3), 347–353. doi:10.1093/bja/ael372

Redman, R. W. (2006). The challenge of interdisciplinary teams. *Research and Theory for Nursing Practice, 20,* 105–107.

Reeves, S., & Freeth, D. (2006). Re-examining the evaluation of interprofessional education for community mental health teams with a different lens: Understanding presage, process and product factors. *Journal of Psychiatric and Mental Health Nursing, 13,* 765–770.

Rice, A. H. (2000). Interdisciplinary collaboration in healthcare: Education, practice and research. *National Academies of Practice Forum, 2*(1), 59–73.

Rodehorst, T. K., Wilhelm, S. L., & Jensen, L. (2005). Use of interdisciplinary simulation to understand perceptions of team members' roles. *Journal of Professional Nursing, 21*(3), 159–166. doi:10.1016/j.profnurs.2005.04.005

Ross, F., O'Tuathail, C., & Stubberfield, D. (2005). Towards multidisciplinary assessment of older people: Exploring the change process. *Journal of Clinical Nursing, 14,* 518–529.

Rossen, E. K., Bartlett, R. B., & Herrick, C. A. (2008). Interdisciplinary collaboration: The need to revisit. *Issues in Mental Health Nursing, 29,* 387–396.

Salmon, D., & Jones, M. (2001). Shaping the interprofessional agenda: A study examining qualified nurses' perceptions of learning with others. *Nurse Education Today, 21,* 18–25.

Schim, S. M., & Raspa, R. (2007). Crossing disciplinary boundaries in end-of-life education. *Journal of Professional Nursing, 23,* 201–207.

Schofield, R. F., & Amodeo, M. (1999). Interdisciplinary teams in healthcare and human service settings: Are they effective? *Health and Social Work, 24,* 210–219.

Seago, J. A. (2008). Professional communication. In R. G. Hughes (Ed.), *Patient safety and quality: An evidence-based handbook for nurses* (Vol. 2, pp. 2-247–2-269). Rockville, MD: Agency for Healthcare Research and Quality (AHRQ Publication No. 08-0043)

Senge, P. M. (1990). *The fifth discipline: The art and practice of the learning organization.* New York: Doubleday.

Sessa, V. (1998). Professional development initiative: Using conflict to improve effectiveness of nurse teams. *Orthopaedic Nursing, 17*(3), 41–46.

Simpson, G., Rabin, D., Schmitt, M., Taylor, P., Urban, S., & Ball, J. (2001). Interprofessional healthcare practice: Recommendations of the National Academies of Practice expert panel on healthcare in the 21st century. *Issues in Interdisciplinary Care, 3*(1), 5–19.

Sincox, A. K., & Fitzpatrick, M. (2008). Lateral violence: Calling out the elephant in the room. *Michigan Nurse, 81*(3), 8–9.

Suominen, T., Savikko, N., Kukkurainen, M., Kuokkanen, L., & Doran, D. I. (2006). Work-related empowerment of the multidisciplinary team at the Rheumatism Foundation Hospital. *International Journal of Nursing Practice, 12,* 94–104.

Townend, M. (2005). Interprofessional supervision from the perspectives of both mental health nurses and other professionals in the field of cognitive behavioural psychotherapy. *Journal of Psychiatric and Mental Health Nursing, 12,* 582–588.

Ubbes, V. A., Black, J. M., & Ausherman, J. A. (1999). Teaching for understanding in health education: The role of critical and creative thinking skills within constructivism theory. *Journal of Health Education, 30*(2), 67–72.

Valdez, G. M., Boswell, C., & Vickers, P. (2007). Planning and implementing an interdisciplinary diabetes workshop for healthcare professionals. *Journal of Continuing Education in Nursing, 38,* 232–237.

Verma, S., Paterson, M., & Medves, J. (2006). Core competencies for health care professionals. *Journal of Allied Health, 35,* 109–115.

Weaver, J. E. (2008). Enhancing multiple disciplinary teamwork. *Nursing Outlook, 56,* 108–114. doi:10.1016/j.outlook.2008.03.013

Wheelan, S. A., Burchill, C. N., & Tilin, F. (2003). The link between teamwork and patients' outcomes in intensive care units. *American Journal of Critical Care, 12,* 527–534.

Williams, J., Vares, L., & Brumbaugh, M. (2006). Education to improve interdisciplinary practice of health care professionals: A pilot project. *Medicine & Health Rhode Island, 89,* 312–313.

Critical Thinking and Evidence-Based Practice

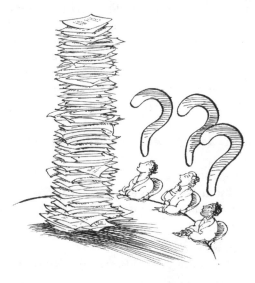

"All this research and we still have questions."

Evidence-based practice (EBP) is a very important paradigm shift in how health care is practiced and taught. Publications on EBP have exploded in the past few years. Various definitions of EBP and its "cousins" (e.g., evidence-based medicine, evidence-based nursing) have emerged. Common among the many definitions of EBP is the idea of moving away from practice based merely on tradition—doing things the way they've always been done without questioning whether that is the best approach—toward practice decisions based on the best available knowledge (evidence). This chapter is designed to introduce nurses, nurse educators, and nursing students to the thinking required to base practice on evidence.

The Institute of Medicine (IOM) described EBP as "the integration of best research evidence, clinical expertise, and patient values in making decisions about the care of individual patients" (2003, p. 56). The IOM clarified "best research evidence" as quantitative evidence such as that obtained through clinical trials and laboratory experiments, evidence from qualitative research, and evidence from experts in practice. "Clinical expertise" comes from knowledge and experience over time. "Patient values" are those unique circumstances of each patient. The IOM enumerated several tasks necessary to EBP: (1) knowing where and how to find best evidence, (2) formulating clinical questions, (3) searching for answers to those questions with the best evidence and determining the validity and appropriateness of that evidence for patient populations, and (4) determining how and when to integrate those new findings in practice. Each task is primarily a thinking process. Specifically implied is the use of the critical thinking (CT) skills of *analyzing, applying standards, discriminating, information seeking, logical reasoning, predicting,* and *transforming knowledge,* and habits of the mind, such as *contextual perspective, inquisitiveness, intellectual integrity,* and *open-mindedness.*

Increasingly, we are seeing links between thinking and EBP in the literature; even when the links aren't explicit, there is an implication that the very nature of EBP necessitates CT. A collection of some of those statements is in **Box 8-1**. The history of this movement is very helpful for understanding its importance and how closely aligned with CT it has been since its inception.

BOX 8-1	**Links Between EBP and Thinking in the Literature**

Avis and Freshwater, 2006:
"Critical analysis of the concept suggests that EBP overemphasizes the value of scientific evidence while underplaying the role of clinical judgement and individual nursing expertise" (p. 216).

Bucknall and Hutchinson, 2006:
"The use of evidence in practice is dependent upon cognitive competence" (p. 137).

Scott-Findlay and Pollock, 2004:
"We hope to improve clinical decision making by increasing practitioners' reliance on research findings while acknowledging the important part played by other forms of knowledge in the decision-making process" (p. 96).

Fonteyn, 2005:
"Nurses' ability to think well and understand research is essential to evidence-based practice and, correspondingly, involvement in evidence-based practice and scholarly activities is important for honing nurses' thinking skills and enhancing their ability to comprehend research" (p. 439).

Hancock and Easen, 2006:
"As both the extension of nursing practice and the demand for evidence-based practice increase, the quality of the decision making of nurses becomes imperative" (p. 694).

Harbison, 2006:
"What turns 'information' into 'evidence'? A process of reasoning is undergone, whereby information is selected and assessed in relation to its relevance and weight in the individual case" (p. 1490).

BOX 8-1 (Continued)

Holmes, Murray, Perron, and McCabe, 2008:
"The BPG [Best Practice Guideline] movement is ideologically driven, giving us 'ready-made tools,' 'rules' and 'guidelines' that ultimately impede nurses' critical thinking and serve as disciplinary technologies to govern nursing work" (p. 395).

Hudson, Duke, Haas, and Varnell, 2008:
"Multiple ways of knowing, or evidence, for informed clinical decision making must be considered based on situational context" (p. 409).

Mantzoukas, 2008:
"EBP is a decision-making process that enables the practitioner to consciously and explicitly choose the best treatment option for individual patients" (p. 221).

McWilliam, 2007:
"As evidence-based practice gains momentum, continuing education practitioners increasingly confront the need to develop and conduct events promoting the uptake of research findings. Recently this challenge has changed . . .[;] the current expectation is one of knowledge translation" (p. 72).

Pierce, 2007:
"A prerequisite to becoming an evidence-based rehabilitation nurse is to become a reflective professional" (p. 203).

Profetto-McGrath, Hesketh, Lang, and Estabrooks, 2003:
"Nurses who have the attributes consistent with the ideal critical thinker, and especially those who are open-minded, inquisitive, and systematic, are more likely to use research findings in their work as nurses" (p. 334).

Rycroft-Malone, 2008:
"Evidence-informed practice is a problem-solving process in which practitioners are active stakeholders" (p. 407).

Sams and Gannon, 2000:
"Evidence-based practice is well suited to the information age because it demands critical thinking, integration of work efforts, ongoing knowledge-based queries, continual outcome improvement, and interdisciplinary work" (p. 126).

Sandelowski, 2004:
"Qualitative health research offers the best chance of producing truly transformative knowledge and fully activating the knowledge transformation cycle foundational to the evidence-based practice paradigm" (p. 1382).

Stetler, Brunell, Giuliano, Morsi, Prince, and Newell-Stokes, 1998:
"Inherent to EBP are critical thinking and research utilization competencies" (p. 49).

Historical Overview of EBP

Nurses have a quintessential picture of EBP in their founder, Florence Nightingale, who collected and analyzed evidence to show how deaths of Crimean War soldiers could be drastically reduced. Using that evidence, she enabled a change in health care that persists even today (Hayes, 2005). It is too bad that more references don't put Nightingale at the top of the list of those credited with the EBP movement. We nurses must remember to brag about her more.

More often, the historical roots of EBP are credited to the forward thinking of Archie Cochrane, a British physician who, in the 1970s, saw a need to examine the economics of health care and determine the cost/benefit of treatments. In 1993, Cochrane and others founded the Cochrane Collaboration, which has become the core of EBP ("Archie Cochrane," n.d.). The Cochrane Collaboration focuses on interventions, precise and thorough searches for and evaluation of evidence, and considers the randomized controlled trial (RCT) as the gold standard of research evidence (Jennings & Loan, 2001).

On this side of the ocean, coining the term *evidence-based medicine* in the 1980s were Canadians at McMaster Medical School in Hamilton, Ontario, who made this new critical approach to medical education and practice a reality (Straus, Richardson, Glasziou, & Haynes, 2005). The McMaster approach heralded a move away from valuing authority to valuing research as a basis of learning.

Meanwhile, in the United States, the federal government committed money in the early 1990s to set up the Agency for Health Care Policy and Reform (AHCPR), which established interdisciplinary teams to gather and assess available literature and develop evidence-based clinical guidelines for several important areas of health care. Examples of early guidelines were *Pressure Ulcer Treatment*, *Depression in Primary Care*, and *Management of Cancer Pain*. Those of us who grabbed these guidelines as if they were gold soon realized that we had reached a new era of practice. It wasn't just up to us to keep up with the latest research; someone else valued our desire to provide the best care using the best evidence. Nurses were prominent members of the interdisciplinary teams who did this early work. AHCPR became the Agency for Healthcare Research and Quality (AHRQ) in the mid-1990s (http://www.ahrq.gov); it now has a clearinghouse for clinical guidelines (http://www.guideline.gov) and has established 14 EBP centers in the United States (AHRQ, 2008).

Other aspects of nursing history are also very important to the EBP movement. In the late 1970s and early 1980s, nursing groups started focusing on research utilization. Of particular note is the Conduct and Utilization of Research in Nursing project in Michigan. Seventeen hospitals in Michigan participated in developing research-based protocols in pre- and postoperative teaching, in reducing diarrhea in tube-fed patients, and in several other areas (Haller, Reynolds, & Horsley, 1979). Unfortunately, although this group and its many followers pushed for increased use of research in nursing, a gap between research and practice in the field persisted. However, the research utilization movement provided fertile ground for nursing to wholeheartedly embrace the EBP movement.

In 1994, Sigma Theta Tau International started publishing *Worldviews on Evidence-Based Nursing*. In 1998, the *Evidence-Based Nursing Journal* was published by a Canadian and British group. In Australia, the Joanna Briggs Institute (JBI) became a model of nursing-focused EBP, conducting systematic reviews, developing evidence-based best practice guidelines, and maintaining an excellent Web site used by nurses all over the world (http://www.joannabriggs.edu.au). The Registered Nurses of Ontario have developed a similar online nursing resource, creating and posting evidence-based best practice guidelines (http://www.rnao.org).

Today, one can find vast amounts of material on the Internet relative to EBP. We have compiled in **Box 8-2** a few of our favorite sites; others can be found in Chapter 9, "Critical Thinking and Informatics." If you look at these sites, you can find links to hundreds more. Because the EBP and informatics movements are growing so rapidly, by the time you read this book, there likely will be many other sites to be found, and some may no longer exist. A general Internet search with the words "evidence-based practice" will give you lots of strong hits. You need very little *information-seeking* ability to find EBP resources. However, you will need all your other thinking dimensions to sift through them intelligently.

A recent trend in nursing literature is an EBP debate focused on the interpretation of "evidence." On one side, you have the advocates of EBP, who define evidence in terms of hierarchies, with randomized controlled studies on top. On the other side, you have the deconstructionists, who question the assumptions that controlled trials are the epitome of evidence (Rolfe, 2005). These debates have great value because they force readers to think about their interpretation of EPB. With our view through CT-colored lenses, we believe many of the debates would be mollified by keeping this thought topmost: EBP is a thinking process! Once you remove or deemphasize the thinking part, the polarization over evidence becomes greater.

Why Is EBP So Important?

It really doesn't require much *logical reasoning* to see why EBP is so important. It just makes sense to base health practices on the best evidence because most of the time, it costs less, and almost all the time, there are better patient outcomes. You'll note that we don't say it's always less expensive; sometimes the best approaches are costlier because they are newer. However, when we factor in costs of not using the best evidence in practice, the few times it costs more will be far outnumbered by the overall cost savings. What constitutes better patient outcomes must be clarified with caution—we must always take into account the patient's wishes, values, and so forth. Once in a while, for all kinds of reasons, patients will refuse what providers see as the best evidence-supported approaches. Ultimately, we must respect patient wishes as long as we know that their decisions are based on the best available information. For more discussion on patients' roles in this thinking journey, look back to Chapter 6, "Critical Thinking and Patient-Centered Care."

BOX 8-2	Some Favorite Internet Sites for EBP

National Guideline Clearinghouse:
http://www.guideline.gov

Registered Nurses' Association of Ontario:
http://www.rnao.org

Centers for Disease Control and Prevention:
http://www.cdc.gov/CDCForYou/healthcare_providers.html

Evidence-based Practice Center (McMaster University):
http://hiru.mcmaster.ca/epc/default.asp

The Joanna Briggs Institute:
http://www.joannabriggs.edu.au

Agency for Healthcare Research and Quality:
http://www.ahrq.gov/

Centre for Health Evidence (University of Alberta):
http://www.cche.net

American Diabetes Association:
http://professional.diabetes.org/

Evidence Based Nursing:
http://www.ebn.bmj.com

University of Minnesota Evidence-Based Practice:
http://www.biomed.lib.umn.edu/learn/ebp/

Medical Library Association:
http://www.mlanet.org/resources/consumr_index.html

Turning Research Into Practice:
http://www.tripdatabase.com/index.html

The Cochrane Collaboration:
http://www.cochrane.org/index_practitioners.htm

Cochrane Consumer Network:
http://www.cochrane.org/consumers/sysrev.htm

**McMaster University Health Sciences Library,
Resources for Evidence-Based Nursing:**
http://hsl.mcmaster.ca/education/nursing/ebn/index.htm

Cochrane Qualitative Research Methods Group:
http://www.joannabriggs.edu.au/cqrmg/about.html

The AGREE Collaboration:
http://www.agreecollaboration.org/

Clinicians: On What Is Your Practice Based?

Before we launch into details of the thinking that accompanies EBP, stop for a minute and think about your practice arena. Is your practice and that of clinicians around you based on knowledge you learned in school? How long ago was that? Is your practice based on your unit's protocols? What are those protocols based on? How many nursing journals do you read? What drives you to read them? What determines when you consider a change in your practice? Does it come from you or from some outside source? How often do you search the Internet for medical and nursing information? What are your sources of information?

Many clinicians will admit that they often do things because of past practice. Something stuck in their minds that worked. We are all very influenced by extreme events that stand out vividly in our memories—those in which something very positive or very negative occurred. Nursing practice is often directed by such events. Although learning from past peak experiences is important, there is danger in allowing those critical events to direct our practice too much, as you will see in TACTICS 8-1.

TACTICS 8-1

Clinicians, On What Evidence Do You Base Your Practice?

Reflect on these issues:

1. What in your past has been a "critical event" in your nursing practice? (Examples: A patient fell after you gave him a vaccination. A patient started to yell loudly when you touched her arm. A patient told you he could always breathe better after drinking a glass of cold water. A clogged percutaneous endoscopic gastrostomy (PEG) tube opened up miraculously when you flushed it with Coca Cola.)
2. Was it a positive or negative event?
3. When and under what circumstances did it occur?
4. How much has this event influenced how you practice in similar situations?

After answering those questions, think about the CT dimensions you used and why. Then, for even more detailed thinking, consider how to search for evidence to support or negate what you are doing in that area of practice. You may want to read the rest of this chapter and Chapter 9 before you start your search because we'll discuss the thinking that will help you with that search.

Discussion

Without *reflection* such as this, we can go merrily along without realizing what a tenuous basis there is for our actions. We have a saying that you've probably used yourself: "She's basing that practice on an 'N of one.'" The danger, of course, in basing actions on an "N of one" is that the event may have been a fluke. Flukes are definitely not part of EBP (except perhaps to fishermen? . . . Groan . . .). What worked well for one patient does not provide evidence for generalizing to other patients.

Educators: On What Evidence Do You Base the Information You Teach?

Just as we've asked clinicians to reflect on their practice, we ask educators to consider the knowledge base they use for teaching. How old is it? Are you teaching the most current evidence, and are you encouraging your students to seek out the best evidence?

TACTICS 8-2

Educators, On What Evidence Do You Base the Information You Teach?

How are you doing with promoting EBP? Look at your last teaching plan and answer these questions:

1. Am I handing down information, or helping students seek knowledge?
2. How old is the information I'm using?
3. How many times do I use the word *evidence* or *EBP*?
4. Have I searched for the latest evidence on this topic?
5. If I searched, how did I evaluate the evidence I found?
6. Do any of my course objectives address EBP and thinking?

Discussion

Most educators would like to think that they teach the most up-to-date information, but it is easy to get in a rut and use the same notes year after year. That can no longer be an option. If we expect clinicians to access and use the best evidence for practice, we need to teach them how to do just that. We need to demonstrate how we are finding and evaluating new information. In the next section, which links CT with EBP, you will see how teaching can promote that thinking.

If you really want to embrace basing teaching on the best evidence, ask yourself not just about the content you teach but also these questions about your teaching methods: How is my teaching? Am I simply teaching with strategies I've used for years? Where is the research on teaching and learning that could enhance my process of teaching? Reflection on evidence-based teaching as an equal partner with teaching evidence-based content is essential for developing the nurses of today and tomorrow.

BOX 8-3	Comparing Old and New Thinking

Old Thinking	New Thinking
Follow usual practice until an authority hands down a new policy.	Question practice constantly. Is this the best, most efficient, most cost-effective, safest way to do _____?
Knowledge is static.	Knowledge is dynamic. There's always something new being discovered.
Practice is discipline specific.	Practice is interdisciplinary.
Practice guidelines and policies are developed by management.	Practice guidelines and policies are developed by all nurses and other disciplines too.
Searching for evidence to support practice is someone else's job.	Searching for evidence to support *my* practice is *my* job.
Knowledge is factual information.	Evidence-based practice means *transforming knowledge*—judging and adapting it.

Links Between Critical Thinking and EBP

Not only are there specific thinking strategies involved in EBP, but the whole notion of practice based on evidence is a shift of thinking. Consider this comparison of old and new thinking in **Box 8-3**. Once you have the new thinking mindset, you can think about the tasks and link them with CT dimensions.

A clear connection between all dimensions of CT and EBP can be made. In **Figure 8-1**, eight steps as thinking "landings" on the path of EBP are identified, and superimposed on the path are all the CT skills and habits of the mind. Because CT skills and habits of the mind are used in harmony, there is no absolute step or stop in the EBP process in which only one or two CT dimensions are used alone. However, certain parts of the EBP process demand more of some skills and habits of the mind than do others. Look back to the beginning of this chapter (pp. 191–192) to the four tasks set forth by the IOM (2003) as necessary to EBP. There are many such lists of tasks or steps to this process; most have a sequence of asking questions, looking for evidence, appraising evidence, using the evidence to improve practice, and evaluating the effectiveness of the practice revision. Although such lists appear linear, EBP is not simple; it's a set of complex tasks, all of which require CT. We have simplified the task list a little in Figure 8-1 to superimpose the thinking dimensions onto the components of EBP. Let's walk through that process. Before continuing, look again at Figure 8-1 to appreciate the whole, and then start at the bold **Questioning Practice** point on the left.

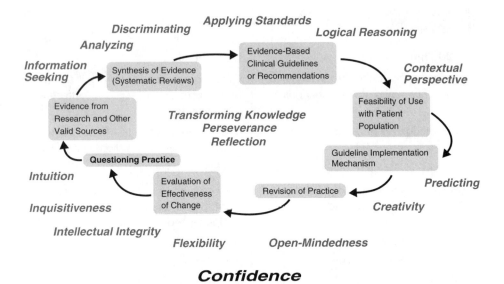

Confidence

FIGURE 8-1 Inter-relationships of CT skills and habits of the mind and components of EBP.

Questioning Practice

This questioning is the absolute essential starting point on the path of EBP; one must approach health care, specifically nursing practice, as a dynamic process that changes as our knowledge base grows and patients' situations change. The initial question might have to do with almost anything—an intervention (e.g., what's the best way to flush PEG tubes?), a specific patient population characteristic (e.g., what's the ideal blood pressure for this diabetic patient?), a potential complication (e.g., if I turn this patient more often than every 2 hours, can I prevent a pressure ulcer?), an expected outcome (e.g., what is the likelihood of this patient getting a urinary tract infection?), or a specific task (e.g., do I need to do this dressing as a sterile procedure?).

Once a question arises, it is important to ask it in a way that will help you search for answers. Straus et al. (2005) have helpful lessons for this task. First, use your *discriminating* skill to distinguish between *background questions* and *foreground questions*. A background question is the kind that one asks in a new situation—for example, *how does acetaminophen work?* An answer to that question could be found in a drug reference book. Foreground questions are more specific and are those posed for EBP—for example, *which works best to reduce fever, acetaminophen or ibuprofen?*

To help one's thinking while formulating foreground questions, many authors (e.g., Melnyk & Fineout-Overholt, 2005) advocate arranging thoughts in the PICO format: P—Patient population of interest; I—Intervention of interest, which could be a treatment, patient perception, test, prognosis, and so on; C—Comparison of interest, for example, the usual practice or another intervention; and O—Outcome of interest.

So, are you ready to try your hand at these kinds of questions? Down with passivity! Use these CT habits of the mind: *inquisitiveness* (be curious), *intellectual integrity* (look for answers even if they might go against what you're presently comfortable with), and *intuition* (listen to your gut). For a simple start, think about your area of practice and consider this question: Is there a better, more efficient, safer, less expensive way to do _____? Here are some examples to help you get in the groove: (1) For elderly patients (P), does exercise (I) work as well as laxatives (C) to decrease constipation (O)? (2) How do women (P) with fibromyalgia (I) perceive changes (C) in their quality of life (O)? (3) For elderly patients with pressure ulcers (P), are wet-to-dry dressings (I) as effective as mechanical debridement (C) in time of healing (O)?

Inquisitiveness makes that questioning process come alive when clinicians wonder if they are practicing in the best possible way. Nurses who are eager to know and seek knowledge and understanding because they are naturally curious will more than likely seek the best knowledge/evidence all the time. They are the seekers of knowledge, not the takers. Seeking is an active process; taking is a passive process.

Intellectual integrity augments that *inquisitiveness*; nurses who value EBP will seek the truth of best practice evidence even when that questioning makes more work and increases discomfort as the status quo is shaken up. Nurses with strong *intellectual integrity* will give up traditional care approaches when there is clear evidence for considering changes in practice. An "N of one" will not be considered a legitimate source of evidence.

Another part of questioning practice is *intuition*. Think about nurses who have "gut feelings" that there must be a better way to do something. It's a fairly common phenomenon that is often not acknowledged because on the surface, it seems not to be part of EBP. However, those vague feelings that there should or might be better approaches often drive nurses to go further, searching for those improved possibilities.

Only after clinicians' questions become focused can they look for the best evidence to find answers. Although we have the CT dimension *discriminating* a little further along the path, clinicians definitely use it to help them hone the question. Remember our discussion of problem-based learning in Chapter 4—that focusing on a problem or question makes way for the exploration and learning that follows in this EBP process.

Thinking While Searching for and Evaluating Evidence

Move to the next EBP "landing" in Figure 8-1. We have listed three sources of evidence that require thinking. The search for evidence can be approached in many different ways. Some start with information in its most synthesized, usable form, which for nurses is usually an evidence-based clinical practice guideline. Others build up from specific reports of research studies. The search process and its accompanying thinking can be a convoluted path.

The best evidence doesn't magically appear in front of each clinician; there must be some effort at *information seeking*. In the old way of thinking, nurses practiced one way until a manager came along and handed out a new policy. Today, with EBP, there will be management-level mandates for change, but each individual nurse cannot wait for that information to be distributed to him or her. There is too much evidence appearing constantly. Nurses must individually and collectively exercise professional role accountability and promote *information seeking* to find the best practice standards. They must move beyond expecting to find answers in their immediate environments—a book or a colleague—and learn how to find for themselves the best information from multiple sources. Did you catch that? Don't be tempted to stop after finding one source!

This *information-seeking* process seems at first very complex and may be overwhelming to nurses with limited backgrounds in research language and methods. However, increasingly there are excellent resources that offer assistance in how to find, analyze, and critique the quality of evidence (for example, DiCenso, Guyatt, & Ciliska, 2005; Melnyk & Fineout-Overholt, 2005). We also have lots of help from technology today as we do online searches for new evidence. We will discuss this more in Chapter 9, but for now, think about your abilities relative to search technologies. Have you searched a CINAHL or MEDLINE database on a computer? Can you define a topic narrowly or broadly enough to be successful in finding articles?

Beyond the availability of computer searches and new technology, nurses must approach gathering evidence with their *analyzing* skills in top form. The process of searching for evidence is easier when the question has specific parameters. The best search techniques must be sought and used, and when difficulties in finding evidence arise, the searcher must again turn to *analysis* to figure out how to break down the search problems further. Librarians, especially those with health sciences or medical specialties, are a wonderful resource to help with searches.

Evidence from Research and Other Valid Sources

We're sure our readers have all done some searching for articles. Nevertheless, to illustrate this process, let's look at an example: Say you're a nurse on a surgical floor, and you're interested in decreasing post-op infections and finding the best way to do wound dressings. You might frame the question in PICO language as this: In adult patients, which postoperative wound care results in low infection rates? You could take a traditional approach to searching that you probably learned in school. Go to a health-related database (PubMed is our current favorite) and do a literature search. What words would you search under? We did just that by logging on to our university library, pulling up the PubMed database, and typing in these subjects:

"wound care" and "nursing." A total of 1,090 results came up, with article titles as diverse as "hemi-pelvic amputations" and "risk factors for thromboembolism." Using *analyzing* to break things down more, we added a time frame of the past 2 years and took out options for letters and editorials (leaving research, clinical guidelines, and so on). A total of 46 articles were then listed. Subjects were still pretty diverse, such as "healthcare-associated pneumonia" and "evaluation of lower extremity arterial circulation." Nevertheless, we were able to scan through 46 titles, marking those that seemed to relate to wounds and nursing. After downloading and reading a couple of articles, we did not feel we had a good grasp on the body of evidence out there, but we certainly were using our thinking dimensions of *information seeking* and *analyzing*. Using more analysis, one decides if articles are research based and, using *discriminating* and *applying standards*, one decides on the quality of that research. **Box 8-4** contains a simple set of criteria for judging a research article.

BOX 8-4	**Judging the Quality of Research Articles**

Is the study valid?

> What type of study is it?
>> Did the researchers clearly state their purpose?
> What do I know about this method of study?
>> Did the researchers follow the rules of the method?
>> Were there factors that may have interfered with the integrity of the research?
> What resources do I need to help me determine if this is a valid study?

What does the study tell me?

> What are the results?
> Are there clear links between the data collected and the conclusions reached?
> What resources do I need to interpret the results?
> How do these results compare with results found in similar studies?

Can I use the results of the study?

> Can the results be generalized?
> Is the study population similar to my patient population?
> What do the researchers say about applicability of results?

Source: Adapted from Cullum & Guyatt, 2005.

As an aside here, we need to note that we are assuming that most readers have a working knowledge of the scientific research process and are able to recognize a research study and read it critically. It is obviously beyond the scope of this book to go into all of that. If you need to refresh that part of your knowledge, we recommend you review a research textbook and/or find a colleague with more experience and/or education, such as a clinical nurse specialist, and ask for help analyzing the article.

Continuing with our searching example, we decided that our quest to find the best evidence on wound care should focus on infections. Our next step was to visit the Cochrane Library to look for systematic reviews of evidence related to postoperative infections. We'll discuss the thinking surrounding systematic reviews and then come back to this example as we move through our critical thinking skills and habits of the mind.

Evidence from Synthesized Sources (Systematic Reviews)

Fortunately, today there are many professional groups that collect research findings, do analyses, and compile syntheses of evidence bases, often called systematic reviews. Some of these sources we mentioned earlier—AHRQ and the Cochrane Collection are popular examples. These groups are doing the time-consuming job of collecting the evidence (articles and so forth), making judgments about the quality of that evidence, and compiling it into reports.

The Cochrane Collaboration is currently the largest organization that produces and maintains systematic reviews in health care, and its library can be accessed by any organization with a subscription. In the Cochrane Collection, we found, for example, one systematic review on dressings and topical agents for surgical wounds (Vermeulen, Ubbink, Goossens, de Vos, & Legemate, 2004), and another on removal of nail polish and rings to prevent surgical infection (Arrowsmith, Maunder, Taylor, & Sargent, 2001).

So, where does that take us relative to EBP? Can we shut down our thinking a bit because we have found reviews by the prestigious Cochrane group? You know that the answer to that must be "no," of course. Whether nurses are finding specific research reports or finding compilations of research (systematic reviews), those sources must be read with *discrimination*. Nurses must *analyze* reports and *discriminate* the quality of the evidence. There are standards to help clinicians do just that, and nurses are *applying standards* as they judge the quality of the evidence and the conclusions reached by those conducting reviews.

A very important part of understanding and *discriminating* systematic reviews is determining how the evidence was gathered and judged for strength. There are standards that should have been applied, and you need to look for them. Systematic reviews, if they are indeed "systematic," must report how the evidence was collected so that you, the reader, can judge whether it was thorough and systematic. Theoretically, you should be able to reproduce what they found by following the report of their search process. You must be able to see the strength of the evidence and how that strength was judged. The Cochrane Library has a reputation

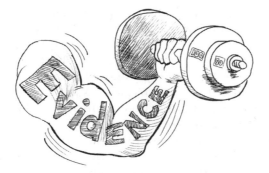

for excellence in doing reviews that is equaled by no other group, so you might be able to trust their reviews a bit more than those of other organizations. Nevertheless, keep that keen *analytical* and *discriminating* ability in high gear at all times.

Now, how about the issue of "strength of evidence"? There are heated debates over what constitutes legitimate and/or best evidence. All systematic reviews should report the evidence hierarchy used. There are no universal evidence hierarchies, but one similar to this example from Stetler et al. (1998) is commonly seen:

I. Meta-analysis of multiple controlled studies
II. Individual experimental study
III. Quasi-experimental study
IV. Nonexperimental study (for example, descriptive, qualitative, and case studies)
V. Systematically obtained, verifiable quality improvement program evaluation of case report data
VI. Opinions of nationally known authorities based on their experience or the opinions of an expert committee, including the interpretation of non-research-based information; regulatory or legal opinions

You will note that this hierarchy has meta-analysis of multiple controlled studies at the top. Many groups, such as the Cochrane Collaboration (Higgins & Green, 2008), have specified RCTs as the gold standard for the best evidence. Recently, methods of judging evidence have been questioned because in some areas of practice, we have only expert opinions and no research; also, there is a vast amount of research that is noncontrolled, descriptive, qualitative, and so forth. Groups such as the Cochrane Collaboration, with stringent standards for "evidence," therefore include fewer nursing studies in their reviews. The danger of evidence hierarchies that place controlled, quantitative research findings at the top is that other forms of evidence may be eliminated (Holmes, Perron, & O'Byrne, 2006). Caution in being too rigid is being advocated (Romyn et al., 2003). Some nurses advocate revised hierarchies because there are few RCTs in nursing (Cesario, Morin, & Santa-Donato, 2002). Hudson and colleagues (2008) went so far as to say, "Nursing is too contextual to have a fixed hierarchy" (p. 414).

In response to the challenge to include qualitative research in systematic reviews, the Cochrane Collaboration set up a Cochrane Qualitative Research Methods Group in conjunction with the JBI (http://www.joannabriggs.edu.au/cqrmg/about.html). The 2008 Cochrane reviewers' handbook had this to say, while acknowledging that they focus primarily on systematic reviews of RCTs: "evidence derived from qualitative studies complements systematic reviews of quantitative studies" (Higgins & Green, 2008, Part 3: Special Topics, 20.1 Introduction).

We are still at a point of debating the issue of evidence and its relative strength. We are not at the point at which we have widely accepted standards. Perhaps we will have more standardization by the time you read this, but more than likely, because nursing is always *contextual* and evidence comes from many sources, several approaches will remain for determining strength of evidence.

Ultimately, readers of systematic reviews must always look for criteria used to determine the strength of evidence. Because there are no hard and fast rules about what constitutes the "best" evidence, the reader's thinking is crucial. Readers must have *discriminating* abilities to see similarities and differences in the various studies and the conclusions about the body of evidence. They must look for and *apply standards* while thinking. We have provided a set of standards in **Box 8-5** to start this thinking process.

Evidence from Clinical Guidelines or Recommendations

Ultimately, because EBP is all about improving practice, clinicians need evidence translated into practice recommendations or clinical guidelines. Many groups that do systematic reviews go the next step and develop those guidelines. If you visit some of the Web sites in Box 8-2 on page 196, you will find lists of evidence-based clinical guidelines and/or links to sites with guidelines. However, you can't turn off your brain after you find a guideline. You must use those thinking dimensions we discussed in the preceding section and add logical reasoning. All conclusions reached about what should be done in practice must be supported

---

| **BOX 8-5** | **Judging the Quality of Systematic Reviews** |

- Did a reliable, qualified person or group conduct the review?
- Is the method used for collecting and including studies clearly stated?
- Is a hierarchy of strength of evidence clearly described?
- What is the likelihood that valid studies were missed?
- When was the review done? What studies may have occurred since then?
- What conclusions were made?
- Can the conclusions be tracked back to specific studies?

by the evidence and your logical reasoning. When using prepared guidelines, one must look to see if the trail from evidence to recommendations can be easily tracked. Only after that are you ready to consider if these guidelines fit with your patients' situations.

Many groups offer standards for evaluating clinical guidelines. We've compiled a list of them in **Box 8-6** using the references we included in that box. We recommend that our readers access The AGREE Collaboration project (2001) for a more comprehensive instrument that has been tested for validity and reliability (The AGREE Collaboration, 2003). One must never assume that guidelines are based on the best evidence, even if a seemingly trustworthy group developed them. We have to use *analyzing* and *logical reasoning*, and *apply standards* to make our own judgments about how evidence-based those guidelines are. There is much potential for harm if guidelines are used without their careful evaluation (Woolf, Grol, Hutchinson, Eccles, & Grimshaw, 1999).

BOX 8-6	**Judging Clinical Practice Guidelines**

- Is the guideline too vague to be usable?
- Is the guideline too specific to be practical with your patient group?
- Who developed the guideline?
- Are the developers qualified to develop this guideline?
- How broad is the representation of the group?
- Were healthcare consumers part of the group?
- Are there any potential conflicts of interest because of developers or sponsors of the guideline?
- Is there a clear explanation of the evidence used to develop the guideline?
- Is there an explanation of how the strength of evidence was determined?
- Could you retrieve the evidence easily?
- How strong is the evidence supporting the guideline's recommendations?
- What is the date of this guideline? Is it current?
- When was it last updated? Is there a reasonable pattern of updates?
- Has it been tested? By whom?
- Are there other guidelines available in the same area? If so, how consistent are they?

Sources: The AGREE Collaboration, 2001; Centre for Health Evidence, 2001; Grol, Dalhuijsen, Veld, Rutten, & Mokkink, 1998; National Guideline Clearing House, n.d.; Shekelle, Woolf, Eccles, & Grimshaw, 1999; Thomson, Lavendere, & Madhok, 1995.

Feasibility of Use with Patient Population

Once evidence-based clinical guidelines are found or established, one must determine the feasibility and desirability of using those guidelines in a specific practice setting. This activity certainly requires a *contextual perspective*. One must consider the patient population, their preferences, and their values. One must consider the institution in which the guidelines are to be used. How feasible is it to implement those guidelines? What resources are available for implementing them?

Considering the feasibility of using evidence-based guidelines with specific patient groups is best done by those providers working directly with patients and by patients themselves. Academics cannot stand afar and say that certain guidelines must be used with all patients. People who know patients best should make these decisions. However, those folks—providers and patients—must be educated about EBP and what constitutes good, better, and best evidence. Making decisions about feasibility of evidence-based guidelines is a CT process.

Some might say that EBP is the antithesis of CT, viewing EBP as following the recommendations/guidelines that are formulated (often by groups outside one's personal arena) in cookbook fashion. Sackett, Rosenberg, Gray, Haynes, and Richardson (1996) responded to this best: "Evidence-based medicine is not 'cookbook' medicine. Because it requires a bottom-up approach that integrates the best external evidence with individual clinical expertise and patient-choice, it cannot result in slavish, cook-book approaches to individual patient care" (para 6). We need to be cognizant of the temptations, however. More and more, we can find quick references that tell us they have the best evidence (e.g., Slawson, Shaughnessy, Ebell, & Barry, 2007). Taking such a reference and changing practice based on its recommendations without CT will result in cookbook approaches. Such behaviors cannot be called EBP.

If, in the ideal world, we had evidence-based guidelines that appeared in front of us in a timely manner, there still would be a need for the *contextual perspective* of CT. As with any "standardized" approach, such as assessment guidelines or clinical pathways, there will always be those who have an image of patient assembly lines and who just "do the job and go home." However, as most nurses realize, thankfully, the individuality of patients supersedes all such imagery and forces even the most slothful nurse to think. Evidence-based guidelines actually provide clinicians with tools that augment rather than impede CT. Consider this example: You go to the JBI Web site and find a best practice sheet, Management of Constipation in Older Adults (JBI, 2008), and you see that increasing fiber in the diet is recommended as a first-line intervention. Now, if you don't look at the context of your patient, you may do more harm than good. Have you considered the patient's other health issues? Can the patient drink enough fluid to keep the fiber from hardening? If you haven't considered the whole *context*, you may be worsening the problem and causing an impaction.

Guideline Implementation Mechanism

Predicting as a CT skill is imperative as nurses move toward a specific plan or mechanism to implement evidence-based guidelines. As anyone who has promoted change will quickly tell you, this process also requires *creativity*. How do you get clinicians, educators, and patients to value evidence-based guidelines enough to commit to implementing those guidelines? How do you devise a system easy enough to follow that the system of implementation doesn't bog down? Sometimes it's as simple as thinking about the people who will be implementing the guideline and talking to them about what they think is the best mechanism.

Recently at a conference on EBP, one of the speakers was discussing such mechanisms. Being gung-ho informatics advocates, we expected this educator to say that he was developing some elaborate plan for his medical students to download guidelines onto their personal digital assistants. When asked, he replied, "Oh no, I'm thinking along the lines of a laminated card for students and residents to carry in their pockets." It's hard to predict at this point in time, but maybe the old-fashioned approaches still work the best; because we are asking people to change what they do, maybe we will have more luck if we keep the mechanism of implementing that change simple.

Revision of Practice

Ultimately, if practice is to be revised to be consistent with best evidence, all those involved in the process must be *open-minded* and *flexible* in their thinking. The persons advocating the change in practice must not demoralize those who would prefer to hang on to tradition, but use *creativity* to help them increase their *flexibility*. This is, of course, no easy task. It is beyond the scope of this chapter and this book to describe all the dynamics of the change process, but certainly anyone contemplating a true commitment to EBP will want to think about all the nuances and strategies for successful change. We discuss the thinking involved in change in Chapter 11, "Thinking Realities of Yesterday, Today, and Tomorrow," but before we leave this subject, we'd like you to reflect on your reaction to the last change proposed at your institution.

TACTICS 8-3

How Have You Reacted to Past Practice Changes?

Clinicians and Educators

Take a few minutes and think about a practice or teaching/curriculum change that you either supported or resisted—the ban on acrylic nails, moving IV flushes from heparin to saline, changing skills checkoffs to a less rigid format, moving from sterile to clean techniques for dressings, and so on. Use these questions to guide your reflection.

1. Did I support this or not?
2. If I did, how did I show that support?
3. If I didn't, how did I react?
4. Were my comments and actions proactive or reactive?
5. Was my response emotional or based on my thinking, or a combination of both?
6. How much knowledge did I have in making my decision to support or not support this?
7. How confident was I in my reasoning?

Discussion

Although we haven't talked much about the change process in this chapter, it is clear that approaching practice and education with an evidence-based perspective requires some change on our parts. Neither practice nor education is static; both are dynamic. It behooves us all to think about how we deal with change generally, and how we deal with practice changes specifically. Change not only requires effort in thinking, but it also takes time. Change can be uncomfortable; discomfort will interfere with thinking and decision making. Recognizing this fact of life helps in planning changes.

Evaluation of Effectiveness of Change

Evaluating the effectiveness of a specific change of practice based on evidence is very important. Besides showing us if this was a good move, the evaluation process reminds us to continue questioning practice. We should no more go on our way thinking that a new approach to practice allows us to rest on our laurels than we should continue blindly doing what we've always done. We must critically evaluate what's been done and how it can be done even better.

Judging the effectiveness of a change requires planning ahead (*predicting*) to determine important data to collect, when to collect them, and for how long. It requires *logical reasoning* as one makes conclusions about this change. The skeptics will sit up and take notice when we can show, with objective data, why this change saved money, increased patient satisfaction, decreased complications or length of stay, and so forth.

Back to the Whole Picture of CT and EBP

EBP is not for the fainthearted. That's why CT *confidence* is written across the bottom of Figure 8-1 as the "sine qua non" of this process. It is hoped that you have developed *confidence* in your thinking skills as you have learned to embrace EBP. Three other CT dimensions cross over and are used through the entire EBP process: *transforming knowledge, reflection,* and *perseverance.*

EBP **is** *transforming knowledge*: The whole EBP process is the quintessential example of that CT skill. We are taking evidence and adapting it to our uses. McWilliam (2007) described the role of continuing education in EBP as one of "transformative knowledge translation."

EBP is also a process of *reflection* at each stop along the way. One must constantly *reflect* on practice, the need for change, the change process, the results of the change, and so forth. And, as anyone who has tried to practice nursing with an EBP approach realizes, *perseverance* in one's thinking processes is also essential. There will certainly be obstacles, some big and some small, depending on how large a change is required based on the evidence available. Ultimately, although the picture of the interrelationships of the CT components and the components of EBP might look like a neat oval process, it is, of course, not that clean, nor are the "steps" mutually exclusive. Just as happens when nurses use the nursing process, there is a lot of back and forth, modifying, adjusting, thinking, and rethinking along the way.

Big, Small, Individual, and Group Moves Toward EBP

As we have been discussing EBP so far, aside from our little foray into searching for information on wound care, we have not specified examples of EBP in action. Individual nurses can move to EBP thinking as a daily process and/or can focus on moving their teams in that direction. It is certainly ideal to work with a team that values EBP. That group will share evidence they find; they will plan changes together and support each other in the process. We often think that CT is an individual phenomenon, but look at the thinking points in Figure 8-1 from the perspective of your group. Then, if you're really brave, keep your EBP hat on and look at it from the perspective of interdisciplinary teams as described in Chapter 7.

Now, consider EBP in terms of magnitude. Sometimes a major change in policies and procedures is called for as we get new evidence. Take, for example, the recent strong evidence that tight control of glucose post-op for cardiac patients drastically reduces sternal infections (Clement et al., 2004; The ACE/ADA Task Force on Inpatient Diabetes, 2006). Many institutions are working on new protocols for glucose control via IV insulin. Here in Michigan, for example, Marcia Hegstad, clinical nurse specialist for diabetes at a large teaching hospital, has done extensive work with an interdisciplinary team to develop guidelines for physicians and nurses to follow based on this evidence (M. Hegstad, personal communication, July 20, 2004). That change in practice has been hugely effective in reducing the incidence of sternal infections post–cardiac surgery. Extensive interdisciplinary team thinking went into that EBP area. Look at Chapter 11 for more details of Marcia's story.

Here's an example of a smaller nature—one nurse with an EBP mindset. Imagine this scenario: A nursing assistant on an adult medical-surgical unit takes vital signs on all patients. Nurse A glances at the results, sees nothing very far above 140/90 (the traditional "normal"), tells the aide to record them, and goes on with the day.

Now, using *analysis* and a *contextual perspective*, Nurse B might think about the data as they relate to the specific patient, evaluating the normalcy of each reading.

If Nurse B is thinking about EBP, the diabetic patient with a blood pressure of 140/90 will stand out as in need of attention because that nurse will be aware of the best evidence to direct practice and will apply that knowledge to the patients she is taking care of. The American Diabetes Association (ADA; 2008), in its recommendations for hypertension management in diabetics, used strong research evidence from the UK Prospective Diabetes Study (UKPDS) (Adler et al., 2000), which showed that for each 10-mmHg decrease in systolic blood pressure, there was a 12% decrease in risks for any complication, a 15% decrease in the risk for diabetes-related death, an 11% decrease in the risk for myocardial infarction, and 13% decrease in the risk of microvascular complications. Citing the UKPDS and other strong evidence, the ADA developed guidelines (easily accessible on its Web site, http://www.diabetes.org) recommending that blood pressures of less than 130/80 be maintained for diabetics.

Any nurse working with diabetics—and these days, that includes virtually all nurses—must vow to keep abreast of the enormous body of diabetes research evidence that has exploded over the past few years and that continues to change. Fortunately, groups such as the ADA continually review that research systematically and translate the evidence into clinical guidelines that are reviewed and updated yearly. All guidelines are freely available on the ADA Web site. Nevertheless, many clinicians who work with diabetic patients continue to practice with information they learned in school or with 5-year-old protocols. We should question why that is so.

In this example, we used the CT skill of *analyzing* and the habit of the mind, *contextual perspective*, to illustrate a first step toward EBP. However, nurses in similar situations would need to use far more CT skills and habits to fully accomplish a goal of EBP. As we discussed earlier, two of the most important habits of the mind to promote those early steps toward EBP are *inquisitiveness* and *intellectual integrity*.

TACTICS 8-4

Clinical Practice "Question of the Month"

Clinicians

Try this on your unit: Each month, create a contest for the best clinical practice question. You might want to make cards with an explanation of the PICO components to help people word their questions succinctly. Encourage nurses to search for guidelines or evidence to support or negate usual practice, and post them in a specific place such as the gathering room. Rewards can be whatever is most coveted by that group—time off, money for conferences, a new uniform, or "chits" that can be saved and turned in for things such as being taken off the float list for 6 months. Such behavior could be built into performance evaluation criteria.

Take that a step further and post criteria for evaluating the strength of evidence of a summary report or a clinical guideline. (Consider using the AGREE instrument described earlier.) Have a contest for who can most accurately judge the strength of evidence for changing practice. If you want to really take it further, have nurses identify the thinking skills and habits of the mind used in this activity.

Educators

Use the same strategy with students. Whatever course you're teaching, build into your syllabus credit for students formulating questions about practice, finding the latest evidence, evaluating it, and discussing if and how that evidence should be used.

Discussion

As educators, we have used this tactic to teach EBP principles. In our nursing research classes, we have students write their major paper on a clinical issue that they explore for the latest evidence. They show their knowledge of the research process in discussing the evidence they found. **Box 8-7** has several other general suggestions for activities to promote EBP, both in clinical and classroom situations. We hope that they will help you think of specific TACTICS that will work for you.

BOX 8-7 | **Suggestions for Promoting EBP in Clinical and Classroom Settings**

- Incorporate reflection activities into assignments that require thinking about EBP.
- Have students or nurses work in groups to do an EBP activity of their choice and identify how the 17 dimensions of CT were used in that activity.
- Create an EBP Tracking Thinking Diagram modeled after Figure 8-1, or let students create one.
- Build EBP expectations into evaluation criteria for promotions or grades.
- Make a list of how you can socialize a group to emphasize not only EBP but also the underlying thinking skills needed to operationalize EBP.
- Take a guideline that would be familiar to most students and nurses, such as the *Guideline for Hand Hygiene in Health-Care Settings* (Centers for Disease Control and Prevention, 2002); have them find several of the studies used as evidence for the recommendations, and discuss how the Centers for Disease Control and Prevention (CDC) decided on strength of evidence.
- Develop a rubric for assessing evidence-based guidelines in your setting.

One Nurse's Story of Successful EBP

Before we end this chapter, we'd like to share an EBP thinking story. Judy Meyers is a clinical nurse specialist in gerontology who has successfully cultivated EBP on her inpatient unit at a large teaching hospital in Michigan (J. Meyers, personal communication, December 5, 2008). She has, over the past few years, instituted changes in several areas of practice: use of fewer indwelling Foley catheters, a protocol to assess and treat agitation, decreasing the number of orders for bed rest, liberalized diets for the elderly, and an activity project to get older people up and moving. She is now working on a plan to improve nurse–physician communication. Here are some excerpts from our conversation, especially those in which she revealed her thinking as she planned and instituted these innovations. You will also note that she makes reference (without prompting, we might add) not only to EBP but also to the other four IOM competencies: interdisciplinary practice, patient-centered care, quality improvement, and use of informatics.

▶ TACTICS 8-5 ──────────────────────────────

Find the Thinking and EBP Components in Judy's Story

Clinicians and Educators

As you read the story, take a pen and circle the parts that illustrate thinking dimensions and those that exemplify EBP. You might also see signs of the other four IOM competencies.

I knew the problems caused by Foley catheters, and so many of our patients had them. I prepared a self-learning module for the nursing staff on bowel and bladder management for older people and, in the bladder part, discussed reasons why you don't want indwelling catheters. I did a literature review and a proposal to change our policy. I found the CDC guidelines for judging when Foleys are necessary and, along with Dr. Alan Dengiz, a geriatrician, we developed a protocol outlining the CDC criteria and four others that we added, such as terminal illness, severe perineal excoriation, etc.

We educated the physicians. I went to the Medical Section meeting to get the support of all the department heads, and they took the information back to their peers. Most of them were in favor of the protocol. We put the protocol into the computer for nurses to follow. They could assess patients and discontinue catheters without waiting for an order from an MD.

In another example, I noticed that we had a lot of patients with orders for bed rest. I worked with physicians on this and tried to get them to understand that this was bad. We audited charts for 3 months to check how many patients had orders for bed rest or bathroom privileges only. We found the older patients were, the more likely they were to have those orders; 52% of patients over 70 had an initial order for bed rest. When questioned, the physicians said they were ordering bed rest because they didn't know what the patient could do.

I did a review of literature and took a proposal to the MDs. I worked with people in electronic data entry and had them take out "bed rest," which was at the top of the order options, and put it at the bottom with a required write-in section for the reason to justify the bed rest order. We also added an option to discontinue bed rest. The percentage of patients with bed rest orders went from 52% to 5%; those who have the orders have things like hip fractures, so those orders are appropriate.

I'm always thinking, what do our patients need? What do we need to be doing better? If I notice something, I collect data. If you want MDs to buy into something, you need data. I check the literature, and I let staff know what I find. They are much more apt to go along with something if they can see why we should be doing it, especially if it's an uncomfortable thing. I think ahead to what's going to be difficult in doing this. I make things as easy as possible. I educate staff, go out and role model what I'm talking about, and I specifically work with people who are resistant.

I also have a great nurse manager who is good at creating the expectations of quality. She is right there in the thick of things. She is committed to excellent care and needs to be doing what is state of the art. She goes to conferences and brings ideas back to me.

Right now we're working on improving nurse–physician communication. Physicians want nurses to give concise, pertinent information; they want nurses to know the patients well. Nurses tend to use narrative approaches and focus on relationships. Some physicians come on the floor and leave without ever talking to a nurse; nurses have to call them more frequently than they should. Right now I'm doing a review of the literature on this subject and planning a quality improvement project for this fall. We'll start small, and most of the initiatives will come from nurses. One idea is to have laminated cards for nurses to use when calling physicians; those cards would have reminders of important information to include in their reports. Another is to institute MD/RN rounds to facilitate sharing information.

Physician geriatricians tend to be EBP advocates. For example, several years ago, one of them saw a bladder scan used in a nursing home and asked me if we could look into getting one. We did, and now every unit in the hospital has one. We did it first. One of the biggest aids to EBP is constant curiosity.

Discussion

We'll bet many of you would like to work with Judy. Are you fortunate enough to work with nurses like her? Are you a nurse like her? She exemplifies EBP, doesn't she?

PAUSE _____

and Ponder

Where Should Our EBP Thinking Go?

OK, so you're totally convinced that EBP is the bandwagon you should be on, right? We hope you can approach this not as a bandwagon but as a thinking journey for excellence in practice. It is a more enlightened and exciting approach that gets us away from tradition as a driving force. However, it is changing very fast, and we must be clear on what we are promoting when we say EBP. As Estabrooks (2003) cautioned, there is a lot of jargon—"research utilization, knowledge utilization, innovation diffusion, technology transfer, evidence-based practice, knowledge translation, knowledge transfer and knowledge mobilization" (p. 62). It is all about using the best thinking and knowledge we have for practice and that knowledge will not just be handed down. Knowledge must be sought actively. Recognizing when we need it, accessing it, evaluating it, using it, and evaluating its usefulness is a constant cycle requiring CT. CT also helps us recognize that not all current knowledge is "bad." We need to be careful that we don't throw the baby out with the bath water. But we have to apply the standards of EBP to support what we keep, what we pitch, and what we update.

Reflection Cues

- EBP is an important paradigm shift away from practice based on tradition to one based on the use of the best knowledge available.
- The IOM envisioned EBP as several tasks—knowing where and how to find best evidence, formulating clinical questions, searching for and evaluating the evidence to answer those questions, and determining how and when to integrate that evidence into practice.
- Links between CT and EBP can be easily tracked.
- The history of EBP shows an international movement that primarily started in the 1980s and continues today.
- There is increasing focus on health consumers' part in the EBP movement.
- EBP is important because most of the time it saves money and other resources and promotes better patient outcomes.
- Clinicians and educators need to reflect on how they use evidence in their daily practice.
- EBP requires the use of all 17 dimensions of CT.
- Questioning practice is augmented by *inquisitiveness, intellectual integrity,* and *intuition*.

- Searching for evidence necessitates the use of informatics and the thinking dimensions of *discriminating, information seeking,* and *analysis.*
- Synthesis of evidence in systematic reviews is done by several groups today, notably the Cochrane Collaboration.
- Users of systematic reviews must evaluate them with *discrimination,* use *analyzing* skills, and *apply standards* for judging quality.
- Mechanisms to judge strength of evidence are currently being studied extensively.
- Using evidence-based clinical guidelines requires *logical reasoning* so that recommendations for practice can be traced back to the evidence.
- A *contextual perspective* is imperative when considering the feasibility of using evidence-based guidelines with patient populations.
- EBP is not cookbook health care.
- Implementing EBP requires *predicting* and *creativity.*
- Revising practice is best done with *open-minded, flexible* thinking.
- Evaluating effectiveness of practice changes requires *logical reasoning* and *predicting.*
- The whole process of EBP requires *confidence* in one's thinking, *reflection,* and *perseverance.*
- EBP is a process of *transforming knowledge.*
- EBP can be done with large innovations or in small, day-to-day increments.
- One nurse's story about how she is using EBP helps us appreciate how this is possible and how important CT is to this process.
- Clinicians and educators must take care not to approach EBP with a bandwagon mentality, but with CT fully engaged.

References

The ACE/ADA Task Force on Inpatient Diabetes. (2006). American college of endocrinology and American Diabetes Association consensus statement on inpatient diabetes and glycemic control. *Diabetes Care, 29,* 1955–1962. doi:10.2337/dc06-9913

Adler, A. I., Stratton, I. M., Neil, A. A., Yudkin, J. S., Matthews, D. R., Cull, C. A., et al. (2000). Association of systolic blood pressure with macrovascular and microvascular complications of type 2 diabetes (UKPDS 36): Prospective observational study. *British Medical Journal, 321,* 412–419.

Agency for Healthcare Research and Quality. (2008, November). *Evidence-based practice centers overview.* Retrieved November 15, 2008, from http://www.ahrq.gov/clinic/epc/

The AGREE Collaboration. (2001). *Appraisal of guidelines for research & evaluation: AGREE instrument.* Retrieved May 14, 2009, from http://www.agreecollaboration.org/pdf/agreeinstrumental.pdf

The AGREE Collaboration. (2003). Development and validation of an international appraisal instrument for assessing the quality of clinical practice guidelines: The AGREE project. *Quality and Safety in Health Care, 12,* 18–23.

American Diabetes Association. (2008). Standards of medical care in diabetes: 2008. *Diabetes Care, 31*(Suppl. I), S12–S54. Retrieved August 18, 2008, from http://care.diabetesjournals. org/content/vol31/Supplement_1/

Archie Cochrane: The name behind the Cochrane Collaboration. Retrieved August 19, 2008, from http://www.cochrane.org/docs/archieco.htm

Arrowsmith, V. A., Maunder, J. A., Taylor, R., & Sargent, R. J. (2001). Removal of nail polish and finger rings to prevent surgical infection. *Cochrane Database of Systematic Reviews* 2001, Issue 1. Art. No.: CD003325. DOI: 10.1002/14651858.CD003325.

Avis, M., & Freshwater, D. (2006). Evidence for practice, epistemology, and critical reflection. *Nursing Philosophy, 7*, 216–224.

Bucknall, T., & Hutchinson, A. M. (2006). Editorial. *Worldviews on Evidence-Based Nursing, 3*, 137–138.

Centers for Disease Control and Prevention. (2002). Guideline for hand hygiene in health-care settings: Recommendations of the healthcare infection control practices advisory committee and the HICPC/SHEA/APIC/IDSA hand hygiene task force. *Morbidity and Mortality Weekly Report, 51*(RR-16), 1–47.

Centre for Health Evidence. (2001). *How to use a clinical practice guideline.* Retrieved August 15, 2008, from http://www.cche.net/usersguides/guideline.asp

Cesario, S., Morin, K., & Santa-Donato, A. (2002). Evaluating the level of evidence of qualitative research. *Journal of Obstetric, Gynecologic, and Neonatal Nursing, 31*, 531–538.

Clement, S., Braithwaite, S. S., Magee, M. F., Ahmann, A., Smith, E. P., Schafer, R. G., et al. (2004). Management of diabetes and hyperglycemia in hospitals. *Diabetes Care, 27*, 553–591.

Cullum, N., & Guyatt, G. (2005). Health care interventions and harm: An introduction. In A. DiCenso, G. Guyatt, & D. Ciliska (Eds.), *Evidence-based nursing: A guide to clinical practice* (pp. 44–70). St. Louis, MO: Elsevier Mosby.

DiCenso, A., Guyatt, G., & Ciliska, D. (2005). *Evidence-based nursing: A guide to clinical practice.* St. Louis, MO: Elsevier Mosby.

Estabrooks, C. A. (2003). Translating research into practice: Implications for organizations and administrators. *Canadian Journal of Nursing Research, 35*(3), 53–68.

Fonteyn, M. (2005). Guest Editorial: The interrelationships among thinking skills, research knowledge, and evidence-based practice. *Journal of Nursing Education, 44*, 439.

Grol, R., Dalhuijsen, J., Veld, C., Rutten, G., & Mokkink, H. (1998). Attributes of clinical guidelines that influence use of guidelines in general practice: Observational study. *British Medical Journal, 317*, 858–861.

Haller, K. B., Reynolds, M. A., & Horsley, J. A. (1979). Developing research-based innovation protocols: Process, criteria and issues. *Research in Nursing and Health, 2*, 45–51.

Hancock, H. C., & Easen, P. R. (2006). The decision-making processes of nurses when extubating patients following cardiac surgery: An ethnographic study. *International Journal of Nursing Studies, 43*, 693–705.

Harbison, J. (2006). Clinical judgement in the interpretation of evidence: A Bayesian approach. *Journal of Clinical Nursing, 15*, 1489–1497. doi:10.1111/j.1365-2702.2005.01487.x

Hayes, R. A. (2005). Introduction to evidence-based practices. In C. E. Stout & R. A. Hayes (Eds.), *The evidence-based practice methods, models, and tools for mental health professionals* (pp. 1–9). Hoboken, NJ: Wiley.

Higgins J. P. T., & Green, S. (Eds.). (2008). *Cochrane handbook for systematic reviews of interventions* Version 5.0.0 (updated February 2008). Retrieved May 14, 2009, from http://www.cochrane-handbook.org

Holmes, D., Murray, S. J., Perron, A., & McCabe, J. (2008). Nursing best practice guidelines: Reflecting on the obscene rise of the void. *Journal of Nursing Management, 16,* 394–403. doi:10.1111/j.1365-2834.2008.00858.x

Holmes, D., Perron, A., & O'Byrne, P. (2006). Evidence, virulence, and the disappearance of nursing knowledge: A critique of the evidence-based dogma. *Worldviews on Evidence-Based Nursing, 3*(3), 95–102.

Hudson, K., Duke, G., Haas, B., & Varnell, G. (2008). Navigating the evidence-based practice maze. *Journal of Nursing Management, 16,* 409–416. doi:10.1111/j.1365-2834.2008.00860.x

Institute of Medicine. (2003). *Health professions education: A bridge to quality.* Washington, DC: National Academies Press.

Jennings, B. M., & Loan, L. A. (2001). Misconceptions among nurses about evidence-based practice. *Journal of Nursing Scholarship, 33,* 121–126.

Joanna Briggs Institute. (2008). Management of constipation in older adults. *Best Practice, 12*(7), 1–4. Retrieved May 14, 2009, from http://www.joannabriggs.edu.au/pdf/BP_Book_Vol12_7.pdf

Mantzoukas, S. (2008). A review of evidence-based practice, nursing research and reflection: Leveling the hierarchy. *Journal of Clinical Nursing, 17,* 214–223. doi:10.1111/j.1365-2702.2006.01912.x

McWilliam, C. L. (2007). Continuing education at the cutting edge: Promoting transformative knowledge translation. *Journal of Continuing Education in the Health Professions, 27*(2), 72–79. doi:10.1002/chp

Melnyk, B. M., & Fineout-Overholt, E. (2005). *Evidence-based practice in nursing and healthcare: A guide to best practice.* Philadelphia: Lippincott Williams & Wilkins.

National Guideline Clearinghouse. (n.d). *Guideline comparison description.* Retrieved August 16, 2008, from http://www.guidelines.gov/about/GuidelineComparisonDescrip.aspx

Pierce, L. L. (2007). Evidence-based practice in rehabilitation nursing. *Rehabilitation Nursing, 32,* 203–209.

Profetto-McGrath, J., Hesketh, K. L., Lang, S., & Estabrooks, C. A. (2003) A study of critical thinking and research utilization among nurses. *Western Journal of Nursing Research, 25,* 322–337.

Rolfe, G. (2005). The deconstructing angel: Nursing, reflection and evidence-based practice. *Nursing Inquiry, 12*(2), 78–86.

Romyn, D. M., Allen, M. N., Boschma, G., Duncan, S. M., Edgecombe, N., Jensen, L. A., et al. (2003). The notion of evidence in evidence-based practice by the nursing philosophy working group. *Journal of Professional Nursing, 19,* 184–188.

Rycroft-Malone, J. (2008). Evidence-informed practice: From individual to context. *Journal of Nursing Management, 16,* 404–408. doi:10.1111/j.1365-2834.2008.00859.x

Sackett, D. L., Rosenberg, W. M. C., Gray, J. A. M., Haynes, R. B., & Richardson, W. S. (1996). Evidence-based medicine: What it is and what it isn't. (Article based on editorial from the *British Medical Journal, 312,* 71–72.) Retrieved August 18, 2008, from http://www.cebm.net/ebm_is_isnt.asp

Sams, L., & Gannon, M. E. (2000). Evidence-based practice and clinical work assessment. *Seminars in Perioperative Nursing, 9*(3), 125–132.

Sandelowski, M. (2004). Using qualitative research. *Qualitative Health Research, 14,* 1366–1386. doi:10.1177/1049732304269672

Scott-Findlay, S., & Pollock, C. (2004). Evidence, research, knowledge: A call for conceptual clarity. *Worldviews on Evidence-Based Nursing, 1,* 92–97.

Shekelle, P. G., Woolf, S. H., Eccles, M., & Grimshaw, J. (1999). Developing guidelines. *British Medical Journal, 318,* 593–596.

Slawson, D., Shaughnessy, A., Ebell, M., & Barry, H. (2007). *Essential evidence: Medicine that matters.* Hoboken, NJ: Wiley.

Stetler, C. B., Brunell, M., Giuliano, K. K., Morsi, D., Prince, L., & Newell-Stokes, V. (1998). Evidence-based practice and the role of nursing leadership. *Journal of Nursing Administration, 28*(7/8), 45–53.

Straus, S. E., Richardson, W. S., Glasziou, P., & Haynes, R. B. (2005). *Evidence-based medicine: How to practice & teach EBM* (3rd ed.). New York: Elsevier Churchill Livingstone.

Thomson, R., Lavendere, M., & Madhok, R. (1995). Fortnightly review: How to ensure that guidelines are effective. *British Medical Journal, 311,* 237–242.

Vermeulen, H., Ubbink, D., Goossens, A., de Vos, R., & Legemate, D. (2004). Dressings and topical agents for surgical wounds healing by secondary intention. *Cochrane Database of Systematic Reviews* 2004, Issue 1. Art. No.: CD003554. DOI: 10.1002/14651858.CD003554.pub2

Woolf, S., Grol, R., Hutchinson, A., Eccles, M., & Grimshaw, J. (1999). Potential benefits, limitations, and harms of clinical guidelines. *British Medical Journal, 318,* 527–530.

CHAPTER 9

Critical Thinking
and Informatics

The computer, the telephone, the Web, video—these, and all that is still to
come, are unquestionably powerful tools. Used badly, they waste time and
money, and dehumanize our interactions with each other. Used well, guided
by a clear understanding of basic informatics principles, they are neither to
be feared, loved nor loathed. They are simply to be used. In the next century, the study of informatics will become as fundamental to the practice of
medicine as anatomy has been to the last.

That poignant statement is from Enrico Coiera's paper, based on an article he
wrote for the *Medical Journal of Australia* in 1998 and posted on the Internet as *10
Essential Clinical Informatics Skills* (1999). He is referring to *informatics*—a term
that is now as much a part of nursing and healthcare delivery as the bedpan.
Although it is commonplace, informatics is not a natural subject for most nurses;
however, it is being thrust upon us as a necessity because computer technology
and the information it processes are here to stay.

Health informatics is about how we process, use, and share information relative
to healthcare delivery. The Institute of Medicine (IOM), with its conjoint emphasis
on patient-centered care, evidence-based practice (EBP), quality improvement, and
interdisciplinary practice, described the competency of utilizing informatics as

"communicate, manage knowledge, mitigate error, and support decision making using information technology" (2003, p. 46).

Informatics, in this definition, is a broad concept covering a wide range of technology—from simple e-mail to complex clinical information systems, from the familiar EKG machine to electronic medical ordering systems, from Power-Point presentations to complete computer-assisted instruction, to high-fidelity simulation learning in the laboratory setting. You get the idea. One can become narrow in view depending on what aspect of informatics one is most involved with. For example, if you are a nurse working in an institution going "paperless," you are focused on the electronic health record; if you are a nurse working in a rural clinic, you might be focused on telehealth; if you are a nursing student, you might be focused on doing a thorough electronic search for evidence.

At any level of involvement, and clearly evident in the IOM definition and Coiera's statement, is that critical thinking (CT) needs to be an integral part of using informatics. Coiera's 10 skills almost all started with words that imply thinking—"understand," "search for and assess," "interpret," "analyze and structure clinical decisions," "adapt and apply knowledge," "access," "assess," "select and apply," "structure and record data," and so forth. The IOM statement included "manage knowledge" and "support decision-making." Using informatics has great potential; it will require a whole lot of thinking, but it will improve our thinking, too. CT's relationship with informatics will be this chapter's focus.

The Context of Old Nurses and Young Informatics

Some of you may be tempted to skip this chapter because you think you won't understand informatics. Maybe it's something you're just not interested in. You probably get really angry at all the cell phone conversations in restaurants and stores, and the exorbitant prices you pay for cable TV and computer games for your teenagers. Stick with us and you'll see you are not alone in your frustration over informatics. We sympathize with you on a personal as well as professional level because we're also "old" nurses dealing with "young" informatics.

If you remember when we didn't use computers every day, you are possibly our age. When we started out in nursing in the late 1960s and early 1970s, computers were props in science fiction movies—big, cumbersome things that filled whole buildings, whirring and whizzing to help the spies. Thirty-some years later, we're unable to imagine life without these machines—now small as peas—that we love and hate. (Yes, Dr. Coiera, in spite of what you say, we do love and hate them.) We love them because they make access to information so easy. We hate them because when they go down, freeze up, flash blue screen messages, lose our last 3 hours of writing, get viruses, and cause other situations too numerous to list, we are left with the realization that we are way too dependent on them. For most of us, that dependency is not only frustrating but also scary because so much of today's technology is mysterious. However, information technology is here to stay, and it's evolving more rapidly than we can fathom. As McBride (2005) said, "There is no aspect of nursing that will be untouched by the informatics revolution in progress" (p. 188).

Those of us in the Baby Boom generation have lived through the birth and rapid growth of computers. We've learned this foreign language later in life. For several years, we wrote with a pen and then typed things into the computer—the old typewriter mentality. (Don't worry; we've grown up; we're now typing original ideas here sans yellow pad.) We oldsters have had to change our ways to keep up with computers. For younger generations, computers are as common as electricity was for most of us back then. However, many nurses are our age and older. The average age of doctorally prepared nursing faculty today is 54.3 years, and for master's-prepared faculty, it is 49.2 (American Association of Colleges of Nursing, 2005). The average age of the working nurse is 46.8 years, and registered nurses (RNs) younger than 30 represent only 8% of our ranks (Health Resources and Services Administration [HRSA], 2007). The majority of nurses did not grow up with computers in their homes; many used a computer for the first time in their places of employment. Many still anxiously stumble along using computers every day.

In an editorial in the *Online Journal of Nursing Informatics*, McGonigle (2006) hit the scary nail on the head when she wrote the following paragraph to illustrate the "abbreviation frenzy" that makes the language of informatics so foreign to many of us:

> When we speak of BI and look for VAP from the VAN it is not so surprising that we crunch IEs on our HPCs. Sometimes we use a DSS. At other times, we look for help from as many people as we can by using VNC, our VM or enlisting VOIP to contact the people "in the know" at the NHIN or RHIOs. Now doesn't that make it as clear as MUD with MOO (para 4).

She gave an abbreviation translation taken from the Biomedical Abbreviation Server (2003): BI = business intelligence; VAP = value-added process; VAN = value-added network; IE = information element; HPC = handheld personal computer; DSS = decision support system; VNC = virtual network computing; VM = virtual machine; VOIP = voice over Internet protocol; NHIN = national health information network; RHIO = regional health information organization; MUD = multi-user dimension/domain; and MOO = MUD, object oriented. We've given you this example not to scare you off, but to help you realize that you're not alone in thinking this new language is beyond you. Others are realizing the challenges and helping with the transition—for example, the Biomedical Abbreviation Server by Chang, Schutze, and Altman (2002).

Almost everyone around us uses computers in some way—if not directly, at least indirectly. We have a U.S. government mandate that all Americans have electronic medical records by 2014, making computer competency an immediate reality (Ornes & Gassert, 2007). In Chapter 6, we discussed patients surfing the Internet to find out things such as what medications they want, the best treatment options, and current standards of care. Consumers of health care have more access to information than they have ever had before. People who think they can survive in this world without integrating informatics into their lives are dinosaurs trying to survive in the 21st century. We're getting ahead of ourselves here, but we want to show you that reading this chapter is worth the effort even though it may be scary to some of us with middle-aged eyes. We apologize to our youthful readers, but, according to the statistics, you are a minority. Let's go back and set up more groundwork.

Healthcare Informatics Evolution

Lest we lead you down a confusing path, and before we join CT with informatics, we'll detour here to discuss the evolution of health informatics more. It used to be that informatics meant computer technology, and so far, we have focused many of our comments in that direction. Because computers were the instigators of this field, we often equate them with informatics. Today, however, the focus of this burgeoning field is more on information and the meanings of information in communicating, sharing knowledge, and decision making.

As you may deduce from that statement, not everyone defines informatics in the same way. The term *informatics*, coined in the 1970s, initially referred to computers and their immediate context (Saba, 2001). Since that time, people have broadened descriptions, some doing it according to discipline. For example, *nursing informatics*, according to Saba and McCormick (2001), is:

> the use of technology and/or a computer system to . . . process . . . and communicate timely data and information in and across healthcare facilities that administer nursing services and resources, manage the delivery of patient and nursing care, link research resources and findings to nursing practice, and apply educational resources to nursing education. (p. 226)

The American Nurses Association (ANA) supports the movement toward informatics in the practice arena and has developed a document, *Nursing Informatics: Scope and Standards of Practice* (2008). The ANA defined the specialty of nursing informatics in this way:

> Nursing informatics (NI) is a specialty that integrates nursing science, computer science, and information science to manage and communicate data, information, knowledge, and wisdom in nursing practice. NI supports consumers, patients, nurses, and other providers in their decision-making in all roles and settings. This support is accomplished through the use of information structures, information processes, and information technology. (ANA, 2008, p. 1)

You may notice that the newer definition from the ANA has a broader focus than the earlier Saba definition. This change reflects the move from computers as the central idea to that of information.

The National League for Nursing (NLN) focused its support on the education arena as demonstrated by its 2008 position statement titled, *Preparing the Next*

Generation of Nurses to Practice in a Technology-Rich Environment: An Informatics Agenda. The position statement was triggered by an NLN survey indicating that:

1. Only 50–60% of respondents identified informatics as being integrated into their curricula, and most of that was primarily in the clinical setting.
2. Only 60% of the programs surveyed had computer literacy as a program requirement.
3. Only 40% of the programs surveyed had an information literacy requirement.
4. Content on informatics was more commonly found in baccalaureate degree programs and higher.

The NLN (2008) concluded that

> there was considerable confusion as to what nursing informatics entails and what constitutes the necessary knowledge to practice in an informatics-rich environment. . . . . (para 4) [and] faculty, deans, administrators, and the NLN itself [must] advocate that all students graduate with up-to-date knowledge and skills in each of three critical areas: computer literacy, information literacy, and informatics. (para 3)

Perhaps because of the published results of that survey, or perhaps in spite of them, it seems that nurses in academic settings are embracing informatics in a big way. Nursing courses are being taught, national conferences are being held, articles, whole journals, and books are emerging, and nursing curricula across the country are integrating informatics with gusto. For example, in Michigan, Oakland University offers NRS 830: Health Care Informatics (Giordana, 2008). Grant dollars are becoming available. A 5-year $1.5 million federal grant from the HRSA—Faculty Development: Integrated Technology into Nursing Education & Practice Initiative—was awarded collectively to five university programs (University of Kansas School of Nursing, University of Kansas Center for Healthcare Informatics, University of Colorado Denver School of Nursing, and Indiana University School of Nursing) and the National League for Nursing to implement the Health Information Technology Scholars Program (2007).

In spite of this mushrooming focus in nursing, there are still debates about informatics being discipline specific—for example, medical informatics versus nursing informatics (Masys, Brennan, Ozbolt, Corn, & Shortliffe, 2000) and the problems with these narrow foci (McBride, 2005). We have broader interdisciplinary definitions, such as biomedical informatics (Columbia University, n.d.), and recently adding to the terminology conundrum are the terms *patient informatics* (e.g., Bader & Braude, 1998; Williams, Gish, Giuse, Sathe, & Carrell, 2001) and *consumer health informatics* (e.g., Eysenbach & Jadad, 2001). *Health literacy* (Kutner, Greenberg, Jin, Paulsen, & White, 2006; Weiss, 2007), *health information literacy* (Medical Library Association, 2005), and *information literacy* (Saranto & Hovenga, 2004) have emerged as close cousins of *informatics* because we are increasingly concerned with how well consumers understand the vast amounts of information available to them.

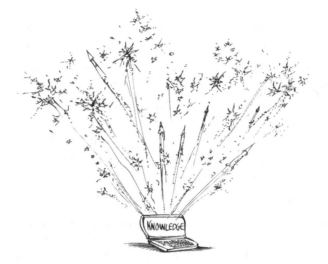

The British folks, in what seems like a commonsense move, have adopted the term *health informatics*. The UK Health Informatics Society (formerly the British Medical Informatics Society) had what seems to be the most straightforward but comprehensive interdisciplinary description of health informatics on its Web site: "[Health informatics] . . . can be best understood as the understanding, skills and tools that enable the sharing and use of information to deliver healthcare and promote health" (2004, para 1). They noted that the term *health informatics* is replacing the term *medical informatics*. The broader term, focused on health, allows all healthcare disciplines and consumers to be part of this important field.

Clearly evident from these various descriptions is that informatics has to do with managing information/knowledge, communicating, and making decisions—all direct links to thinking. The IOM specifically noted its value in preventing errors, which fits with its emphasis on increased safety in health care. The subject of safety and reducing errors in health care was addressed in more detail in Chapter 5.

The Changing Nature of Informatics

In considering how to approach the subject of CT and informatics, we were struck by the real probability that anything we said about informatics would be out of date by the time this book was published. Indeed, as one reads about informatics, one can readily see that unless informatics information has been posted on a Web site in the past 6 months, it is out of date. This rapid rate of change, of course, is due to the increasing sophistication of the technology we use to share and use information.

We're trying to get a feel for where informatics will be going in the near future, but by the time we sit down to write that, the future has become the present. Nevertheless, we'll try to keep as much of a "futuristic" view as possible in our comments about CT and informatics. The IOM, in its Quality Chasm Series, *Patient Safety* (2004), called for three important foci for informatics that can contribute to increased quality in health care. It proposed increased support from government agencies and healthcare systems to accelerate improvement of (1) data exchange formats, (2) structured terminologies, and (3) knowledge representation. These three areas will facilitate recording and accessibility of information, increase the intersystem and interdisciplinary communication, and facilitate decision making. For example, the IOM (2004) would like to see the Agency for Healthcare Research and Quality, the National Institutes of Health, the Food and Drug Administration, and similar agencies support the development of generic clinical guideline models in computer-executable formats to help with EBP and clinical decision support (CDS). You will recall from Chapter 8 that implementation of clinical guidelines is still a challenge, largely because of inadequate mechanisms to facilitate their use in daily practice.

Another interesting view of the present and near future of informatics was articulated by Ball and Lillis (2000). Even though they published this article in 2000, which by informatics standards is very old, their observations about trends remain relevant. Using information from the Gartner Group Research Review, Ball and Lillis discussed eight trends in healthcare information technology, which are paraphrased in **Box 9-1**.

BOX 9-1	**Eight Trends in Healthcare Information Technology**

1. **Data to decisions:** Technology will automate more decision-making processes (for example, decision trees or algorithms).
2. **Communication to collaboration:** There will be more knowledge sharing across cultures, and geography will become irrelevant.
3. **Information to knowledge:** Information will be more integrated via technology (for example, Internet vs. books; e-mail vs. snail mail).
4. **Network computing to ubiquitous computing:** Specifically where the information is stored or processed will become unimportant (for example, desktop computers to laptops to PDAs to pocket whatevers).
5. **Graphical to cognitive user interfaces:** Technologies such as speech recognition and natural language processing will enhance ease of using technology. (This will dramatically change the nature and speed of dictation into medical records, for example.)
6. **Situated to mobile:** We will need to meet the needs of people on the move and in remote locations. (Imagine this example: You work at a small rural center, but you can link to larger facilities easily.)
7. **Physical to virtual:** Technologies such as "smart cards" and "e-commerce" will make things simpler. (I can't wait for my virtual colonoscopy, can you?)
8. **Business to customer:** We will need to consider the needs of users beyond our immediate environment.

Source: Ball & Lillis, 2000.

As you look at the box, you can probably see yourself in the middle of those trends right now, and maybe even past them. The constant rapid rate of change of informatics and our panting as we run alongside to keep up ultimately are reasons why addressing the thinking involved in informatics is so critical. All healthcare providers need to have a CT frame to go along with the rapid changes. That thinking frame will have built into it ways of dealing with the changes in those mechanisms that can enhance our thinking. Linear or dualistic thinking must be minimized; thinking must be primarily *contextual* and relativistic. Thinkers who are uncomfortable with uncertainty will either give up, or they will suffer extreme stress. Stop for a minute and assess (*reflect*) on your style of thinking. Where are you on a continuum, with dualistic thinking (seeing the world dichotomously, such as only black or white, right or wrong) at one end, and relativistic thinking (able to recognize many shades of gray depending on the circumstances and the situation) at the other end? Many of us may be closer to the dualistic end, which helps explain the next paragraph.

It seems that nursing is lagging in its informatics competency (Fetter, 2008; NLN, 2008). Several initiatives have begun to focus on how we can catch up. The Technology Informatics Guiding Education Reform (TIGER) Initiative (2007) hopes to close the gap by providing recommendations for, among other stakeholders, academic institutions and professional organizations. The Canadian Nurses Association has an "E-Nursing Strategy" (2006). Nursing is not alone in its perceived need to get going to increase its informatics competency. The U.S. federal government has set up the Office of Health Information Technology within the Department of Health and Human Services (Health Information Technology AHIC Workgroups, n.d.) with work groups to focus on consumer empowerment, chronic health care, electronic health records, and biosurveillance.

Critical Thinking and Health Informatics

We may be biased, but it doesn't seem like a leap to see that CT must be part of the informatics picture. Mastrian (2008), echoing Wang (2003), proposed "cognitive informatics" as a branch of informatics bridging artificial and natural intelligences. Turley's (1996) model showed nursing informatics as the overlap of three science circles—cognitive, information, and computer sciences. Our merging of thinking and informatics may be a bit simplistic when compared with the models by Wang or Turley, but we envision the merger coming from two directions. As seen in **Figure 9-1**, one can augment one's CT with informatics, but one must use CT to best choose and use informatics. Informatics is only slightly akin to a new piece of equipment (for example, needle-less needles) that, once mastered, can be used to augment work. Informatics includes many processes, changing daily, that are there for our use if we know enough about them and are open-minded enough to choose them.

In **Figure 9-1**, we have listed several CT dimensions on the left side that help us choose and use informatics. The list on the right side indicates the dimensions augmented by informatics. There is some overlap of those dimensions, and we will address the reasons for that overlap shortly. You will also note that we have

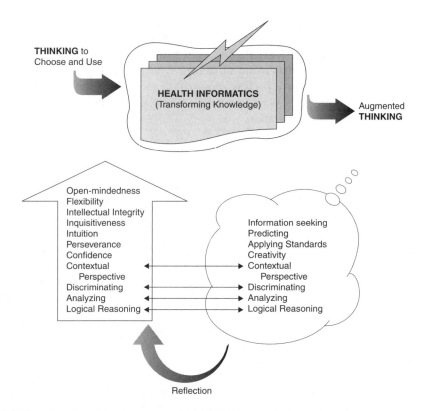

FIGURE 9-1 Relationship Between Critical Thinking and Health Informatics

the dimension of *transforming knowledge* up at the top with health informatics and *reflection* as the connecting dimension with the arrow at the bottom. Why have we done that?

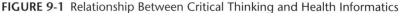

TACTICS 9-1

Use Your *Creativity* and *Logical Reasoning*

Clinicians and Educators

Before reading further, stop a minute and look at Figure 9-1 and reflect on the 17 CT dimensions that we have revisited frequently throughout this book. Test your *creativity* and *logical reasoning* to consider why we might have placed the dimensions where we did.

Discussion

The next section will give you our explanation, but this TACTIC encourages you to construct your own meanings first. Then, compare your meanings with our explanation to see if you thought of things that we forgot. It's quite possible that you put all 17 dimensions on both sides. As you realize by now, artificially separating CT dimensions is just that—artificial. In reality, we use all dimensions in most thinking situations. What we've done here is try to tease out those that are especially important to each side of the picture. Rest assured, there are other ways to interpret this; you may have come up with a much different configuration.

Informatics as Transforming Knowledge

Earlier (remember Dewey in Chapter 4) we talked about the difference between information and knowledge. Informatics allows us to transform information into knowledge and allows us to *transform knowledge*—"changing or converting the condition, nature, form, or function of concepts among contexts" (Scheffer & Rubenfeld, 2000, p. 358). That's why we have highlighted *transforming knowledge* in Figure 9-1. As an aside, have you noticed that *transforming knowledge* comes up frequently as a core thinking skill? We asked you to think of EBP as *transforming knowledge*, for example. EBP and informatics have a very symbiotic relationship. It is through the use of informatics that we can transform the evidence into practice.

Consider a computer application used by a nurse practitioner for prescribing medications. In the old days, the practitioner would have to consider other medications that the patient was taking and try to think of any potential interactions. She would spend time looking up such things, and there was a good chance that something could be missed because there were several places that could, and should, be checked. Today, when using a program like Epocrates (see http://www. epocrates.com), for example, information on each drug is made available so that, in one fell swoop, all potential interactions are noted, dosing for certain conditions is listed, and so on. The drug information has been transformed into usable knowledge and in a very timely manner.

How about a staffing example? In the old days, doing staffing plans by hand meant long hours of figuring out numbers and acuity of patients on units at various times of the day, week, or month and then projecting needs accordingly. There were lots of places where thinking could go awry. Today's computer programs can transform all the information we give them into patterns that tell us with a greater degree of certainty what our staffing needs will be (Hyun, Bakken, Douglas, & Stone, 2008).

The very act of communicating within an informatics framework allows for the transformation of knowledge much more easily. Let's take a really simple example: writing on a computer as opposed to writing on a typewriter or on a pad of paper. Anyone who writes as we do—stream of consciousness first, and then moving things around and editing next—will definitely say that transforming information and knowledge is so much easier on a computer. You get the idea, right? Using informatics is *transforming knowledge*—sorting it, *analyzing* it, communicating it, and converting it into a practical, usable form.

CT for Choosing and Using Informatics

On the left side of Figure 9-1 is a list of 11 CT dimensions that are particularly used to choose and use informatics. The last four on the list (*contextual perspective, discriminating, analyzing,* and *logical reasoning*) are repeated on the right side of the figure because, in addition to helping thinkers choose and use informatics, those dimensions are augmented by informatics. Those dimensions will be discussed here and in the "How Informatics Augments CT" section later in this chapter (p. 242).

Open-Mindedness and Flexibility

First and foremost are the *open-mindedness* and *flexibility* CT dimensions. Using informatics means changing from how one has been doing things, either using applications for the first time or keeping up with newer applications. We'll bet that many of you can remember, as we do, the first year we moved our teaching materials over to PowerPoint programs. It seemed like such a big deal, and it would have been so much easier to stick with our handwritten notes and overhead transparencies. Today, we expect PowerPoint presentations and are shocked when someone doesn't use them.

Another area for *open-mindedness* and *flexibility* in the education arena is the movement toward high-fidelity simulations in the nursing clinical skills laboratory. There are growing numbers of "adult," "child," and "infant" simulators that are considered state-of-the-art necessities for nursing skills laboratories these days. These highly sophisticated devices can talk, breathe, react to medications, and even die (Leigh & Hurst, 2008).

Learning how to use these devices has not been easy for nurse educators. Leigh and Hurst (2008) discussed the challenges of helping faculty to be *open-minded* and *flexible* in order to embrace these new teaching tools and maximize their benefits. Maintaining a flexible and open-minded approach to new methods of gathering, storing, sorting, *analyzing,* and using information and technology is a challenge because it seems that we are always at the start of a learning curve. In case you haven't caught on yet, that will never change; nursing and health care are too dynamic. Change is the name of the game!

Intellectual Integrity

Related to *open-mindedness* and *flexibility* is *intellectual integrity*—"seeking the truth through sincere, honest processes, even if the results are contrary to one's assumptions and beliefs" (Scheffer & Rubenfeld, 2000, p. 358). This is a tough one because it is so much easier to maintain the status quo: *The way I do things now works just fine; I don't want to learn a new way; I don't have time or energy.* We've all said those things, especially on a Friday after a long week. But *intellectual integrity* nudges us to think beyond our own needs and consider what is best for our patients and our students in the long run.

Just how does one maintain an *open mind*, the *flexibility*, and the *intellectual integrity* to embrace informatics? For starters, it helps to receive positive reinforcement for those thinking habits of the mind. Second, it's important to tell yourself that you can't survive in this field without informatics. (You can't, you know; it's definitely a force to be reckoned with.) Third, start talking about informatics to the people you work with and those who work at institutions like yours. Ask them what they know—their visions, fears, and reality—when it comes to information technology. Fourth, make yourself sit down at a computer and do something you haven't done before. To get you started with those four suggestions, try TACTICS 9-2.

TACTICS 9-2

Think How Informatics Could Ease Your Life

Clinicians and Educators

Take some time and reflect on informatics, and then think about your daily activities. Even if you know nothing about computers or information technology, where do you think you could improve your job efficiency and accuracy with technology? Don't allow yourself to think about the specifics of changing over to such technology; that will shut down the open-minded side of your brain. Be a divergent thinker; let your thoughts expand!

Discussion

What did you come up with? Did you let your creative juices flow? As clinicians, we'd want voice-activated recording devices and handheld computer "terminals" that we could put in our pockets to access and record information. We'd want all patients to have a "smart card" with their health data on it—one that we could insert into our handheld device and retrieve and record information. Perhaps by the time you're reading this book, you'll laugh because you have such devices with you. Maybe you'll laugh even more because what you have goes far beyond our old-fashioned vision.

As educators, we would want teaching aids that "talk" to each other more easily. We'd want instant, surefire Internet access in every classroom. We also would want those handheld devices that we can carry around and use easily. We'd want functioning virtual classrooms where people can talk to each other around the world, all at the same time. We'd want students to have these handheld resources so that, if they have to do tracheostomy care, for example, they can pull up a virtual demonstration anytime and anywhere. We want to explore the use of simulation technology in the clinical laboratory, where students can learn from critical mistakes but can bring patients back to life after an "oops." You get the idea, right? Let your mind soar; almost anything our limited minds can envision will most likely be a reality very soon.

Inquisitiveness

Getting back to our dimensions for choosing and using informatics, it will help your *intellectual integrity* if you engage your *inquisitiveness* habit of the mind. Are you naturally inquisitive? If so, you've probably already explored the various information technologies available to you. If you are less inquisitive, try to tweak it more—but do it with fun activities. For example, go to the video store and get some movies that deal with informatics—not necessarily science fiction stuff, but stories about people who are touched by technology. If you need suggestions, here are some examples (in no particular order) listed by Tyler, one of our sons who is a movie buff: *Jumping Jack Flash, LOL, Being There, The Conversation, Blow Out, Apollo 13, Enemy of the State, The Net, Eternal Sunshine of the Spotless Mind, You've Got Mail, Something the Lord Made,* and *Wag the Dog.*

Need more suggestions to get your *inquisitiveness* going? Get a computer program that's fun—a game or drawing program that you can really "get into." Talk to kids about technology. Consider where you are first, though—that could scare you off because kids are really knowledgeable; they grew up with this stuff. Find the person in your environment you secretly call the "techno-geek" and strike up a conversation about why he or she is so into technology. Go on the Internet and look up people you know; you may be surprised what you find. Try to find friends from your past whom you've lost track of. Write e-mails to those persons. One of us, because of a simple e-mail request, has had a wonderful renewed friendship with a childhood friend after being out of touch for 30 years. The point of these activities is to immerse yourself in technology and information exchange. It's hard for some of us to be *inquisitive* about something that we've never played around with. Start by "putting your toes in" the technology waters, and it won't be long before you'll love diving in so much, you'll lose track of time, even days!

Intuition

Intuition can help enhance one's choice and use of informatics. That may seem a bit strange at first glance because *intuition* seems so subjective and informatics seems so objective, but it really isn't that dichotomous. Computers can't be intuitive, but we can be. Without *intuition*, we wouldn't be able to use technology, including computers, as well as we can. Just because the computer program dictates that we do something a certain way doesn't necessarily mean it's the best or only thing to do in that situation. If it doesn't feel right, chances are it isn't.

To illustrate more subtle connections between *intuition* and informatics, let's get away from computers and use a simple, more familiar technology example: a computer order-entry program used by a physician to order enoxaparin. The enoxaparin comes from the pharmacy already loaded in its syringe—technical aids to your work. You double-check the dose (*applying standards*), and you go to administer it. How do you know how much pressure to use when you inject the short needle? Can you remember the first time you gave a subcutaneous injection? You may have not punctured the skin, or you may have done it so hard that you were almost past the hub. What guides you to know how much pressure to exert? That doesn't come from the instrument. Effken (2001) would call that "prospective control"—intuitive visual information. That information is so taken for granted by experts that many would not call it thinking. However, without that *intuitive* part of the process, the technology part cannot be fully used. Because *intuition* usually comes with experience, and because most of us are new to informatics, it's easy to forget about *intuition*. With repeated use of informatics and openness to "gut" responses, we allow *intuition* to help our CT.

Intuition can certainly help us identify areas in which we need technological interventions. A hospital that we have frequented as faculty used a carbon-copy medication order system; checking an order became a guessing game as one worked with partially visible orders, messy handwriting, etc. Every time we used it, we knew intuitively that this was a mistake waiting to happen. Fortunately, that system has now moved to a computer-based ordering system.

Perseverance

Perseverance is an absolute necessity for using informatics, especially if this field is new to you. Recently, in one of our early classes on EBP, students complained about the amount of time they spent searching the Internet to find the evidence reports they needed. They had horror stories of spending hours in one area, only to discover they could have saved that time if they had gone to another Web site first. Some students gave up, thinking that 8 hours on the computer was excessive.

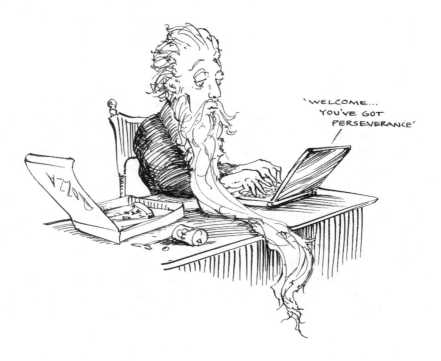

'WELCOME...
YOU'VE GOT
PERSEVERANCE'

Many were surprised when we didn't bat an eyelash and they heard similar stories from their classmates. We discussed the realities of time when using new technologies and how important *perseverance* is, especially in doing something new like evidence searches.

In our old ways of getting information—asking someone, finding a book, searching library index cards—there were fewer options for search paths. Less *perseverance* was needed to think from question to answer. Today, we noodle around on the computer/Web for hours before finding what we're looking for. (That's our favorite description—"noodle"—implying that this is not a straight, linear process.) Because we are new to computers and their mechanisms to address information, we are slower than we think we should be.

It's an interesting position to be in—most nursing leaders, as noted at the start of this chapter, were not raised in homes where computers were commonplace. We are learning a new language and a new set of skills constantly. Because we are experts in our fields already, we have trouble accepting that when it comes to today's technology, we are just novices. Look at teenagers and young adults today—they can maneuver around a computer program so fast that we're left in the dust. Part of the reason youngsters can maneuver so well is their experience with computers and computer programs. They have developed an *intuitive* sense of where to move that cursor to get to the screens they want. We take much longer to do everything because it's still so new to us. We often say we don't have enough RAM to do things fast. (You can tell how in-the-know about computers your listeners are when they either laugh or don't at that remark.) We must maintain *perseverance* and accept our novice status relative to informatics.

Confidence

Related to our novice technophile status is *confidence*. It is hard to have confidence in one's thinking in unfamiliar territory. This is an area in which it is helpful to separate confidence in doing something from *confidence* in one's thinking ability. We can accept our novice states and the reality of our clumsiness and anxiety when using new information technology, but still have *confidence* in our ability to think. Actually, the latter will help the former. A confident thinker can often figure out unknown computer commands just by relying on his or her own logic, and sometimes *intuition*. Computer programs are, in spite of what we think sometimes, very logical (or at least as logical as the people who have programmed them ☺). However, they don't "think" as such; they only follow our commands or the commands of the programmer. In that area, we are superior. Having a little sign over your desk that says "Computers can't think, but I can" is helpful to confidence-building. Advances in computers with sophisticated artificial intelligence are growing, but for right now, your brains and CT are still what we want to count on for quality, safe nursing care.

So what interferes with your thinking *confidence* besides lack of experience? We cannot underestimate the negative effects of anxiety on our thinking *confidence*.

If you are choosing and directing the implementation of a new technology for your work unit, for example, consider how you might decrease the anxiety of the staff as they begin this difficult process. First and foremost, we must acknowledge the negative effects of anxiety on thinking and that working with a new technology produces anxiety. There is nothing more anxiety-producing than to anticipate looking stupid. We tend to respond in anger and use pretty low-level thinking skills. Let's get that on the table and acknowledge that we're all in that boat when we try something new.

Second, we must set up support services. Nurses take pride in their self-sufficiency; we have strong thinking skills and manage on our own quite well. Well, it's time to swallow that pride and accept the fact that we all need help with informatics. A technology or informatics expert should be available at all times to staff using something new. That person should be in place before the initiation of a new system. If you work in a system without this, demand one. You could also come up with rules to avoid technology-driven frustration. For example, Koeniger-Donohue (2008), while starting a project for students and faculty to use personal digital assistants (PDAs), had a 15-minute rule: They wouldn't struggle for longer than 15 minutes on a technical problem before calling in help.

We need to broaden our view of our teams when we increase our use of informatics. One thing we say to our students frequently is, "The librarian is your friend." As we set out to do things, such as finding evidence-based clinical guidelines or discovering what computer programs are available for our consideration, we forget that librarians are expert in such searches. Older people (we) often have this old-fashioned view of librarians as bespectacled, quiet people who stamp and sort books. Much as nursing has had to fight the old stereotypes, so too have librarians. Our cartoon illustrates this change in vision that we'd like to see for nurses and librarians. Have you talked to librarians recently, especially those with a specialty in healthcare informatics? They are phenomenal resources, and we need an updated vision of who they are and how they can be critical to our use of informatics.

Crumley and Koufogiannakis (2002) listed six domains of librarianship. Three of those six are providing service and access to information; helping users with library resources; and creating better methods to retrieve and access information. "The librarian's role has expanded to include the role of teacher or consultant as well as that of expert mediated searches" (Calabretta, 2002, p. 34).

An excellent example of the recognition of this new collaboration between faculty and librarians is the Mellon Library/Faculty Fellowship on Undergraduate Research at the University of California, Berkeley. This project, funded by the Andrew W. Mellon Foundation, promoted joint planning for course assignments to improve use of informatics. At the April 4, 2006, annual meeting of the Higher Learning Commission, the university librarian acknowledged that "academic librarians are crucial partners in heightening students' awareness of resources and research processes . . . and cultivating the habits of mind of successful learners" (Dupuis, 2006, para 3).

THEN   NOW

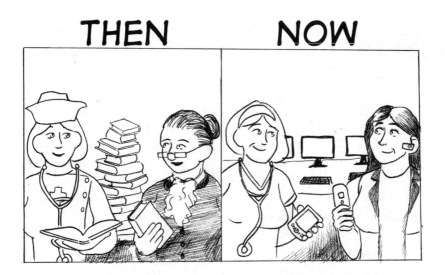

TACTICS 9-3

Take Your Librarian to Lunch

Clinicians and Educators

OK, this may seem a bit hokey, but bear with us here. If you know your librarian well and he or she often helps you, then you probably can skip this TACTIC. But, if you've never thought of your institution's librarian in Calabretta's terms (just mentioned) or those of the University of California, go to the library, send an e-mail, or call the librarian and ask that person to lunch with you. Tell him or her that you would like to pick his or her brain about health informatics.

Discussion

If you did this, we'll bet you were pleasantly surprised in terms of what you learned about that person's knowledge and willingness to help you. You will feel more *confident* in your thinking relative to informatics once you know you have this resource. You may also find someone who would be delighted to come to your unit or classroom to help with informatics. That's what we found when we started working more closely with our wonderful health sciences librarian, Elizabeth Bucciarelli, at our university. We talked to her about her relationship with nursing students and faculty in this time of informatics explosion. We have summarized some of her words of wisdom in **Box 9-2**.

BOX 9-2	**Words of Wisdom from Academic Health Sciences Librarian Elizabeth Bucciarelli**

- Librarians are seekers of knowledge; they enjoy the whole research process, not just finding information. Roy Tennant, a keynote speaker at the Michigan Library Association's Academic Libraries Day, said it this way: "Librarians like to seek, most people like to find" (Tennant, 2008).
- The best approach for teaching library research skills is a tiered one, in which the librarian has multiple sessions with students. Each session builds on the previous ones, with some overlap to reinforce learning.
- Information literacy is a shared responsibility of faculty and librarians.
- Librarians need to meet with and be part of the teaching team to:
  - Better understand the subject
  - Better identify how to weave new technology into courses
  - Make volumes of information streamlined and useable
  - Appreciate the necessity of leveling research skills for all students, from beginners to graduate students
  - Acknowledge the librarian's role as a guide for both students and faculty in the seeking process, not just finding things for them
  - Clarify that helping students synthesize knowledge is usually a teaching faculty, not a librarian, responsibility
- Handing information to students is not the best way for them to learn how to navigate research tools, but we have to realize that everyone learns differently. Sometimes we have to "get to the end of their sidewalk" and meet them.
- The librarian's job is to weave in new technology and streamline the extreme number of resources.
- Key areas for nursing faculty and librarians to address when they meet:
  - Expectations for the course, including topics and, in particular, assignments that will require searches
  - Syllabi with due dates for projects
  - Learning objectives for the library research session
- Key areas that librarians should address during a library research session:
  - Role of librarians today and how it differs from yesterday
  - Student fears and concerns about using technology and searching
  - Glossary of terms related to searching
  - Search process, including research databases and keyboard skills
  - Time-saving "tricks-of-the-trade"

BOX 9-2	(Continued)

- Help students understand that searching is not a "quick and dirty" process, but takes a significant amount of the total time needed to complete a project or paper
- Pass along the theoretical concept regarding the stream of information created and disseminated in nursing (e.g., a conference paper may become a journal article, which may become a review article, which may become a book)

- Thinking dimensions most needed with informatics and library searches:
  - *Information seeking*
  - *Analyzing* to evaluate the content of an article
  - *Discriminating*—goes hand and hand with *analyzing* and determining quality
  - *Flexibility*—you can't be linear; searching is very relational, going from one idea to another, such as with following up on bibliography references to gain more information.
  - *Inquisitiveness*—going beyond the basics
  - *Intellectual integrity*—both academic and professional
  - *Perseverance*
  - *Open-mindedness*—you have to let go of an idea, and get broader in thinking and move on

Contextual Perspective

We have now arrived at the four dimensions that are on both sides of Figure 9-1. *Contextual perspective* is a thinking habit of the mind that is important to choosing and using informatics, and it is augmented by informatics. Here we focus on the choosing and using part: If you are the person choosing computer applications for your office or unit, for example, you need to think about the whole picture. Who will be using them? What will they cost? How easy is it to use the hardware? How easy is it to access program information, such as patient records, student records, etc.? How much training will staff need? What information technology support is available? Is the support available 24/7? Is the support a living, breathing person in your facility, or will it be in the form of a phone call to who knows where? Will your computer system be able to "talk" to other computers (programs) in the system to share information, or will they each work in "silos"? What security systems are needed to protect computer information? What will computers and technology add to or subtract from your resources? Take time to explore all these possibilities.

Better yet, get a knowledgeable information technology person to help examine the full *contextual perspective*; we can't think of it all alone.

Keep in mind that, just as they aren't intuitive, computers and their programs are noncontextual; we, however, have to use them with our *contextual perspective*. If you are using a staffing program that says you need a staff of 10 people for Saturday, it will not tell you to think about the forecasted sunny day and the big party someone is having (factors that might very well influence how many call-ins you have). If the computer tells you that each practitioner should be able to see four patients every hour, you can't be a slave to that; you must look at the context of who those patients are (sometimes older people take 5 of their 15 minutes just to walk back to the exam room).

Discriminating

Another thinking dimension that will be augmented by informatics is also needed for choosing and using informatics: It is *discrimination*. One of the biggest drawbacks to information technology is the issue of reliability. Anyone can post anything on the Internet. People can identify themselves by any title. There is very little *discrimination* as to quality. This is a problem for all of us, but particularly for patients, who may make health decisions based on indiscriminate information, and students, who are quick to accept written information as authoritative.

Some attempts are being made to help consumers *discriminate* quality information today. For example, the National Library of Medicine has lists of reliable health-related resources (http://medlineplus.gov). You can find several others in **Box 9-3**. Most of these Web sites have links to many others that they have checked out. However, a word of caution about using any Web site in a list in a book: Web sites can change quickly, disappear, move, and so forth. We have also discovered, to our chagrin, that a slight typo in a Web site address (either in print or when typing) can lead to some undesirable sites.

For students and other library users, criteria for judging the quality (*discriminating*) of information can increasingly be found. Such guidelines have become standards in the library world (E. Bucciarelli, personal communication, September 3, 2008). Our library has posted A^3BCD; this acronym represents six categories of criteria, the details of which are available easily on our library Web site (Stanger, 2008). A summary of the six criteria follows:

- **A**uthority of Source (judging information about the organization or author)
- **A**ccuracy (documentation of facts)
- **A**udience (appropriateness of information for the intended audience)
- **B**ias/point of view (purpose of document, distinguishing fact from opinion)
- **C**urrency (creation date and updates)
- **D**esign/site navigation (ease of site navigation)

For healthcare providers looking for evidence-based clinical guidelines, you will recall from Chapter 8 that we suggested evaluation criteria for *discriminating* quality.

BOX 9-3	Consumer Health Internet Sites That Maintain Standards and Have Links to Similar Sites

(These are not meant to be recommendations, merely a list from which to start searching.)

http://medlineplus.gov/

http://www.healthfinder.gov/

http://www.medweb.emory.edu/

http://www.healthgrades.com/

http://www.leapfroggroup.org/

http://www.informedhealthonline.org/

http://www.guideline.gov/

http://www.who.int/en/

http://www.paho.org/

http://www.ahcancal.org/

http://www.mlanet.org/resources/healthlit/

Keeping such things in mind is very important as you exercise your *discrimination* thinking skills. You must constantly question what you see and read. You must also educate patients to be discriminatory in their thinking. People who have limited knowledge of a subject have more difficulty *discriminating* the relative importance or validity of information. Walji et al. (2004) made a startling discovery when they analyzed 150 Web sites on alternative medicine: Thirty-eight sites (25%) had statements that could cause harm if acted upon, and 145 sites (97%) had omitted information. Walji et al. cautioned consumers to use other means of validating information found on Web sites.

In another example, a clinician recently told this story: A depressed patient was started on Lexapro and stopped taking it within 2 days because she felt worse. When the clinician questioned this, the patient said, "Well, I went on their Web site, and it said this drug may worsen depression, so I figured that's what was happening to me." What the patient didn't do was read further to see the remainder of the explanation of how this drug's action builds over time. This example may remind you of a discussion in Chapter 6 and what we said about our responsibilities to help patients develop their CT skills.

Analyzing and Logical Reasoning

The last two CT dimensions on both sides of Figure 9-1, *analyzing* and *logical reasoning*, are augmented by informatics and used for the nitty-gritty work of choosing and using informatics. Get away from looking at informatics as a whole—a scary, big field—and break things down (*analyze*) into manageable units. If you're in a position of choosing a new information technology, ask these types of questions:

- What is it you are trying to accomplish?
- How are you doing it now?
- What's available as an alternative?
- What resources are needed to get something new?
- How will it work? What will be the surrounding issues? How long will a transition take?
- What are the external support systems I may need after the fact (e.g., software or hardware customer support and troubleshooting)?
- What are the costs and benefits?

If a new technology is thrust upon you, ask these questions:

- What is the goal of this change?
- What do I need to know?
- What do I know already that I can use during this change?
- How long will this take?
- Why am I angry?
- How anxiety-producing is this?
- What about it is making me anxious?
- How can I deal with my anxiety?
- Who and what do I have as resources?

Logical reasoning will help you make the best decisions, ones based on evidence rather than emotional responses alone. If you've come to a conclusion that a new technology forced on you by your manager is a bad idea, on what have you based that conclusion? If you're gung ho to have a particular e-mail system in your institution, on what is your enthusiasm based? It's easy to be critical or overly enamored of new technology if we don't know much about it. Knowledge is power; not having knowledge about something thrust upon us makes us feel powerless and potentially frustrated in our actions. (Should we start looking for a new entry in the DSM-IV-TR: "Informatics Rage"?)

How Informatics Augments CT

There is no question that when used well, informatics can significantly help our thinking. Let's look at the CT dimensions listed on the right side of Figure 9-1. We'll start with the four we just discussed, which are listed on both the left and the right sides—those that are both augmented by, and necessary to choose and use, informatics (*contextual perspective, discriminating, analyzing*, and *logical reasoning*). Then we'll discuss the four listed at the top (*information seeking, predicting, applying standards*, and *creativity*).

Contextual Perspective

The communication ability that is afforded by informatics has broadened our *contextual perspective* enormously. The Internet has broadened our patients' perspectives, but we don't yet have enough research to determine the full effect (Murray et al., 2003). Although the system is still not without wrinkles—such as liability, confidentiality, and payment—some providers are using e-mail with patients (Forkner-Dunn, 2003; Patt, Houston, Jenckes, Sands, & Ford, 2003). According to Forkner-Dunn (2003), about 100 million Americans obtained health information from the Web in 2002. They can broaden their perspective and their resources by e-connecting with others who have the same medical conditions.

Discriminating

Not only does informatics broaden our *contextual perspectives* and those of patients, but it also helps us with our *discrimination* of information. Remember, as we discussed in the preceding section, you also need sharp *discrimination* skills to use informatics. Now we're focused on how informatics can help that cognitive skill. We can access much more information and broaden our field so much that we can begin to see patterns and differences in information. We can begin to distinguish and differentiate the information in order to make decisions that are the best fit for the situation. Ahh, more *contextual perspective* here too! We can have computers link information for us to see if patterns exist; as educators, we can predict where our students will have trouble on the National Council Licensure Examination by looking at patterns in their other tests. We can *discriminate* any list of things according to rank with the touch of one button. As an example, the National Guideline Clearinghouse (n.d.) has a way to compare multiple clinical practice guidelines with the click of a mouse.

Analyzing

It is easy to miss the forest for the trees, and vice versa, with our natural cognitive abilities and emotions. Informatics allows for ease of *analyzing*—breaking things down into manageable units.

We're going to veer off a bit here and look at *analyzing* relative to standardized language. For computer programming, we must have information broken down and described in standardized descriptors—but there are still many challenges to standardizing healthcare and nursing terminology (Bakken, Cimino, & Hripcsak, 2004). Hannah (2007) saw us as having a long way to go with standard language; according to her, "we have built our profession's own Tower of Babel" (p. 19). To standardize anything, one must break it down (*analyze* it) and give it a consistent designation (name, number, and so forth). Informatics has forced and helped nursing to define itself—to *analyze* the parts of our profession and standardize our nomenclature. These taxonomies, among others, have become standard in the United States and in many countries around the world: nursing diagnoses (North American Nursing Diagnosis Association), nursing interventions (Nursing Interventions Classification; NIC), and nursing outcomes (Nursing Outcomes Classification; NOC).

Back in the 1970s, when the first talk of describing components of nursing according to nursing diagnoses began, it was triggered by the need for us to keep up with informatics. The first conference to classify nursing diagnosis was called in 1973 by two nurses from St. Louis, Gebbie and Lavin, for two reasons. One reason was related to clinical issues, and the other was that they had been "offered space on a computerized record-keeping system" (Gordon, 1982, p. 2). You can't put something that has several names and definitions into a computer; it must be specific and broken down clearly. This need to specifically define our profession in terms of our diagnoses, interventions, and outcomes has already benefitted nursing practice, education, and research, and will continue to do so. We transform data into nursing knowledge and build our theoretical frameworks in the field (Bakken & Constantino, 2001).

Look at the first chapter of the latest edition of the NIC (Bulechek, Butcher, & Dochterman, 2008), and you will see the long list of information systems that endorse the use of NIC; it is licensed for inclusion in the Systematized Nomenclature of Medicine, for example. Look at the NOC (Moorhead, Johnson, Maas, & Swanson, 2008), and you'll see a similar focus on this classification fitting into information systems; for example, it meets the American Nurses Association Standards from the Nursing Information and Data Set Evaluation Center. This need for a specific classification that can work with the systematic nature of information technology has been a large driving force for nurses in defining their discipline.

Logical Reasoning

Just as *analyzing* is both necessary for choosing and using informatics and augmented by it, so too is *logical reasoning* used on both sides of the picture in Figure 9-1. Remember, *logical reasoning* requires that conclusions be clearly supported by raw data or evidence. Human logic, of course, is always influenced by emotions. We see things that don't necessarily exist because we want to see them. We ignore things in front of us because we don't want them to influence our decisions. Computers don't have that emotional component (except in some movies, like HAL in *2001: A Space Odyssey*). A computer can only deal with what's been put into it. Any "conclusion" reached by the computer is less likely to be influenced by human bias (taking into account the programmer); it has a logical progression back to the raw data put into it. Although we must acknowledge the value of *contextual perspective* and *intuition*, those cannot stand alone if we are to be safe, effective, and efficient providers. The logic that informatics promotes is the balance for our human biases.

We are seeing much more in the literature about clinical decision support systems (CDSSs). These are programs that help us make *logical* decisions; however, these are still in their infancy and have very little research support to date (Randell, Mitchell, Dowding, Cullum, & Thompson, 2007). Nursing is lagging behind medicine in developing and using CDSSs (Anderson & Willson, 2008). However, there are encouraging reports; for example, Warren, Connors, Weaver, and Simpson (2006) reported that an electronic simulated clinical information system helped students think in a more data-driven way. Saleem et al. (2007) reported on the usefulness of a clinical reminder system in an ambulatory clinic. This is certainly an area to watch closely in future years.

Information Seeking

Probably the easiest benefit to see from informatics is in *information seeking*. It's hard to imagine how we wrote papers and books before electronic searches, isn't it? You can find something about almost any subject on the Internet; you can access libraries around the world, and you can ask a question of someone in Taiwan as easily as you can ask it of the person in the office next door—sometimes more easily. With a PDA, one can carry virtually a whole library in one's pocket. Think of how electronic health records will ease our information seeking in patient care situations. According to MacDonald (2008), we will know our patients better and more quickly. We will have, at the click of a mouse, health histories, lab results, and so forth. In terms of *information seeking* and access, we in our 50s frequently are in awe of this new ability we have. Of course, as we discussed earlier, *information seeking* without *discriminating* skills can be very problematic and even dangerous.

Predicting

Because of the help we can get with our *information seeking* and *discriminating*, we are also better at the cognitive skill of *predicting*. Because informatics allows us to see patterns, it is easier to predict how patterns will continue. Think about the move to prospective reimbursement (Beyers, 1985) if you need an "in-your-face" example of the predictive capabilities of informatics. Using diagnosis-related groups for prospective reimbursement was a method of predicting how long patients would stay in the hospital, based on certain diagnosis-related data that were analyzed by a computer program. Budget programs help us predict what we'll need for the future. Computer scheduling applications help us *predict* how many nurses we'll need for the Saturday shifts in the summer. Tracking medication errors with adverse event documents and seminal event data helps *predict* problem medications, as well as relationships between things like acuity or time of year associated with those medication errors.

Applying Standards

Applying standards is sort of related to the earlier discussion of standardized language. In the same way that labels for nursing diagnoses, interventions, and outcomes are specified in information systems so that we're all on the same wavelength, so, too, can professional standards be unified and easily available.

To avoid being duplicative, we remind you to go or think back to the previous chapter on EBP. Our ability to access evidence-based clinical guidelines is justification enough that informatics helps with *applying standards*. We can practice with the best, most current standards because technology allows for their availability to all clinicians. Joining an e-mail list gives us nearly immediate updates without even having to search. Faculty can apply standards in their teaching by accessing the most current and accurate information on their teaching topics. We can find all kinds of help with teaching methodologies in informatics. Standards to protect human subjects in research situations can be accessed easily through government Web sites.

Imagine yourself as a clinician on a hospital unit, and you have to use an intervention you haven't used in a long time. In the old days, you could ask other nurses and possibly get the best standard of care, or you could go through the policy and procedure manual—that dog-eared book in the conference room whose updates were often nebulous. In most institutions today, you can pull up a computer program and find just what you need.

Creativity

Because we have tools such as computers at our fingertips, informatics can help our *creativity* thinking habits. Ask artists how their tools affect *creativity*, and most will say that those tools augment their *creativity*. It is easier to be creative and individualize your patient teaching, for example, if you have videotapes, computer-based learning modules, and written materials to work with. If you are an educator, are you using technology and assignments designed to get students to embrace the Internet in order to be the most creative thinker and teacher?

TACTICS 9-4

Using Informatics to Improve Teaching *Creativity*

Educators

Reflect on your teaching methods. When was the last time you updated them? Do an inventory of the available informatics that you may not be using to spice up your teaching. Have you considered any of these?

- Podcasts
- Teleconferencing with nursing experts and leaders to engage students in critical dialogue on a particular topic
- In-class activities that require students to search the Internet
- Demonstrations of searching techniques on the Internet with the help of liquid crystal display projectors
- Mannequin simulations in the clinical laboratory to demonstrate the effects of medications on blood pressure
- Enhancement of your classroom activities with e-learning and threaded discussions

Clinicians

Do a mental inventory of the things you repeatedly teach patients. Are you using standardized materials? Is it the most current information? How many options are available to you to teach that material? Are you using the most efficient teaching methods? The most creative ones? Have you used informatics to help you with this? Have you downloaded pictures or diagrams from the Internet to help illustrate concepts for patients? Has your hospital or organization developed a "telehealth" system for patient information?

Discussion

Creativity is not something we think of as a companion to informatics because one seems so right-brain and the other so left-brain. However, when you think of informatics as a tool, what it has to offer is boundless. Sometimes just using the tools forces a fresh look at content and how we teach. Magnussen (2008) noted that when she moved from face-to-face instruction to e-courses, she became less content centered and more learning centered. This was our realization also as we moved to online teaching last year. Creating meaningful e-learning experiences forced us to think about ways to help students engage in critical dialogue, reflect, justify their thinking, and teach themselves and others (real learning); we couldn't rely on the old-fashioned content-laden lecture.

Reflection on CT and Health Informatics

We have now covered all the CT dimensions on the left and right sides of Figure 9-1. Obviously, dividing CT dimensions is somewhat false and awkward. However, keep in mind that you have to use CT with informatics, and you also augment CT with informatics. It is time now to reflect on how it all fits together.

Reflection is the big arrow at the bottom of Figure 9-1. It's down there to remind you that there's nothing static about thinking when it comes to incorporating informatics in health care. You will constantly need to reflect on where you're going. As we have said many times now, informatics is constantly changing. While using the same 17 dimensions repeatedly, you will need to keep all the doors and windows of your mind open to let in the new ideas and seize the new opportunities that informatics has to offer. You will always use *logical reasoning*, for example, but the data you have available to make decisions will certainly change. You will always need *perseverance* because unfamiliar pieces of informatics that you have to slog through will keep cropping up. A friend of ours likes to say "get over it" when people voice disgruntled opinions about the rapid change of technology. Your thinking will *persevere* because it will have to if you are to achieve the quality level of nursing care you want to provide.

An overarching *reflection* focus involves being open to the future of informatics. According to Ball and Lillis (2000), whose trends we cited at the start of this chapter, new technology goes through three phases: replication, innovation, and transformation. Health care is lagging behind other systems—such as those used by banks and airlines—in that its informatics is still between the first and second phases. The first, replication, occurs when a manual job is replaced by a machine, and the second, innovation, is a new way of doing something. The last phase, transformation, in which an industry is completely transformed by informatics, has not yet occurred in health care. Ball and Lillis projected the three most important emerging technologies in health care to be "the computer-based patient record (CPR), Internet/intranet/extranet applications, and clinical decision support (CDS) systems" (p. 389).

Just since the publication of the Ball and Lillis (2000) article, great strides have been made in CPR, but we are still a distance away from the full implementation of CPRs that can be used at the bedside with voice activation. Most institutions use Internet and intranet communication applications; however, many issues, such as patient privacy, must be dealt with before these applications are widely used by patients and providers. CDS systems are also not yet widely used. As those of us who live and breathe topics like CT are quick to point out, the nuances and complexities of human decision making can be augmented by computers, but we don't see how computers will replace that thinking. We might have telephone, e-mail, voice mail, or video mail available, but we still need a caring, thinking person to decide which one is best to use.

Challenges of Informatics

There are many challenges facing us in health care, and many of them can be helped with informatics. Critically thinking clinicians and educators must try to *predict* those challenges and use *creativity* along with the other CT dimensions to overcome the challenges. The overarching challenge, of course, is dealing with change and the magnitude of the change. Embracing informatics in health care qualifies for the high end on any change adaptation scale; this change requires not only that individuals change but that two huge systems change as well. Those two systems are, of course, the healthcare system and the educational system that prepares future healthcare providers.

A frequently cited challenge is, of course, the cost of innovative technologies. Even though many of the changes will ultimately save large amounts of money, an enormous outlay of resources is still required to get new and better systems going.

The politics of informatics can be a barrier for nursing. Some nurses want to avoid dealing with informatics; others wish they were more in the loop when it comes to choosing and planning for information technology (Simpson, 2007). McBride (2005) echoed these issues and added the challenges of an ill-prepared academia responsible for teaching future nurses. As cited earlier, the NLN, among other educational organizations, is keenly aware of the need to better prepare the 21st-century nursing workforce when it comes to technology and informatics.

Politics overlaps human factors that affect accepting, choosing, and using informatics. We have several times touched on the difficulties folks in our age group have with informatics. Ironically, because of our age, we are leaders in our professions, and therefore we are making decisions about informatics. Kaminski (2005) pointed out the need to address the culture of nursing when addressing informatics:

> The professional nurse is now expected to function well within a technologically advanced healthcare environment, carry out higher-level, complex activities, and are held responsible and accountable for. . . . humanistic nursing care. . . . This is expected to occur within a system plagued by a nursing shortage, heavy workloads and long shiftwork hours. . . . Technology does not function in a vacuum but within a social matrix (para 13).

This *contextual thinking* reminds us that there are no simple answers to choices about informatics. That's why we must constantly rely on our CT.

The human factor context must also be considered as we look to healthcare consumers. Repeatedly, we see the need to work on quality evaluation tools for consumers of electronic information. Health search improvements, especially consumer-directed tools, are strong themes in Greenberg, Andrea, and Lorence's (2004) online health action agenda. We need research in these areas, but we also need to develop education models for finding and intelligently using information.

Health professions are moving to meet the challenges of informatics. Specialists in informatics are increasing rapidly. The American Nursing Informatics Association (ANIA) has over 1,000 members (ANIA, n.d.). Canada's Health Informatics Association has more than 1,450 members from many health disciplines, including nursing (Canada's Health Informatics Association [COACH], 2008). **Box 9-4** has a listing of some informatics societies; look for a growth of these in the future.

BOX 9-4   **Health Informatics Associations**

American Medical Informatics Association:
   http://www.amia.org/
American Nursing Informatics Association:
   http://www.ania.org/
Healthcare Information and Management Systems Society:
   http://www.himss.org/ASP/index.asp
Health Information Management Association of Australia:
   http://www.himaa.org.au/
International Medical Informatics Association:
   http://www.imia.org/
Nursing Informatics Europe:
   http://www.nicecomputing.ch/nieurope/
Ontario Nursing Informatics Group:
   http://www.onig.on.ca/

Before we leave our challenges behind, we'd like you to hear from a nurse who is, on a daily basis, facing the challenges of leading other nurses in a move toward an electronic medical record in a large healthcare system that includes several geographically disperse centers. Kate Kimmet is, in our minds, a very brave and resilient RN clinical liaison for this massive project. We asked her to talk about some of the challenges, and we've included excerpts from our fascinating conversation with her. We'd like you to actively think while you read her story.

TACTICS 9-5

Finding Kate's Critical Thinking

Clinicians and Educators

After reading Kate's story, make yourself a grid similar to **Table 9-1** and fill it in. (Those of us who are more linear thinkers appreciate this style of organizing our thinking.) You may want to refer to the tear-out card in the front of this text for the 17 critical thinking dimensions and their definitions if you haven't already got them memorized.

TABLE 9-1 Critiquing Kate's Critical Thinking

CT Dimension Used by Kate	What did Kate do that demonstrated this CT dimension?	What would you have done differently to demonstrate this CT dimension?

Kate's Story

Time has been a big issue. We started this project several years ago. It was to have been in place in 2006, but there was a long pause, and now going live is to be in 2009. It's hard to keep people excited and moving when there's a gap like this. I've had to adapt what I was meant to do; other duties were added to my job description, so I've had to deal with a larger area. Time is also a factor for the nurses. If I could take back all the minutes of people saying, "I don't have the time to do this. . . " ["this" being learning and practice sessions for the new system]. Nurses are so busy; they have to do these things on top of their usual duties.

Anxiety is also an issue. This is a new set of skills; nurses are used to being experts in their practice areas, but they are beginners with the electronic system. Basically, everyone feels incompetent, and that's scary. There is daily uncertainty. Another challenge is communication. We have teams of nurses set up, but it is difficult dealing with lots of groups. It is hard to get information. I ask a question and someone says, "We'll find out. . . ." and then they don't get back to you. Then there's the whole new language to learn. It was very difficult for me at first. I asked why I was in this position since I really didn't know anything about computer systems or even the language. They told me it was important to have nurses who have been taking care of patients using their critical thinking to be in on the planning phase of this project. Once I learned the language, I was more comfortable; it was a metamorphosis. I had to have confidence in my thinking; I could learn this.

Then, of course, there's the issue of change. It is huge and very complex; every part is a domino that bumps into something else. The staff mix is different from site to site, and each site has a different reputation for strengths and weaknesses. We have to come up with a transition system that can work for each unit. Also, things haven't shut down while this is going on; there are many other mandates that must be implemented at the same time. The "go live" date looms its huge and scary head.

Discussion

How many CT dimensions were you able to identify? Many of you probably realized how some of the dimensions overlap, merge, and work together. That is how CT works in real life and real nursing, so don't be distressed that things don't always fit into nice, neat boxes. If you want some additional challenges, compare your thinking about this task with that of a nurse colleague or a fellow nursing student; discuss differences and similarities and your reasoning behind your thinking. Talk about how you might combine your thinking to create some new ideas that neither of you thought about originally but that might help Kate's organization achieve its transition to an electronic medical record system.

PAUSE _____

and Ponder

Health Informatics and the Future

We'll leave you with one parting challenge to consider: Dare we even envision a healthcare future without a wholehearted embrace of informatics? Of course not. Just what that future will look like we're not able to fathom yet. Will we someday see healthcare information managed as it was by Dr. McCoy in his *Star Trek* infirmary or with his "tri-corder"? Cox (2007) envisioned 2050 as a time when we may never meet a patient face to face to provide care, robots will do surgery, and patients will have embedded computer chips and will be housed in virtual reality pods. Turley, Murray, Saranto, Ehnfors, and Seomun (2007) allowed that "the future will be stranger than we think" (p. 55). Whatever emerges as the future of informatics, we should not embrace it without sharp thinking in order to determine the best technology and the best uses of it. Kleiman and Kleiman (2007) expressed these cautionary steps best: "Technology is not a neutral phenomenon and as such requires attention in our world of radical technologization" (p. 158). They warn us about using terms like "the computer says" and about "the extent to which our reliance on computers has disenfranchised us from our status as . . . unique beings capable of rational thought who make choices" (p. 160). For a sobering consideration, read Eysenbach's 2003 article on severe acute respiratory syndrome and population health technology. This physician from Toronto General Hospital outlined the many technologies used that both helped the crisis and negatively fueled fear during the 2002–03 outbreak of this scary new, deadly disease. Eysenbach cautioned us to learn lessons for future public health emergencies: "Population health technology clearly has a vast potential to increase our preparedness for the next public-health emergency, but it also raises many questions related to ethics, libertarian values, and privacy, and has the potential to fuel an epidemic of fear and collective mass hysteria." (last para)

Reflection Cues

- Informatics has to do with managing information/knowledge, communicating, and making decisions.
- There are clear links between CT and health informatics.
- Healthcare technology is a vast, constantly changing force to be reckoned with.
- For baby-boom generation healthcare workers, informatics does not come as easily as it does, and will, for generations who grew up with computers.

- Healthcare informatics has been defined by discipline—for example, medicine and nursing—but today, there is a move toward the interdisciplinary idea of health informatics.
- Almost anything said to describe the current state of informatics in a textbook is out of date by the time the book is published; that's how fast things are changing.
- Having a futuristic perspective is helpful when considering informatics and the thinking surrounding it.
- Informatics is moving from data to decisions, communication to collaboration, information to knowledge, networking to ubiquitous computing, graphical to cognitive user interfaces, situated to mobile, physical to virtual, and business to consumer.
- The relationship between thinking and informatics comes from two directions; one's thinking will be augmented by informatics, but one needs CT to choose and use informatics.
- Informatics is a process of *transforming knowledge*.
- The primary CT dimensions needed for choosing and using informatics are *open-mindedness, flexibility, intellectual integrity, inquisitiveness, contextual perspective, intuition, perseverance, confidence, logical reasoning, analyzing,* and *discriminating*.
- Informatics particularly augments these CT dimensions: *information seeking, contextual perspective, discrimination, predicting, logical reasoning, analyzing, applying standards,* and *creativity*.
- *Reflection* is the CT dimension that must always be used to study where we are and where we're going with informatics.
- CPRs, Internet/intranet applications, and CDS are three areas where emerging technologies are particularly active today.
- Challenges of informatics today include the magnitude of the change in the healthcare and academic systems; costs; human acceptance factors; and the need for better tools to judge quality of information.
- We have organizations, such as ANIA and COACH, to meet some challenges.
- One nurse's story illustrates challenges of implementing a new technology in her healthcare institution.
- An important challenge is to embrace the rapid advances of informatics without doing it blindly and without ignoring quality, ethics, and values.

References

American Association of Colleges of Nursing. (2005). *Faculty shortages in baccalaureate and graduate nursing programs: Scope of the problem and strategies for expanding the supply.* Retrieved August 25, 2008, from http://www.aacn.nche.edu/publications/whitepapers/facultyshortages.htm

American Nurses Association. (2008). *Nursing informatics: Scope & standards of practice.* Silver Spring, MD: Author.

American Nursing Informatics Association. (n.d.). *About ANIA*. Retrieved August 27, 2008, from http://www.ania.org/About%20ANIA.htm

Anderson, J. A., & Willson, P. (2008). Clinical decision support systems in nursing: Synthesis of the science for evidence-based practice. *CIN: Computers, Informatics, Nursing, 26*, 151–158.

Bader, S. A., & Braude, R. M. (1998). "Patient Informatics": Creating new partnerships in medical decision making. *Academic Medicine, 73*, 408–411.

Bakken, S., Cimino, J. J., & Hripcsak, G. (2004). Promoting patient safety and enabling evidence-based practice through informatics. *Medical Care, 42*(2), II-49–II-56. doi10.1097/01.mir.0000109125.00113.f4

Bakken, S., & Constantino, M. (2001). Standardized terminologies and integrated information systems: Building blocks for transforming data into nursing knowledge. In J. M. Dochterman & H. K. Grace, *Current issues in nursing* (6th ed., pp. 52–59). St. Louis, MO: Mosby.

Ball, M. J., & Lillis, J. C. (2000). Health information systems: Challenges for the 21st century. *AACN Clinical Issues, 11*, 386–395.

Beyers, M. (Ed.). (1985). *Perspectives on prospective payment: Challenges and opportunities for nurses*. Rockville, MD: Aspen.

Biomedical abbreviation server. (2003). Retrieved August 23, 2008, from http://abbreviation.stanford.edu/

Bulechek, G. M., Butcher, H. K., & Dochterman, J. M. (Eds.). (2008). *Nursing interventions classification (NIC)* (5th ed.). St. Louis, MO: Mosby.

Calabretta, N. (2002). Consumer-driven, patient-centered health care in the age of electronic information. *Journal of the Medical Library Association, 90*, 32–37.

Canada's Health Informatics Association. (2008). Retrieved August 26, 2008, from http://www.coachorg.com/Default.asp?id=367.

Canadian Nurses Association. (2006). *E-Nursing strategy for Canada*. Retrieved August 23, 2008, from http://www.cna-aiic.ca/CNA/documents/pdf/publications/E-Nursing-Strategy-2006-e.pdf

Chang, J. T., Schutze, H., & Altman, R. B. (2002). Creating an online dictionary or abbreviations from MEDLINE. *Journal of the American Medical Informatics Association, 9*, 612–620.

Coiera, E. (1999). *10 Essential clinical informatics skills*. Retrieved August 23, 2008, from http://www.informatics-review.com/thoughts/skills.html

Columbia University Biomedical Informatics. (n.d.). Retrieved August 11, 2008, from http://www.dbmi.columbia.edu/

Cox, T. (2007). Nursing research in 2050. *Nursing Science Quarterly, 20*, 206–208. doi:10.1177/0894318497303437

Crumley, E., & Koufogiannakis, D. (2002). Developing evidence-based librarianship: Practical steps for implementation. *Health Information and Libraries Journal, 19*, 61–70.

Dupuis, E. A. (2006, April). *Enriching the academic experience through research-based learning*. Paper presented at the Higher Learning Commission annual meeting, Chicago, IL.

Effken, J. A. (2001). Informational basis for expert intuition. *Journal of Advanced Nursing, 34*, 246–255.

Eysenbach, G. (2003). SARS and population health technology. *Journal of Medical Internet Research, 5*(2), e14. Retrieved July 14, 2004, from http://www.jmir.org/2003/2/e14/HTML

Eysenbach, G., & Jadad, A. R. (2001). Evidence-based patient choice and consumer health informatics in the Internet age. *Journal of Medical Internet Research, 3*(2), e19. Retrieved November 17, 2008, from http://www.jmir.org/2001/2/e19/

Fetter, M. S. (2008). Enhancing baccalaureate nursing information technology outcomes: Faculty perspectives. *International Journal of Nursing Education Scholarship, 5*(1), Article 3. Retrieved August 21, 2008, from http://www.bepress.com/ijnes/vol5/iss1/art3/

Forkner-Dunn, J. (2003). Internet-based patient self-care: The next generation of health care delivery. *Journal of Medical Internet Research, 5*(2), e8. Retrieved November 17, 2008, from http://www.jmir.org/2003/2/e8/HTML

Giordana, S. (2008). *NUR 830 Health care informatics* (Course Syllabus). Oakland University School of Nursing, Rochester, MI.

Gordon, M. (1982). Historical perspective: The national conference group for classification of nursing diagnoses (1978, 1980). In M. J. Kim & D. A. Moritz (Eds.), *Classification of nursing diagnoses: Proceedings of the third and fourth national conferences* (pp. 2–8). New York: McGraw-Hill.

Greenberg, L., Andrea, G. D., & Lorence, D. (2004). Setting the public agenda for online health search: A white paper and action agenda. *Journal of Medical Internet Research, 6*(2), e8. Retrieved November 17, 2008, from http://www.jmir.org/2004/2/e18/HTML

Hannah, K. J. (2007). The state of nursing informatics in Canada. *The Canadian Nurse, 103*(5), 18–19, 22.

Health Information Technology AHIC Workgroups. (n.d.). Retrieved March 12, 2009, from http://www.hhs.gov/healthit/ahic/

Health Information Technology Scholars Program. (2007). Retrieved September 12, 2008, from http://www.hits-colab.org/

Health Resources and Services Administration. (2007). *The registered nurse population: Findings from the 2004 national sample survey of registered nurses.* Retrieved August 25, 2008, from http://bhpr.hrsa.gov/healthworkforce/rnsurvey04/

Hyun, S., Bakken, S., Douglas, K., & Stone, P. W. (2008). Evidence-based staffing: Potential roles for informatics. *Nursing Economics, 26*, 151–173.

Institute of Medicine of the National Academies. (2003). *Health professions education: A bridge to quality.* Washington, DC: National Academies Press.

Institute of Medicine of the National Academies. (2004). *Patient safety: Achieving a new standard for care.* Washington, DC: National Academies Press.

Kaminski, J. (2005). Editorial: Nursing informatics and nursing culture. Is there a fit? *Online Journal of Nursing Informatics, 9*(3). Retrieved August 23, 2008, from http:ojni.org/9_3/june.htm

Kleiman, S., & Kleiman, A. (2007). Technicity in nursing and the dispensation of thinking. *Nursing Economics, 25*, 157–161.

Koeniger-Donohue, R. (2008). Handheld computers in nursing education: A PDA pilot project. *Journal of Nursing Education, 47*, 74–77.

Kutner, M., Greenberg, E., Jin, Y., Paulsen, C., & White, S. (2006, September). *The health literacy of America's adults: Results from the 2003 national assessment of adult literacy* (NCES 2006-483). Retrieved August 25, 2008, from http://nces.ed.gov/pubs2006/2006483.pdf

Leigh, G., & Hurst, H. (2008). We have a high-fidelity simulator, now what? Making the most of simulators. *International Journal of Nursing Education Scholarship, 5*(1), 1–9. Retrieved May 26, 2009, from http://www.bepress.com/ijnes/vol5/iss1/art33/

MacDonald, M. (2008). Technology and its effect on knowing the patient. *Clinical Nurse Specialist, 22*, 149–155.

Magnussen, L. (2008). Applying the principles of significant learning in the e-learning environment. *Journal of Nursing Education, 47*, 82–86.

Mastrian, K. (2008). Invited editorial: Cognitive informatics and nursing practice. *Online Journal of Nursing Informatics, 12*(1). Retrieved August 23, 2008, from http://ojni.org/ 12_1/kathy.html

Masys, D. R., Brennan, P. F., Ozbolt, J. G., Corn, M., & Shortliffe, E. H. (2000). Are medical informatics and nursing informatics distinct disciplines? *Journal of American Medical Informatics Association, 7,* 304–312.

McBride, A. (2005). Nursing and the informatics revolution. *Nursing Outlook, 53*(4), 183–191. doi:10.1016/j.outlook.2005.02.006

McGonigle, D. (2006). Editorial: Abbreviation frenzy. *Online Journal of Nursing Informatics, 10*(2). Retrieved May 26, 2009, from http://ojni.org/10_2/dee.htm

Medical Library Association. (2005). *Communicating health information literacy.* Retrieved August 25, 2008, from http://www.mlanet.org

Moorhead, S., Johnson, M., Maas, M. L., & Swanson, E. (Eds.). (2008). *Nursing outcomes classification (NOC)* (4th ed.). St. Louis, MO: Mosby.

Murray, E., Lo, B., Pollack, L., Donelan, K., Catania, J., Lee, K., et al. (2003). The impact of health information on the Internet on health care and the physician-patient relationship: National U.S. survey among 1,050 U.S. physicians. A qualitative exploration. *Journal of Medical Internet Research, 5*(3), e17. Retrieved November 17, 2008, from http://www.jmir. org/2003/3/e17/HTML

National Guideline Clearinghouse. (n.d.). *How to construct a guideline comparison.* Retrieved August 27, 2008, from http://www.guideline.gov/help/ConstructComparison.aspx

National League for Nursing. (2008, May 9). *Position statement: Preparing the next generation of nurses to practice in a technology-rich environment: An informatics agenda.* Retrieved November 17, 2008, from http://www.nln.org/aboutnln/PositionStatements/informatics_ 052808.pdf

Ornes, L. L., & Gassert, C. (2007). Computer competencies in a BSN program. *Journal of Nursing Education, 46,* 75–78.

Patt, M. R., Houston, T. K., Jenckes, M. W., Sands, D. Z., & Ford, D. E. (2003). Doctors who are using e-mail with their patients: A qualitative exploration. *Journal of Medical Internet Research, 5*(2), e9. Retrieved November 17, 2008, from http://www.jmir.org/2003/2/e9/HTML

Randell, R., Mitchell, N., Dowding, D., Cullum, N., & Thompson, C. (2007). Effects of computerized decision support systems on nursing performance and patient outcomes: A systematic review. *Journal of Health Services Research & Policy, 12,* 242–249.

Saba, V. K. (2001). Nursing informatics: Yesterday, today and tomorrow. *International Nursing Review, 48,* 177–187.

Saba, V. K., & McCormick, K. A. (Eds.). (2001). *Essentials of computers for nurses: Informatics in the next millennium.* New York: McGraw-Hill.

Saleem, J. J., Patterson, E. S., Militello, L., Anders, S., Falciglia, M., Wissman, J. A., et al. (2007). Impact of clinical reminder redesign on learnability, efficiency, usability, and workload for ambulatory clinic nurses. *Journal of the American Medical Informatics Association, 14*(5), 632–640. doi:10.1197/jamia.M2163

Saranto, K., & Hovenga, E. J. S. (2004). Information literacy—what is it about? Literature review of the concept and the context. *International Journal of Medical Informatics, 73,* 503–513.

Scheffer, B. K., & Rubenfeld, M. G. (2000). A consensus statement on critical thinking in nursing. *Journal of Nursing Education, 39,* 352–359.

Simpson, R. L. (2007). The politics of information technology. *Nursing Administration Quarterly, 31,* 354–358.

Stanger, K. (2008, June). *Criteria for evaluating resources (Internet- and print-based)*. Retrieved November 17, 2008, from http://www.emich.edu/halle/evaluating_internet.html

Tennant, R. (2008, May). *Virtual libraries/virtual learners: A matter of perspective.* Keynote address at the Michigan Library Association's Academic Libraries Day, Central Michigan University, Kalamazoo.

The TIGER Initiative. (2007). *The TIGER Initiative: Evidence and informatics transforming nursing: 3-year action steps toward a 10-year vision.* Retrieved August 23, 2008, from http://www.aacn.nche.edu/Education/pdf/TIGER.pdf

Turley, J. P. (1996). Toward a model for nursing informatics. *IMAGE: Journal of Nursing Scholarship, 28,* 309–313.

Turley, J. P., Murray, P. J., Saranto, K., Ehnfors, M., & Seomun, G-A. (2007). What if nurses get what they have always sought: Totally personalized care? Trends affecting nursing informatics. In P. J. Murray, H. Park, W. S. Erdley, & J. Kim (Eds.), *Nursing informatics 2020: Towards defining our own future* (pp. 55–72). Fairfax, VA: IOS Press.

Walji, M., Sagaram, S., Sagaram, D., Meric-Bernstam, F., Johnson, C., Mirza, N. Q., et al. (2004). Efficacy of quality criteria to identify potentially harmful information: A cross sectional survey of complementary and alternative medicine web sites. *Journal of Medical Internet Research, 6*(2), e9. Retrieved November 17, 2008, from http://www.jmir.org/2004/2/e21/HTML

Wang, Y. (2003). Cognitive informatics: A new transdisciplinary research field. *Brain and Mind, 4,* 115–127.

Warren, J. J., Connors, H. R., Weaver, C., & Simpson, R. (2006). Teaching undergraduate nursing students critical thinking: An innovative informatics strategy. *Studies in Health Technology and Informatics, 122,* 261–265.

Weiss, B. D. (2007). *Removing barriers to better, safer care—Health literacy and patient safety: Help patients understand. Manual for clinicians* (2nd ed.). Retrieved August 25, 2008, from http://www.ama-assn.org/ama1/pub/upload/mm/367/healthlitclinicians.pdf

Williams, M. D., Gish, K. W., Giuse, N. B., Sathe, N. A., & Carrell, D. L. (2001). The patient informatics consult service (PICS): An approach for a patient-centered service. *Bulletin of Medical Librarians Association, 89,* 185–193.

———————————— **10**

Assessing Critical Thinking

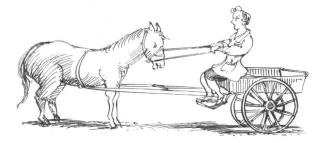

Now for the million-dollar question: "How do we measure critical thinking?" You might think that such a question has a neat answer, such as a list of exams or test questions that provide a picture of thinking. However, the answers are anything but simple. A big complication is the assumption that critical thinking (CT) can be measured, or assessed, without a clear understanding of what CT is. The "cart before the horse" cartoon is meant as a visual reminder of this backward thinking. To get the horse in front of the cart, therefore, we used our *logical reasoning* and saved this topic for the next-to-last chapter of the text, to be read after you've gotten a better idea of what CT is. This chapter focuses on the terminology of measuring/assessing CT; the rationale for discussing measurement/assessment at the end of the book; the challenges of measuring/assessing, including who does the assessing; the linkages among CT teaching, learning, and assessing in both academic and clinical settings; and finally, examples of both evidence-based and practical teaching/learning/assessing "tools" of CT.

Terminology of Measuring/Assessing Critical Thinking

Before we launch into details of determining if CT is occurring, we'd like to discuss why we've used the word *assessing* instead of *evaluating* in our title and why we're going to use the term *assessment* from here on as we discuss measuring CT. First of all, what we call *evaluation* in nursing is often referred to as *assessment* in other fields—education and business in particular. *Evaluation* has a connotation of right or wrong; *assessment* implies data collection or measurement followed by interpretation, but the interpretation is not necessarily a judgment of right or wrong.

The nursing profession may have gone over to the word *evaluation* because of the established description of the nursing process, in which *assessment* means collecting data and interpreting patients' needs, and *evaluation* means determining if the patient has met the goals outlined in our plans of care after the implementation of planned interventions. In reality, our nursing process "evaluation" phase is really another "assessment" with goals as a standard of comparison.

CT is not a right or wrong thing—it just is. Everyone thinks; granted, some do it better and more critically than others, but we rarely come to conclusions that someone's totality of thinking was wrong. Because most healthcare professionals are still discussing what CT actually is, we're a long way from being able to say that this thinking is right and that thinking is wrong. Most people would be hard-pressed to even describe how one person's thinking is better than another's. At this point, we basically see the outcomes of thinking, but not the actual thinking that led to those outcomes. We're hard pressed to say whether the thinking that led to those outcomes was poor, mediocre, good, or top notch.

OK, can we live with *assessment* being the better word for now? We'll assume that you all nodded your heads, so we'll move on to a discussion of the points we laid out in the introduction to this chapter.

Rationale for Discussing Assessing Last

First and foremost, it is essential to understand the vocabulary and the complexity of CT—how difficult it is to talk about CT without a vocabulary for the components of CT; how the dynamic context of health care affects, and is affected by, CT; how it fits with current desired competencies in health care, such as those advocated by the Institute of Medicine (IOM); and how it plays out in real life—before we discuss how it might be assessed. We believe that many of the existing approaches to evaluation of CT have imposed a very reductionist view of CT in nursing; educators and clinicians have been led to believe that CT can be put into boxes to be dichotomously checked off. They have been using instruments that have little validity for nursing because they weren't based on descriptions of CT in nursing.

Second, we believe that nurses (especially in nursing education) jumped on the bandwagon of evaluating CT in the early 1990s, largely in response to accreditation standards, before they really understood what CT was all about. They started evaluating (assessing) something that they probably weren't overtly teaching. At the very least, there was incongruence between what was being taught and what was being assessed. We want to make sure that the horse (understanding and teaching CT) gets in front and is ready to lead the cart (assessing/evaluating), not the other way around.

These issues—understanding CT complexity and pressures to evaluate CT—are interrelated. Quantitative measuring instruments cannot capture the complexity of

CT, but they are popular because of their ease of use. Qualitative processes can capture the complexity, but they are cumbersome and require more resources to use properly. Outside pressures to measure CT have pushed educators to find measurement instruments quickly. No objective measures accurately reflect what anecdotal reports from clinicians and educators show. Finding a suitable measure has been the most difficult problem in meeting the CT accreditation criterion (Stone, Davidson, Evans, & Hansen, 2001). The literature still documents the lack of valid and reliable tools to measure CT (Britton & Wissing, 2006; Walsh & Seldomridge, 2006a, 2006b). Hold your horses! It appears that many authors have not found our research that does exactly that. Shortly we will show you a valid and reliable "tool/protocol" for assessing CT.

Finally, the third reason we saved assessing CT for the end is that we want you to have a solid foundation from which you can view our suggestions for valid and reliable CT assessment processes—processes with a real-life view of CT in nursing.

After completing the research to find a consensus on CT in nursing, we found that although there were many similarities between our statement and other definitions of CT, there were also unique components. Whether these are unique to nursing or characteristic of healthcare disciplines and applied sciences remains to be seen. (You may want to review Chapter 2 to refresh your thinking relative to those unique areas of CT.) Because we are convinced that CT in nursing has some discipline-specific characteristics, we don't believe it can adequately be assessed with nonnursing instruments or instruments that are not based on a nursing definition of CT.

The Challenges of Assessing CT

Just how did we get the cart in front of the horse? There are several reasons. CT is much more complex than most people realize. When it comes to testing, we like standardization and simplicity, and we are apt to grab instruments that are quick and easy to use. We also see assessment as something done only by others, not by the thinkers themselves.

The Impact of the Complexity of CT on the Assessment of CT

Whew! That subheading alone is complex, isn't it? As Walsh and Seldomridge (2006a) noted, "Critical thinking is not one, monolithic thing. . . . We have come to appreciate that the term critical thinking is a shorthand 'umbrella term' . . . to connote the many activities pertinent to good thinking, and specifically here, to the provision of high-quality nursing care" (p. 216).

So, how do you assess something complex? First of all, you need to articulate what that complex phenomenon is, as we have done in the previous chapters. Then you must break it down (*analyzing*) into understandable parts without losing track of the whole (*contextual perspective*).

As you have probably figured out by now, that's no easy task with CT. Our research gave you a set of 17 dimensions that an international panel of nurses arrived at through a long process of consensus (Scheffer & Rubenfeld, 2000). That research-based description is only now starting to be cited in nursing literature by clinicians, researchers, and educators (e.g., Ali, Bantz, & Siktberg, 2005; Allen, Rubenfeld, & Scheffer, 2004; Lunney, 2003; Staib, 2003; Tanner, 2005; Twibell, Ryan, & Hermiz, 2005; Walsh & Seldomridge, 2006a, 2006b).

Rush, Dyches, Waldrop, and Davis (2008) used our nursing Delphi conceptualization of CT in their qualitative study of distance learning for registered nurse (RN)-to-bachelor of science in nursing degree (BSN) students. They demonstrated that simulations via distance learning cultivated the CT of their subjects. Dickieson, Carter, and Walsh (2008) incorporated the 17 dimensions of our nursing Delphi study in a scenario-testing rubric when studying three approaches to integrative thinking and learning. Lunney (2009), in her chapter of *Nursing Diagnoses: Definitions and Classification, 2009–2011*, reaffirmed the importance of using the 17 dimensions of the nursing Delphi study if nurses want to achieve accurate interpretation of data when making nursing diagnoses.

Things are improving, but it does not negate the issue of complexity. So if we accept the complexity of CT in nursing, what does this mean in terms of assessing CT of clinicians and students? To have any validity, assessment instruments must measure (assess) what they purport to measure (remember Research 101!). Multiple-choice tests are very popular because they provide "objective" numerical data that can be analyzed in varying configurations to show results for individuals and groups. They can be used easily and require very few personnel resources, so they are very desirable in fields such as nursing, which require lots of resources anyway. However, measuring/assessing something as complex as CT via quantitative measures is very difficult; items have to be cleaned up enough so that the instrument has reliability, and in that process of "clean-up," it is easy to lose what is important. In the process of reducing a complex concept to achieve reliability, validity can very easily go out the window.

Standardized Instruments

Even though there has been little consistency in the definitions of CT used by nursing over the years, and descriptions of CT have varied across nursing programs (Dickieson et al., 2008; Scheffer, 2001; Walsh & Seldomridge, 2006a; Zygmont & Schaefer, 2006), attempts at assessment have been made. Nurse educators have traditionally gravitated to assessing CT with standardized multiple-choice tests for quite some time. See Staib (2003) for a concise review of these commonly used multiple-choice instruments: the Watson-Glaser Critical Thinking Appraisal, the California Critical Thinking Skills Test, the California Critical Thinking Dispositions Inventory, and the Minnesota Test of Critical Thinking. The National League for Nursing (2007) developed a nursing-based multiple-choice CT instrument. Two of the newer versions of the standardized CT tests are the Assessment Technologies Institute (ATI) Critical Thinking Assessment (2006) and the Health Sciences Reasoning Test (Facione & Facione, 2006).

Standardized tests for CT, however, are frequently not based on descriptions of nursing CT; rather, they are based on more general descriptions of CT. They also have another problem, as noted by Walsh and Seldomridge (2006a): "The use of standardized instruments to measure critical thinking skills is not particularly useful because such tools assess the skills of classic logic, as opposed to the critical thinking skills of clinical practice. . . . [They] do not target such skills as clinical problem solving or decision making" (p. 216). Many of these standardized tests are still used today despite inconsistent research findings as to their value in assessing students' CT ability (Adams, 1999; Dulski, Kelly, & Carrol, 2006; Staib, 2003). The need for discipline-specific CT instruments continues to be addressed (e.g., Allen et al., 2004; Beckie, Lowry, & Barnett, 2001; Britton & Wissing, 2006; Dulski et al., 2006; Stone et al., 2001; Walsh & Seldomridge, 2006a).

Other reasons have been postulated for the inability of standardized tests to show objectively that students learn CT while in nursing school. A major reason for this inability is that these standardized tests lack validity for nursing because they are not based on definitions of CT in the field. When we conduct workshops on CT around the world, we are frequently asked questions about CT assessment instruments. Academic-based educators are particularly frustrated with their present instruments. Practice-based educators haven't been using these instruments but are interested in how they can assess CT in their staff. Clinicians want to know how they can see if their CT is on track.

One final concern regarding the use of standardized tests to assess CT is the potential language barrier for students and nurses who are not native English speakers. This is particularly important as we move toward a more diverse nursing workforce. Whitehead (2006), the director of research at ATI, tested for potential language barriers with ATI's Critical Thinking Assessment test. She compared a sample of 192 native-English-speaking nursing students with 17 non-native-English-speaking nursing students from 21 universities who took the test at entry to and exit from their nursing program. Although the non-native-English-speaking students scored lower than the native English speakers upon entry into the program, on exit, they scored 72%, as compared with 73% for the native English speakers. This led the researcher to conclude that the ATI test was language neutral. Other researchers have explored similar issues; for example, Guttman (2004) studied the cultural and linguistic competence of nurses immigrating to the United States. It will be important to monitor results of other studies and to always consider language as one of the challenges in accurately assessing CT.

The Cart-Before-the-Horse Challenge with Assessing CT

"Incomplete or premature assessment destroys learning" (Senge, 1998, section 4, para 2). This should probably be posted in meeting rooms as academic-based educators contemplate accreditation visits, and it should appear in front of clinicians who look at their colleagues and conclude that there is little CT going on. In the same section of the document just cited, Senge quoted Bill O'Brien, retired chief

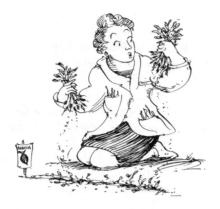

executive officer of Hanover Insurance, as saying that "managers are always pulling up the radishes to see how they're growing."

This is what we've been doing—pulling up the radishes (a.k.a., premature assessment). Some of the push for CT assessment has come from accrediting bodies. The National League for Nursing Accrediting Commission (NLNAC; 2000) had a tradition of being fairly prescriptive in requirements for CT assessment. Their recent accreditation criteria are less specific with regard to CT measurement (NLNAC, 2008). The Commission on Collegiate Nursing Education (2008) asks that *The Essentials of Baccalaureate Education for Professional Nursing Practice* (American Association of Colleges of Nursing, 2008) be used to guide programs; that document lists CT as an assumed outcome for baccalaureate nursing graduates.

We started, at least in academic settings, assessing CT before we articulated what it was, how best to teach it, and indeed, whether we were teaching it at all. We valued CT and have been quite sure that nurses use CT. However, we mistook our valuing of the idea and assumptions about CT; we thought that meant we were teaching it, and we thought that students were learning it. In reality, we were assessing things that we didn't understand well, that we had difficulty articulating, and that we probably were not teaching.

Who Does the Assessing of CT?

Based on the previous discussion, one could assume that assessing CT is a function of education coordinators, nurse managers (in the practice setting), and nurse educators in the academic setting. For the most part, that is true, but we can't leave out one equally important assessor—YOU!

Your ability to self-assess—or, as we say in the language of CT, *reflection*—is as essential to your growth in CT as feedback from authority figures. Remember the definition of *reflection*: "Contemplation upon a subject, especially one's assumptions and thinking for the purposes of deeper understanding and self-evaluation"

(Scheffer & Rubenfeld, 2000, p. 358). This kind of assessment does not require purchased materials or even another person, just you. But it does require time, *open-mindedness,* and *intellectual integrity.*

Harris (2007) addressed the value of critical reflection in a 3-year qualitative study with nurses in South Africa. Scaffolding reflective journal writing was the focus of the study. The project included several support structures for reflection, such as feedback, mutually developed evaluation strategies, and planned dialogue between reflector and reviewer of the reflection. Question prompts were developed. Guidelines for reflective writing, feedback, and critique were established, and a self-evaluation rubric was developed. The nurses who participated found reflective writing quite challenging, but it was worth it for the "transformative learning" (moving to a level of *confidence* in your decision making and learning) that resulted. Harris concluded that the best self-reflection requires preparation, critique, feedback, reinforcement, and assessors/educators who are willing to "develop their own reflexive and facilitative skills" (p. 326).

In preparing this chapter on assessment of thinking, we were inspired by the writings of a nurse from New Zealand (Pothan, 2008). She described how she, an advanced practice nurse, was taking a postgraduate nursing practicum course that required reflective writing. At the beginning of the course, she was skeptical about its value because she already possessed a strong knowledge base and could multi-task from strategic planning to safe patient care with no problem. She could not imagine how reflective writing would make her a better nurse. By the end of the course, however, she had what she labeled as her "eureka" moment. She described the value of reflecting on both the positive and negative aspects of her practice. She acknowledged that the skill of reflection could be taught and learned. Her closing words best describe the transformation she experienced:

> Reflective writing has enabled me to produce some of my best nursing work to date. I describe this new awareness of my own personal/practice development as the final piece of the straight edged, outside frame of a jigsaw [puzzle]. Now this is complete, I feel confident to advance to complete the bigger picture, knowing there is a sturdy frame holding it all together. (p. 23)

Now, not all *reflection* requires writing. Much is done in a less formal way—for example, by simply taking the time to think about your day, a specific incident, a challenging situation, the outcome of a meeting, a grade on a paper assignment, or an interaction with a peer, teacher, or friend. For those who take CT seriously, *reflection* becomes a strong habit of the mind. You are teacher-learner-assessor all rolled into one, and *reflection* becomes a part of your being. We encourage you to reread the Reflection in Practice section in Chapter 4 (p. 84).

So, to summarize before moving on to the linkages among teaching, learning, and assessment, there are some challenges related to assessing CT. Its complexity cannot be ignored if we want valid and reliable assessments. We need to be aware of the advantages and disadvantages of standardized tests that purport to assess CT. We should not assess for CT if we haven't first defined it and taught folks about it. And we must acknowledge that we ourselves are one of the key assessors of CT through reflection.

Linking Teaching, Learning, and Assessing of CT

Figure 10-1 is something we've used in workshops with academic-based educators who struggle to link CT with assessment. It's a simple idea but one that is easily overlooked. We ask educators to look at their expected program outcomes and follow the various steps along the way toward evaluation mechanisms; the steps in between are theoretical and operational definitions of CT, course objectives, CT course content and teaching strategies, and, finally, evaluation. Educators often express surprise when they see that they have gaps or inconsistencies in that sequence; they have course objectives related to CT but no real definition of it. Often, they have CT in the "evaluation mechanisms" box but nowhere else. They know that it is important and that accreditors are looking for it. CT is "tacked on" instead of being integrated into programs.

We see the same tacking-on happening in textbooks. CT exercises have become the norm in most of the big undergraduate texts for adult health, obstetrical, pediatric, and community health nursing. However, if you look closely at many of those texts, you might wonder why those particular exercises are characterized as CT and how the authors are defining CT. There is often an assumption

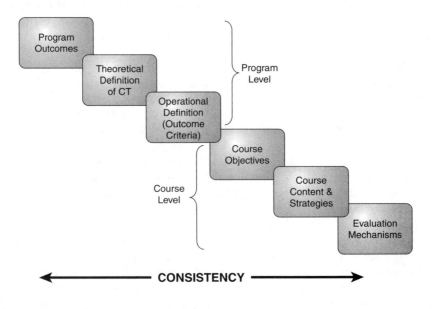

Figure 10-1 Consistency of CT in Academic Programs

that everyone knows what CT is and that everyone defines it the same way. In reality, if you ask many faculty how they are defining CT in their programs, they will have trouble answering (Scheffer, 2001). And most respondents in a randomized sample of 300 full-time nurse educators answered No when asked if they have had any education on CT (Zygmont & Schaefer, 2006).

There is some danger that clinicians will be subjected to the same faulty means of assessment that have occurred in academic settings because increasingly there are messages that nurses must be good critical thinkers to promote safety and increase quality. Administrators and managers will look for quick assessment instruments to give a numerical value, or thinking number, to nurses. We are sometimes asked if we have remedial CT courses for nurses who have made serious mistakes and who need to improve their thinking. (We don't.) That kind of simplistic approach to CT makes it seem like any other tacked-on skill that can be fixed with a refresher course.

Because of our concerns about making the same mistakes in practice settings as in academic settings, we have included **Figure 10-2**, which shows organizational tracking points for looking for consistency in CT. If personnel in practice settings value CT enough to evaluate it, they must be careful to consistently define it in mission statements, aims, objectives, expectations, and so forth.

CT must be integrated throughout clinical and educational programs. All the other things we teach, learn, and practice provide the context for CT. It can't be separated or tacked on. It must be defined, described, taught, and practiced. Clinicians

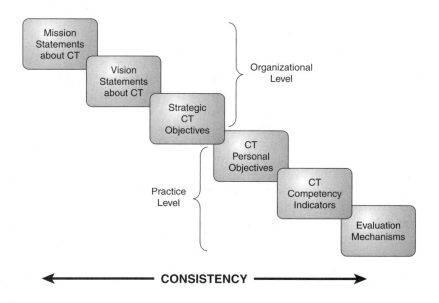

Figure 10-2 Consistency of CT in Practice Settings

and learners must have time to describe their thinking, and practice and demonstrate it before being assessed on how well they've learned it. Assessment of CT must be linked to expectations and behaviors.

Facilitating the Linkages

If we accept that healthcare delivery and education occur in complex, adaptive learning environments, we want to make sure that we assess what is being learned using methods that address complexity and that are also adaptive. Trying to take the complexity out of CT for the purpose of having clean, quantitative tools won't provide a picture of how we, and the people around us, are doing with CT. Likewise, we won't get a picture of CT if our assessment procedures are so vague that no one understands what is being assessed. In **Box 10-1**, we have outlined some considerations for your journey toward valid assessment of CT.

First, have a clear idea of what CT is for your organization. Is it defined as a complex collection of cognitive skills and affective habits of the mind, or is it overly simplified? Beware if it is defined very simply. The definition may have been driven by the assessment method: defined after the fact to fit with an instrument. That's the tail wagging the dog. If there's no description to be found anywhere, then consider if you need one. Is CT important in your organization? It should be in today's complex healthcare delivery and education. You may be the person who needs to develop, adopt, or adapt a description of your organization's thinking model.

If you find a very complex description of CT, is it broken down into manageable components or presented as an operational definition so that it can be assessed? If it hasn't been, then beware, because chances are CT is not being assessed, or there is a misfit between the definition and the assessment process.

If there is no assessment plan in place, should there be one? If your answer is Yes, then, as with finding a description, it may be up to you to develop, adapt, or adopt one. If there is a description and an operational working model of CT, then you can make a list of what should be assessed. Now you have to consider what the assessment results will be used for. Will they be for staff performance evaluations? Self-evaluations? Peer evaluations? Career advancement? Program evaluation? Course grades? Accreditation justification? Obviously, those questions and answers will be largely specific to the institution.

Once you have those answers, you're ready to consider various methods of assessment. We have some suggestions, but first we'd like to address a question that often emerges at this point. Maybe you haven't considered this, but many nurses ask, "Isn't what I do (or my students or staff do) proof enough of CT—that is, isn't it all about actions anyway?" The answer to that is that it depends. Sometimes actions can show CT, sometimes not. You might see the same actions from two people, but the first one just happened to see the second one doing something and mimicked the behavior. The second one might have spent hours thinking to come up with that approach. It's only when you start asking them to describe why they're doing what they're doing that you begin to see the thinking.

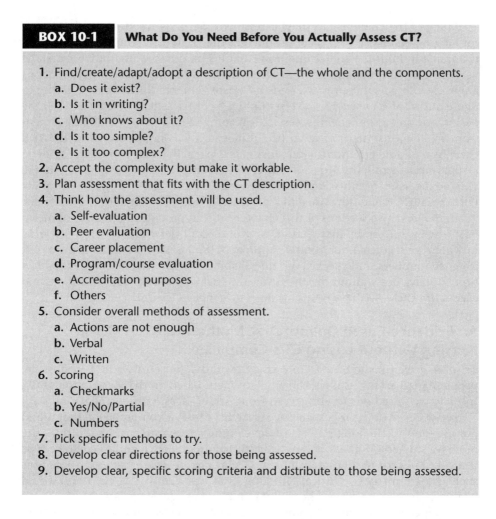

BOX 10-1   **What Do You Need Before You Actually Assess CT?**

1. Find/create/adapt/adopt a description of CT—the whole and the components.
   a. Does it exist?
   b. Is it in writing?
   c. Who knows about it?
   d. Is it too simple?
   e. Is it too complex?
2. Accept the complexity but make it workable.
3. Plan assessment that fits with the CT description.
4. Think how the assessment will be used.
   a. Self-evaluation
   b. Peer evaluation
   c. Career placement
   d. Program/course evaluation
   e. Accreditation purposes
   f. Others
5. Consider overall methods of assessment.
   a. Actions are not enough
   b. Verbal
   c. Written
6. Scoring
   a. Checkmarks
   b. Yes/No/Partial
   c. Numbers
7. Pick specific methods to try.
8. Develop clear directions for those being assessed.
9. Develop clear, specific scoring criteria and distribute to those being assessed.

The mimic will likely have trouble adapting the action to a different set of circumstances because the background thinking hasn't occurred.

To assess thinking, we need the person's descriptions of his or her thinking to judge that thinking. In Chapter 2, we described the necessity of a thinking vocabulary to understand CT (see Box 2-5). That vocabulary becomes equally necessary for assessing CT.

So, you need to either hear or read a person's description of thinking to assess that thinking. Now comes the harder part. How can you do that in ways that will meet all of your needs? Does it always have to be set up like an interview or an essay? No. Do you have to spend hours reading and/or listening to these "answers" to make a judgment about how someone is thinking? No. Can you ever get numerical data from such seemingly qualitative assessment processes? Yes.

Much of the challenge in these assessment methods is setting up the criteria for judging quality. We're so conditioned to the "right or wrong" mentality that is implicit in multiple-choice questions that it's hard to see alternatives. First, be very clear in your directions for assignments used to assess CT. If the directions are fuzzy, the person being assessed will waste valuable thinking time trying to figure out what is expected. Next, set up the "scoring" ahead of time and tell the person how he or she is being assessed. Is it going to be a Yes (the thinking dimension was demonstrated) or a No (the dimension was not demonstrated)? Will there be a middle ground (the dimension was partially demonstrated)? Will you assign numbers or letters to those criteria? Remember, to set up specific criteria, you, as the assessor, must know what you are assessing. Once again, you must know what CT is and how you and your organization define it and its parameters.

In the next two sections of this chapter, we will provide suggestions of methods to assess CT. In the first section, we will report briefly on our latest research, in which we studied a quantitative approach. We assessed all dimensions of CT, assigned numbers, and checked out the reliability of that method. In the final section, we have descriptions of other strategies that we have used in workshops and classes (for these, we have only anecdotal evidence of their success).

An Evidence-Based Quantitative Method to Assess CT in Nursing Without Losing CT's Complexity

As soon as we finished the Delphi study to find a consensus on CT in nursing, people started asking us if we had an instrument based on that description of CT. Initially we raised our forefingers in front of our faces, crossed them, and said, "No way are we doing psychometric research!" Most of you probably understand our aversion to the long process of developing an instrument. In addition, the more we studied CT, the more we realized that an objective multiple-choice-type test could never test all dimensions of CT. We also realized that essay-type tests such as the Ennis-Weir Critical Thinking Essay Test (Ennis & Weir, 1985) would be very time consuming and not helpful in tracking aggregate data.

In our courses, we started giving students reflection assignments to show their CT and to help them learn the vocabulary necessary to articulate their abstract thinking processes. Sometimes we gave them vignettes and asked them to do something to show their thinking. At other times, especially in clinical courses, we asked them to reflect on events from their clinical time to show their thinking. We used the 17 dimensions of CT from our research to give direction so that students could zero in on specific parts of the thinking processes. They wrote about one or two dimensions at a time, not all 17. Over the course of a semester or year, they addressed all dimensions of CT.

As any educator will tell you, grading essays can be extremely time consuming. To save ourselves time, we developed scoring rubrics to give to students ahead of time so that they would know what a 3 or a 2 meant. Then we could just put numerical scores on their papers. After we tried this for a few years, we thought that it might work as a more formal means of assessing CT. We knew that we had some validity going for us because we were basing this work on a research-derived description of CT in nursing. However, we weren't sure if our assessment procedure could be done reliably by others. We decided that it was time for help from someone more knowledgeable about psychometrics and statistics than we were. Enter Dr. George Allen from Michigan State University, up the road from us at Eastern Michigan University. We teamed up with George and told him about our consideration of reflection assignments graded with a scoring rubric as a means to reliably assess CT in nursing students.

We developed a plan and piloted it at four schools with undergraduate nursing students. Because we knew that assessment must be linked with teaching and learning, we conducted workshops for those faculty and described the procedure for assessment. The faculty who agreed to try this in a course assigned the reflections, scored them using the rubric, and sent them to George, who sent them blind to the two of us. We scored them independently and sent them back to George to analyze the results for reliability. We were happy to see that our coefficient alphas for interrater reliability were between 0.70 and 0.80, which, according to most authorities, is quite satisfactory for educational purposes (e.g., Nunnally, 2002). For a detailed report of this research, see Allen et al. (2004).

We learned from this process that short-essay-type CT reflection assignments may be scored quite quickly using a rubric. It took us between 1 and 2 minutes to score each assignment after doing the first few. Remember, we weren't grading things like grammar and writing style, so we did not have to insert written comments as we read; we just used the rubric and assigned numbers. We need to keep that in mind; nursing faculty often feel the need to grade all written projects for writing style. If that is your aim, do it with other assignments, not those for which you primarily want to assess CT.

The final section of this chapter is divided into the two parts listed in **Box 10-2**. List A includes strategies to assess all or selected dimensions of CT, including more details on the Free Response and Vignette protocols researched in the Allen et al. (2004) study. List B contains strategies that fit better with some dimensions than with others. In keeping with our view that assessment must be closely linked with teaching, learning, and practicing CT, all these methods may be used for teaching, learning, and/or assessment purposes.

Examples of Practical Teaching/Learning/Assessing "Tools" of CT from List A in Box 10-2

Free Responses and Vignettes

Both types of reflections are written projects that focus on one or two CT dimensions at a time. In a free response, students are asked to reflect on an activity, such as a clinical encounter, and to describe three things: (1) how they demonstrated one or two of the dimensions, such as creativity and intuition, (2) justification of

BOX 10-2	Practical Teaching/Learning/Assessing "Tools" of CT

List A: Tools That Can Be Used for All or Selected Dimensions
- Written or verbal free-response reflections
- Written or verbal reflections on vignettes
- CT inventories
- Mind maps
- MUDD mapping
- Rubrics

List B: Tools Used for Specific Dimensions
- Developing a new approach to something (*creativity, inquisitiveness, transforming knowledge*)
- Debate from an opposite perspective (*intellectual integrity, open-mindedness*)
- Differential diagnosing (*discriminating, logical reasoning, confidence, contextual perspective, intellectual integrity, intuition*)
- Listing hunches (*intuition*)
- Answering "But, what if. . . ?" questions (*transforming knowledge, flexibility*)
- What is likely to happen to this patient? (*predicting, contextual perspective*)
- What would you assess next? (*information seeking, discriminating, contextual perspective*)
- What is the principle? (*applying standards*)
- Calling the physician (*discriminating, analyzing, contextual perspective*)
- What's wrong with this picture? (*discriminating*)
- Critique of literature (*applying standards, discriminating, analyzing, logical reasoning*)
- Moral dilemmas (*analyzing, intellectual integrity, flexibility*)

why that description represents those dimensions, and (3) expansion—projecting how they could better use those dimensions the next time. These are scored with three numbers, one for each required part of the response, as shown in **Box 10-3**.

This scoring could, of course, be adapted to one's environment. If you worked with one group of students, all of whom were at the same level of expertise, the third part of the score could be simplified to a 2- or 3-point scale. We used an expertise qualifier so we could show students how their level of knowledge naturally affects their thinking of alternatives and details.

Box 10-4 is an example of a junior student's reflection on a clinical situation in which the CT dimension of flexibility was used. This was scored as 8: The

BOX 10-3	**Scoring of Free-Response Reflections**

1. (Identification) Does it represent the dimension?
  a. 2—It is a good representation of the dimension(s).
  b. 1—The description was partially representative of the dimension(s).
  c. 0—The description does not represent that dimension (for example, the description seemed more like logical reasoning than creativity).
2. (Justification) Is there support for the match?
  a. 1—Yes
  b. 2—No
3. (Expansion Level) Is the insight into how to use the dimension(s) better appropriate to student's academic level?
  a. 5—Postbaccalaureate nurse
  b. 4—Senior, second semester
  c. 3—Senior, first semester
  d. 2—Junior, second semester
  e. 1—Junior, first semester
  f. 0—Insufficient for junior-level nursing student

Note: The expansion scoring could be adapted to any group. This was used with baccalaureate nursing students over their last 2 years. Obviously, this could be changed. What is important is to acknowledge the student's or nurse's expected level of nursing knowledge.

description clearly identified thinking flexibility (Identification = 2); the student justified this as flexibility at the end of the second paragraph (Justification = 1); and the expansion was very sophisticated, beyond what we'd expect for a second-semester junior (Expansion = 5).

With vignette responses, students are given a short patient situation/case study and asked to describe how they would do something to demonstrate specified CT dimensions. They are also asked to justify why their description represents those dimensions. These vignette responses are scored with the same scale used for free responses. The expansion (third) part in this case judges the level of detail of the descriptions according to students' class level. **Box 10-5** has an example of a vignette assignment.

Obviously, vignettes could be specific to units, levels, or courses. They could be used as a means of assessment (our focus here) or as a teaching/learning focus. Service-based educators could use unit-specific vignettes to help new staff get used to the thinking needed on that unit, for example. Clinicians could write vignettes and prepare a bank of them for others to use.

BOX 10-4	Example of a Junior BSN Student Free-Response Reflection

*One critical thinking reflection dimension that I used during clinical was **flexibility**, the capacity to adapt, accommodate, modify, or change thoughts, ideas, and behaviors. During an interaction with a patient, several times I had to adapt my approaches to her. She was bipolar, having psychosis, and was in a severely manic acute phase of the disorder, delusional and hearing voices. In my attempts to interact and interview the patient, she displayed disorganized and illogical thought processes. She would jump from one topic to the next and even tried to get me to witness her hallucinations. My attempts to obtain information were constantly being hampered, and it was difficult to keep her oriented and focused. With every attempt at keeping the patient focused, I had to adapt to her various replies. I tried to change my approach and posture in order to find a way to connect with her. When she seemed to be overstimulated by her environment, I moved to the less stimulating atmosphere of the back lounge area. I changed directions in my mind over and over again. I had to appraise the situation and interactions with the patient in my mind.*

*At first I was at a loss as to how to make the interaction successful. Next, I was overly determined to make it work and even felt frustration starting. Consequently, I thought about stopping and trying again later. Something clicked in my mind that made me realize that silence, a break, and maybe just some time and patience would be beneficial. I realized that maybe my thinking of getting goals accomplished was hampering my thought processes and thus my interviewing abilities. I thought about waiting for a time when her anti-psychotic medication was peaking and then implemented this plan of approach. This approach worked much better, and I was able to obtain more information and interact more effectively with my client. Thus, I used **flexibility** in my ability to constantly reevaluate, adapt, and accommodate to the situation by changing my plan of action.*

*In this kind of situation again, I'd still need to consider many different alternatives until one worked, but I'd remember from this experience that I always have to be **flexible** in my thinking and actions with these kinds of patients. I would probably not be so fixated on the goals, and I'd be less frustrated because I'd turn on my flexible thinking right away.*

Both free responses and vignettes can be used as a way to cover all dimensions of CT but allow for a detailed assessment of each dimension one at a time. These can be used to identify areas of strength and weakness; they allow for individual interpretations but require that persons be able to justify why they believe their statements represent the particular dimensions. That justification part is important because it demonstrates logical reasoning. Students must be able to articulate why their described thinking logically demonstrates the dimensions. It's not enough to say that they do; such statements must be justified.

BOX 10-5	**Example of a Vignette with Student Directions**

Directions:

1. Read the clinical vignette that follows.
2. Read the definition of the CT skill or habit that accompanies the vignette.
3. Describe how you would use the designated CT habit or skill to accomplish the proposed nursing intervention. Include in your description:
   a. What you would do, including enough detail of your thinking to show someone who was not there how you demonstrated the designated habit or skill.
   b. Why you believe your actions illustrate the designated habit or skill.

(You will be assessed for your ability to accurately represent the CT skill or habit, your justification of how your actions demonstrate the skill or habit, and the specificity of the description.)

Vignette: Charlotte and Mary's Adoption Plans

Critical Thinking Habit of the Mind: *intellectual integrity* (defined as seeking the truth through a sincere, honest process, even if the results are contrary to one's assumptions and beliefs)

Charlotte Jones and Mary Kelly are partners who have lived together for 2 years. They are considering adopting a child. They are patients in the obstetrics/gynecology practice where another patient, Susan Simone, is 11 weeks pregnant. Susan is unmarried and wishes to carry her child to term and consider adoption even though her partner, Tom, would rather she had an abortion. Susan, a sophomore in college, is very close to her mother, who is supportive of the plan to offer the child for adoption. Susan has no health insurance and has income only from her part-time job as a waitress. When Susan was told that Charlotte and Mary were interested in adopting her baby, she immediately told the nurse that she wanted to go ahead with whatever was necessary to arrange the adoption.

Describe how you, as the nurse in this situation, would use the *intellectual integrity* habit of the mind to help Susan, Charlotte, and Mary **prepare for and interact during their first meeting.**

If you want a numerical assessment of CT so that you can track aggregate data, using scoring rubrics allows you to maintain the complexity of CT but with a time-efficient manageable tool. **Box 10-6** provides several examples of tracking forms for individual and aggregate data.

| BOX 10-6 | Examples of Methods of Tracking CT Dimensions |

Example #1:
Compiling *Individual* **Student Data on CT Skills and Habits of the Mind**

Student Name _____ ID# _____
Undergraduate ❑   Graduate ❑

	Scores		
Dimension	**Course** _____	**Course** _____	**Course** _____
Confidence	_____	_____	_____
Contextual perspective	_____	_____	_____
Creativity	_____	_____	_____
Flexibility	_____	_____	_____
(and so forth for all dimensions)			

Example #2:
Aggregate *Course* **Data on Critical Thinking Skills and Habits of the Mind**

Undergraduate ❑   Graduate ❑   Semester/Year _____
# of Students   _____   _____   _____

	Averages of Scores for All Students		
Dimensions	**Course** _____	**Course** _____	**Course** _____
Confidence	_____	_____	_____
Contextual perspective	_____	_____	_____
Creativity	_____	_____	_____
(and so forth for all dimensions)			

Example #3:
Aggregate Entry/Exit Year Data on Critical Thinking Skills and Habits of the Mind
Undergraduate ❑   Graduate ❑

	Year _____	Year _____
# of students	_____	_____
Dimensions: average scores for all students in year		
Confidence	_____	_____
Contextual perspective	_____	_____
Creativity	_____	_____
Flexibility	_____	_____
(and so forth for all dimensions)		

Critical Thinking Inventory

Using the CT Inventory in Appendix A is another way to assess all dimensions of CT. This inventory has been updated since the first edition of this text. The updated version, which consists of fewer questions with more clarity for each of the dimensions, was based on feedback and its use in multiple nursing courses. The inventory is especially valuable as a self-assessment guide and as a teaching/learning tool to open up minds to the complexities of CT. This is a qualitative approach to assessment; it is difficult to assign numerical points except in terms of clarity, precision, or depth of description. We have used similar instruments for many years, starting with a THINK Inventory in our textbook for beginning-level students (Rubenfeld & Scheffer, 2006). It works best for self-evaluation and peer sharing.

Mind Mapping

We discussed mind maps in Chapter 4 (see Box 4-5 on p. 83) as an active teaching/learning process, but they can be used to assess CT as well. Most nursing literature on mind mapping, or its close cousin, concept mapping, describes its value in teaching and learning CT (e.g., Mueller, Johnston, & Bligh, 2002; Wheeler & Collins, 2003). However, others spoke directly to assessing. For example, Daley, Shaw, Balistrieri, Glasenapp, and Placentine (1999) outlined a method of assigning points for connecting links in concept maps that had good reliability between two scorers. Taylor and Wros (2007) provided examples of concept-mapping grading criteria.

MUDD Mapping

My Understanding through Dialogue and Debate (MUDD) is an active learning strategy designed by two nurse educators from Newfoundland and Prince Edward Island, Canada (Barringon & Campbell, 2008). It is essentially a form of group mind-mapping that is done in stages and that requires ongoing interaction among the participants as the map emerges. The instructor or facilitator considers course objectives and provides the central concept of the map, such as computer-based patient record intervention, and draws a number of spokes extending out from the center concept. This can be done on a white board or flip chart. The learners take turns adding one piece of information at a time, with time given for collaborative discussion of all aspects of that piece of information before moving to the next student's contribution. The authors described the thinking required as "collective . . . corrective . . . improved . . . expanded . . . and supported" (p. 161). The dialogue continues to focus on both new concepts and relationships among the added data. The activity finishes with a debate in which learners are able to state their position and support that position related to the overall components or issues that need to be addressed when considering the concept or intervention.

Rubrics

Have you ever struggled when deciding what grade to assign a student paper or a clinician's project? How do you differentiate between an A– and a B+? Or worse yet, between a C– and a D+? Have your assessments ever been challenged? Are students achieving the learning you want them to achieve on the assignments you give? These questions are more prevalent when we are assessing processes, such as CT, as opposed to more concrete issues, such as administering a subcutaneous injection.

One way to address those questions is with the use of a rubric. Rubrics are assessment scoring tools, and much more (Stevens & Levi, 2005). Designing a rubric requires several aspects of CT on the part of the assessor/educator. Assessors must *analyze* an assignment or project and break it into its component parts. Each component is further *analyzed* for what represents various levels of performance, from acceptable to unacceptable. *Discriminating* and *applying standards* are necessary to separate and level performance variables.

Britton and Wissing (2006), both respiratory care educators, described two kinds of rubrics—holistic and analytic—to achieve "authentic assessment." They cited authentic assessment as a strategy for helping students "develop desirable traits such as critical thinking, problem solving and life-long learning" (p. 21). Holistic rubrics are exactly that: looking at the whole. They examine an overall process or outcome without dissecting the parts. Analytic rubrics analyze the components in detail and score the details. **Tables 10-1** and **10-2** provide examples of each type of rubric as it would apply to learning in nursing.

TABLE 10-1 Example of a Holistic Rubric

The assignment is a 10-page paper designed to engage students' critical thinking regarding the current nursing shortage. Students are advised to (1) compare and contrast the current nursing shortage with shortages in the past, (2) address the impact of this shortage on the quality of patient care, and (3) discuss at least five of the critical thinking dimensions needed to help resolve the problem. Proper American Psychological Association (APA) format is required.

Criteria	Score
All three components of the assignment are clearly addressed and supported with literature.	95
Two of the three components of the assignment are clearly addressed and supported with literature.	80
One of the three components of the assignment is clearly addressed and supported with literature.	70
None of the three components of the assignment is addressed.	0
APA format is accurate.	5
Minor errors in APA format.	3
Significant errors in APA format.	0
Total Score (Maximum possible score = 100 points)	_____

TABLE 10-2 Example of an Analytic Rubric: Grading the Assessment Phase of the Nursing Process

This type of a rubric can be used to assess some of the critical thinking dimensions (*contextual perspective, inquisitiveness, intellectual integrity, perseverance, analyzing, applying standards, discriminating, information seeking, logical reasoning,* and *transforming knowledge*).

	Exemplary (5)	Competent (3)	Needs Work (1)	Score
Data Collection	Included data from interaction, observation, and measurement, as well as multiple sources (patient, family, chart, and other health-care providers)	Included data from two of the following: interaction, observation, and measurement.	Included data primarily from patient's chart.	
Data Analysis	Identified all relevant data. Compared data with population norms as well as personal norms to support conclusions. Listed data gaps.	Identified most relevant data. Compared data with only population norms to support conclusions. Listed some data gaps.	Identified some relevant data. Did not compare data with norms to support conclusions. No data gaps noted.	
Identification of Patient's Strengths	Addressed all strengths re: biopsychosocial-spiritual & environmental issues.	Addressed most of strengths.	Limited determination of strengths.	
Interdisciplinary Problems	Identified all	Identified some	Identified none	
Problems for Referral	Identified all	Identified some	Identified none	
Nursing Diagnoses (N. Dx.)	Identified all N. Dx. using proper NANDA terms. Included all related factors for each N. Dx. and provided defining characteristics for each N. Dx. Described all CT dimensions used during assessment.	Identified most N. Dx. using proper NANDA terms. Included most related factors for each N. Dx. and provided most defining characteristics. Described some of CT dimensions used in assessment.	Identified some N. Dx. using proper NANDA terms. Included some related factors for each N. Dx. & provided some defining characteristics. No CT dimensions ID'd.	

A major advantage of rubrics is that they serve the teaching, learning, and assessment roles all at once. They do this because they provide clear guidance for nurses or nursing students to achieve the learning goals you have identified. Nurses or students can see ahead of time how they will be assessed and work toward achieving those criteria. Rubrics have also been found to work well with both face-to-face and online coursework (Blood-Siegfried et al., 2008). For more information on rubrics, do a Google search with just the term *rubric*, and you might be pleasantly surprised at how much helpful knowledge you gain.

Examples of Practical Teaching/Learning/Assessing "Tools" of CT from List B in Box 10-2

The remainder of the teaching/learning/assessment "tools" from List B in Box 10-2 are a very useful and practical means of assessing parts of CT. We provide a brief explanation of how these might be used, but keep in mind that these methods work best when they are adapted to fit the *contextual perspective* of your teaching/learning/assessment situation.

Developing a new approach to something to show *creativity, inquisitiveness,* and/or *transforming knowledge* may be used to evaluate staff nurses, for example. A career placement assessment could include an innovation criterion. Points could be assigned in accordance with the whole assessment plan when a nurse improves a practice on the unit. This works well with moves toward evidence-based practice (Chapter 8) to reward staff who are innovative in using the best evidence to improve practice.

Debating from an opposite perspective to demonstrate *intellectual integrity* and *open-mindedness* is a valuable exercise for learning and assessment of CT. It is very difficult to debate a controversial issue from a viewpoint opposite your own. Assigning a *reflection* at the end of this exercise can help show the debater's thinking processes. This could be accompanied by a checklist or rubric, and scored. For example, one could assess the number of issues addressed, the depth of study of those issues, the distance of the viewpoints from the debater's true beliefs, strength of expression, and so forth.

Differential diagnosing is a great mechanism to see *discriminating* and *logical reasoning* cognitive skills, as well as *confidence, contextual perspective, intellectual integrity,* and *intuition* habits of the mind. Actually, a case could be made for using all 17 dimensions in this activity. Using case studies and comparing staff nurses' and clinical experts' diagnosing, Margaret Lunney (2001) reported wide variability in the accuracy of nurses' diagnosing. Lunney (2003) proposed 10 CT strategies to promote diagnostic accuracy. A strong case could be made for using her methods and Scale for Degrees of Accuracy (2001, p. 36) as a means to assess CT. Making her point especially poignant, Lunney (2003) shared case examples in which achieving accuracy of nursing diagnoses was particularly challenging. One was a patient with a T5 fracture who presented with symptoms that the nurse interpreted to be decreased cardiac output; in reality, the patient had autonomic dysreflexia. If you look at the signs and symptoms of these two North American

Nursing Diagnosis Association nursing diagnoses (Herdman, 2009, pp. 139, 280), you can appreciate the necessity of CT to make that distinction.

Listing hunches is related to differential diagnosing as part of the diagnostic process. Taken alone, it can be a good measure of *intuition*. Again, case studies could be used; these could be unit specific if this method is used by clinicians, and they could be class-specific in academic settings. "Experts" in those areas could list their hunches, and those lists could be used as a standard for comparison while assessing nurses. Prematurely shutting down one's thinking relative to hunches often leads clinicians to inaccurate conclusions.

Asking and answering "But, what if . . .?" questions is a good way to test for *transforming knowledge* and *flexibility*. At our school, we have been trying this as a component of our skills check-off procedures to add assessment of CT to that process. To use a simple example, think about teaching beginning students to make an occupied bed. Checking their ability to do this merely by watching a demonstration of the classic procedure—turning the patient, pushing the old sheets under him or her, placing new bedding on that side and pushing them under, turning the patient, and pulling everything through to the other side and tucking—does little to show you the students' thinking. What if you add, "The patient has had a right hip replacement"? That allows you to assess CT. The students should, of course, answer with something that indicates that they know not to turn the patient on the unaffected hip, therefore internally rotating the replaced hip and causing problems. You want to hear that they can visualize changing the bed from the top of the bed to the bottom, or some other plan that maintains hip precautions.

Using case scenarios and **asking what is likely to happen to this patient** is a method to assess *predicting* and *contextual perspective*. Again, as with many of these assessment examples, this could be made unit specific if used in practice settings. We often encourage practice-based educators to record case studies for thinking purposes. This is a good thing to have experienced nurses do. In addition, as a way of checking their CT, have them develop the "answers" to whatever questions you'll want to attach to that case study; novice nurses can then benefit from their collective wisdom. In addition, relevant setting-specific cases are available for future assessments.

Similar to *predicting* what is likely to happen to this patient is asking the question, "What would you assess next?" This can be used to assess *information seeking*, *discriminating*, and *contextual perspective* dimensions. We have tried this out with RN-to-BSN students to see what kinds of responses we get. This is a very simple exercise and one that would work well for practice-based educators who want a quick assessment of CT abilities of new nurses. In our trials, we've done this two ways. In the first method, we ask nurses to list the five most important and common patient signs/symptoms found on their units and then to list the parameters that they immediately check upon finding those signs/symptoms. In the second method, we give them a list of signs/symptoms and ask them what they think of right away to check. See **Box 10-7** for some examples. This exercise could easily be

BOX 10-7	Sample Answers to the Question, "What Would You Assess Next?"

Confusion: Check—medications, pulse oximetry, blood pressure, arterial blood gasses, specific neurological signs, temperature, blood glucose, previous mental status patterns, urinalysis, heart rate, headache, weakness

General Complaint of Pain/Discomfort: Check—pain rating, intensity, description, onset, location, duration, history of similar pain, factors that affect pain, last pain medication time, temperature, pulse oximetry, any surgical/dressing sites

Increased Blood Pressure: Check—pain, medications, pulse, cardiac rhythm, anxiety, temperature, past history of hypertension, patterns since admission, headache, IV status, recent patient activity; recheck blood pressure manually

Complaint of Constipation: Check—bowel sounds, abdominal distention, tenderness or pain, last bowel movement, how long constipation, past history, links to medical diagnosis, nausea and vomiting, eating pattern, fluid intake, recent GI tests, medications

Decreased Urine Output: Check—intake and output balance, urine color, blood pressure, pulse, temperature, intravenous fluids, weight change, urinalysis, medications such as diuretics, history of renal problems, edema, bladder distention, BUN, creatinine lab values

Request for Darkened Room: Check—depression, headache, history of headaches, fatigue, light sensitivity, privacy issue, drug use

Angry Responses to Staff: Check—what is wrong, pain, fear, anxiety, stress, loss of personal control, family/significant other issue, conflict with specific staff

scored numerically using expected assessment standards established by setting-specific experts. A rubric could be developed for consistency.

What is the principle? This is a question that promotes *applying standards*. It is also an old assessment technique that was used when we were undergraduates in the 1960s. Asking for standards behind behaviors reveals why someone is doing something and therefore affords the listener a partial picture of that person's thinking. This is an easy assessment method adaptable to almost any setting; it quickly separates those who do tasks without much thought from those who know why they are doing something. The latter group is engaged in thinking.

Calling the physician shows *discriminating, contextual perspective*, and *analyzing* in particular. Incidentally, it also shows communication skills. This could be applied to calling any other healthcare professional; because nurses often have to call physicians, this is a familiar situation. Ask physicians about nurse phone calls, and they will immediately tell you that one of their pet peeves is a nurse who does not seem to have thought through the situation before picking up the phone.

> **Nurse Smith:** Oh, hi, Dr. Jones; thanks for calling back. Mrs. Frank has only had 100 cc's of urine out in the past 6 hours. [Pause. . . . . .]
>
> **Dr. Jones:** She has heart failure, right?
>
> **Nurse Smith:** Yes, she's been on Lasix.
>
> **Dr. Jones:** What was her last dose and when?
>
> **Nurse Smith:** Oh, let me get the med list and check; I just floated down from 700, so I don't know these patients very well.

OK, you get the picture, right? Now, we don't mean to be critical of nurses, and being floated to an unfamiliar unit is all too common in the world of hospital-based nurses. Nevertheless, this kind of conversation is very time consuming and not very helpful because the nurse has not been using much CT.

So, if you were the educator for that unit, you'd probably want to have an in-service on communication and CT. You could use a phone call to a physician as a way of assessing the nurse's level of thinking. Start with a simple situation: Mrs. Frank's urine output has been 100 cc's for 6 hours. "Nurse Smith, would you demonstrate your thinking as you prepare for a call to Dr. Jones?" Once you do this a few times, you can come up with a list of connections that you expect thinking nurses to have made, and you would have your assessment standard.

By the way, you might also invite physicians to your in-service, making it an interdisciplinary session, or model this activity after the situation-background-assessment-recommendation format discussed in Chapter 7. Communication is a two-way street, requiring CT on both sides.

What's wrong with this picture? Asking this question after showing a video-tape or presenting a written or verbal case situation is another simple assessment technique that is especially helpful in showing a person's ability to *discriminate*. Our brains are funny things; it is often easier to see when something is wrong than to figure out how to do it right. But if we can identify what's wrong, we can avoid making that same mistake. Be careful with the "right" or "wrong" messages, though. A better question might be, "How can I do this better?"

A critique of literature is a common assessment method used in academic research classes that shows students' abilities to *apply standards, discriminate, analyze,* and *reason logically.* Unfortunately, literature critiques are less commonplace in practice settings. However, as we discussed in Chapter 8, evidence-based practice requires that all clinicians critique articles, guidelines, Internet reports, and so forth. With the indiscriminate glut of information out there, all healthcare providers have to be able to respond critically to that information, and that response requires CT. It is important to know how well those providers can judge the relative merit of that information, so assessing their abilities is becoming more of an issue. Using words like *critique of a report* can be daunting to clinicians who probably see this as an academic exercise, so we recommend that you stay away from those words. If you want to assess a person's ability to read something critically, use an article/report that you know has some flaws. (It's harder to find one that doesn't.) Use that article as a measure of CT.

The last suggestion we have from List B in Box 10-2 is to **use moral dilemmas** to assess *analyzing, intellectual integrity*, and *flexibility*. Moving to a relativistic thinking perspective and dealing with the realities of ambiguity in health care these days is vital. There are many moral dilemmas today for which there are no easy answers. How long should we keep a baby alive who has a severe brain problem? Should people older than 90 have expensive medical diagnostic tests? How far should we go for stem cell research? Asking individuals to respond to a moral dilemma gives important clues as to how well they can analyze situations to see the various perspectives, what they are willing to see that might go against conventional answers, and how flexible they are with their possibilities.

PAUSE _____

and Ponder

Assessment Is Not an End Unto Itself

There are no simple answers to the challenges in assessing CT. Each approach to judging someone's CT must be scrutinized closely. Remember, this is not something that can be assessed with the same methods that we use to assess skills such as giving an injection. CT is not a set of linear steps, but a process that is adapted in various contexts. Because it is complex and dynamic, it calls for assessment methods that are equally dynamic. It is not an end point with specific criteria that can be judged as right or wrong. We must give credit for pieces of CT—for the process, not just the results of thinking. We all have periods when our CT is sharp, and periods when it waxes and wanes. Assessment parameters should give credit for the CT waxing and allow for coaching when waning.

However, engaging in the whole of teaching/learning/assessing CT is the key to achieving the core competencies of the IOM—patient-centered care, interdisciplinary teamwork, evidence-based practice, informatics, and quality care—addressed throughout this text. The processes of teaching/learning/assessing are essential to the changes necessary in both healthcare practice and healthcare education. We are at a crossroads; CT and managing change will set us in a positive direction. More on change in the final chapter.

Reflection Cues

- The words *evaluation* and *assessment* are often used interchangeably; we have chosen *assessment*, which has less of a right-or-wrong connotation.
- Premature assessment, ahead of clear definitions of CT and teaching CT, is problematic.
- The complexity of CT does not easily lend itself to simple, quantitative means of assessing, such as with standardized tests.
- Nursing education in particular has been prone to premature assessment, largely driven by accreditation expectations.
- Our present approaches to assessing CT in nursing have been reductionistic.
- Because of CT's complexity, measurement instruments that aim for simplicity of scoring often compromise validity and are incomplete measures of CT.
- Current methods to assess CT, for the most part, are unable to show the changes in thinking that are reported anecdotally.
- Teaching/learning/assessing CT must be linked.
- Reflection is an essential aspect of assessing CT.
- One method to assess CT (short essays based on free responses and vignettes) is (1) based on a valid nursing definition of CT; (2) supported by interrater reliability; and (3) quantifiable using a scoring rubric.
- Various methods to combine teaching/learning/assessing CT can be adapted to numerous learning environments.

References

Adams, B. L. (1999). Nursing education for critical thinking: An integrative review. *Journal of Nursing Education, 38*, 111–119.

Ali, N. S., Bantz, D., & Siktberg, L. (2005). Validation of critical thinking skills in online responses. *Journal of Nursing Education, 44*, 90–94.

Allen, G. D., Rubenfeld, M. G., & Scheffer, B. K. (2004). Reliability of assessment of critical thinking. *Journal of Professional Nursing, 20*, 15–22.

American Association of Colleges of Nursing. (2008, October 20). *The essentials of baccalaureate education for professional nursing practice.* Retrieved October 29, 2008, from http://www.aacn.nche.edu/education/pdf/BaccEssentials08.pdf

Assessment Technologies Institute. (2006). *ATI Critical Thinking Test.* Retrieved November 11, 2008, from http://www.ati-international.com/productinfo/CriticalThinking.aspx

Barringon, K., & Campbell, B. (2008). MUDD mapping: An interactive teaching-learning strategy. *Nurse Educator, 33*, 159–163.

Beckie, T. M., Lowry, L. W., & Barnett, S. (2001). Assessing critical thinking in baccalaureate nursing students: A longitudinal study. *Holistic Nursing Practice, 15*(3), 18–26.

Blood-Siegfried, J. E., Short, N. M., Rapp, C. G., Hill, E., Talbert, S., Skinner, J., et al. (2008). A rubric for improving the quality of online courses. *International Journal of Nursing Education Scholarship, 5*(1), Article 34, 1–13.

Britton, L. A., & Wissing, D. (2006). Authentic assessment of learning outcomes. *Respiratory Care Education Annual, 15,* 21–30.

Commission on Collegiate Nursing Education. (2008). *Standards for accreditation of baccalaureate and graduate nursing programs.* Retrieved November 19, 2008, from http://www.aacn.nche.edu/accreditation/

Daley, B. J., Shaw, C. R., Balistrieri, T., Glasenapp, I., & Placentine, L. (1999). Concept maps: A strategy to teach and evaluate critical thinking. *Journal of Nursing Education, 38,* 42–47.

Dickieson, P., Carter, L. M., & Walsh, M. (2008). Integrative thinking and learning in undergraduate nursing education: Three strategies. *International Journal of Nursing Education Scholarship, 5*(1), Article 39, 1–15.

Dulski, L., Kelly, M., & Carrol, V. S. (2006). Program outcome data: What do we measure? What does it mean? How does it lead to improvement? *Quality Management in Health Care, 15,* 296–299.

Ennis, R. H., & Weir, E. (1985). *The Ennis-Weir critical thinking essay test.* Pacific Grove, CA: Midwest.

Facione, N. C., & Facione, P. A. (2006). *Health Sciences Reasoning Test.* Retrieved November 23, 2008, from http://www.insightassessment.com/test-hsrt.html

Guttman, M. S. (2004). Increasing the linguistic competence of the nurse with limited English proficiency. *Journal of Continuing Education in Nursing, 35,* 264–269.

Harris, M. (2007). Scaffolding reflective journal writing—Negotiating power, play and position. *Nurse Education Today, 28,* 314–326.

Herdman, T. H. (Ed.). (2009). *NANDA International Nursing Diagnoses: Definitions & classifications 2009–2011.* Ames, IA: Wiley-Blackwell.

Lunney, M. (2001). *Critical thinking & nursing diagnosis: Case studies & analysis.* Philadelphia: North American Nursing Diagnosis Association.

Lunney, M. (2003). Critical thinking and accuracy of nurses' diagnoses. *International Journal of Nursing Terminologies and Classifications, 14*(3), 96–107.

Lunney, M. (2009). Assessment, clinical judgment, and nursing diagnoses: How to determine accurate diagnoses. In T. Herdman (Ed.), *NANDA International Nursing Diagnoses: Definitions & classifications 2009–2011* (pp. 3–23). Ames, IA: Wiley-Blackwell.

Mueller, A., Johnston, M., & Bligh, D. (2002). Joining mind mapping and care planning to enhance student critical thinking and achieve holistic nursing care. *Nursing Diagnosis, 13,* 24–27.

National League for Nursing. (2007). *Critical thinking in clinical nursing practice-RN 880501* (Test Catalog). Retrieved November 28, 2008, from http://www.nln.org/testproducts/pdf/testcatalog07.pdf

National League for Nursing Accrediting Commission. (2000). *Accreditation manual for post secondary, baccalaureate, and higher degree programs in nursing.* New York: Author.

National League for Nursing Accrediting Commission. (2008). *Accreditation manual: 2008 Standards and criteria: Baccalaureate.* Retrieved November 14, 2008, from http://www.nlnac.org/manuals/SC2008_BACCALAUREATE.pdf

Nunnally, J. C. (2002). *Psychometric theory.* New York: McGraw-Hill.

Pothan, Z. (2008). Reflective practice aids critical thinking. *Kai Tiaki Nursing New Zealand, 14*(8), 23.

Rubenfeld, M. G., & Scheffer, B. K. (2006). *Critical thinking in nursing: An interactive approach* (2nd ed.). Ann Arbor, MI: Huron Valley Publishing, Inc.

Rush, K. L., Dyches, C. E., Waldrop, S., & Davis, A. (2008). Critical thinking among RN-to-BSN distance students participating in human patient simulation. *Journal of Nursing Education, 47*, 501–507.

Scheffer, B. K. (2001). Nurse educators' perspectives on their critical thinking. *Dissertation Abstracts International, 62/2B*, 786. (ProQuest C., No. 3003400).

Scheffer, B. K., & Rubenfeld, M. G. (2000). A consensus statement on critical thinking in nursing. *Journal of Nursing Education, 39*, 352–359.

Senge, P. M. (1998, Summer). The practice of innovation. *Leader to Leader, 9*, 16–22. Retrieved July 21, 2004, from http://www.leadertoleader.org/knowledgecenter/journal.aspx?ArticleID=159

Staib, S. (2003). Teaching and measuring critical thinking. *Journal of Nursing Education, 42*, 498–508.

Stevens, D. D., & Levi, A. J. (2005). *Introduction to rubrics: An assessment tool to save grading time, convey effective feedback and promote student learning.* Sterling, VA: Stylus.

Stone, C. A., Davidson, L. J., Evans, J. L., & Hansen, M. A. (2001). Validity evidence for using a general critical thinking test to measure nursing students' critical thinking. *Holistic Nursing Practice, 15*(4), 65–74.

Tanner, C. A. (2005). What have we learned about critical thinking in nursing? *Journal of Nursing Education, 44*, 47–48.

Taylor, J., & Wros, P. (2007). Concept mapping: A nursing model for care planning. *Journal of Nursing Education, 46*, 211–216.

Twibell, R., Ryan, M., & Hermiz, M. (2005). Faculty perceptions of critical thinking in student clinical experiences. *Journal of Nursing Education, 44*, 71–79.

Walsh, C. M., & Seldomridge, L. A. (2006a). Critical thinking: Back to square two. *Journal of Nursing Education, 45*, 212–219.

Walsh, C. M., & Seldomridge, L. A. (2006b). Measuring critical thinking: One step forward, one step back. *Nurse Educator, 31*, 159–162.

Wheeler, L. A., & Collins, S. K. R. (2003). The influence of concept mapping on critical thinking in baccalaureate nursing students. *Journal of Professional Nursing, 19*, 339–345.

Whitehead, T. D. (2006). Comparison of native versus nonnative English-speaking nurses on critical thinking assessments at entry and exit. *Nursing Administration Quarterly, 30*, 285–290.

Zygmont, D. M., & Schaefer, K. M. (2006). Assessing the critical thinking skills of faculty: What do the findings mean for nursing education? *Nursing Education Perspectives, 27*, 260–267.

———————————————————**11**

Thinking Realities of Yesterday, Today, and Tomorrow

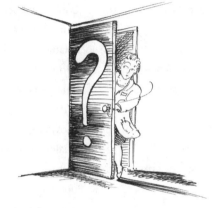

Here we are at the final chapter for our discussions of thinking with the five competencies—patient-centered care, working in interdisciplinary teams, using evidence-based practice (EBP), using informatics, and achieving quality improvement. We introduced these Institute of Medicine (IOM; 2003) competencies in Chapter 4 as we put together the *how*, *where*, and *when* of critical thinking (CT) and suggested some active teaching/learning approaches for educators, and strategies for reflection in practice for clinicians. Now, we step back to look at what all this means to our day-to-day existence as healthcare providers and educators. This existence is certainly not what it used to be 10, or even 5, years ago. We are working in a different world today. As to any significance of this being "Chapter Eleven," we hope our thinking won't be so taxed that we go bankrupt!! (It's OK to groan at that.) An overwhelming theme throughout many chapters, especially Chapters 4–9, has been change. In **Box 11-1**, we've summarized the change messages in those chapters to refresh your memory.

The inevitability of change in health care right now is a timely topic these days. Statements like these abound: "The U.S. healthcare system requires radical, not incremental, change" (Waldman, Smith, & Hood, 2003, p. 5). "It's the end of an era. The type of nursing learned by the average, 47-year-old nurse is ending"

BOX 11-1	Evolving Themes of Change in Health Care
From . . . Provider-centered care	to . . . Patient-centered care
From . . . Giving patients information	to . . . Coaching patients to find information
From . . . Present patient needs/tasks	to . . . Future patient needs/tasks
From . . . Multidisciplinary work	to . . . Interdisciplinary teamwork
From . . . Individual perspective	to . . . Contextual perspective
From . . . Individual CT	to . . . Team/System CT
From . . . Dichotomous thinking	to . . . Relativistic thinking
From . . . Tradition-based practice	to . . . Evidence-based practice
From . . . Change based on anecdotes	to . . . Change based on strong evidence
From . . . Paper and pens	to . . . Informatics
From . . . Information	to . . . Knowledge
From . . . Quality assurance	to . . . Quality improvement
From . . . Culture of blame for errors	to . . . Culture of safety
From . . . Status quo	to . . . Innovation
From . . . Hierarchical power	to . . . Empowerment of all professionals

(Porter-O'Grady, 2003, p. 4). We will discuss the thinking needed to deal with these changes shortly, but first let's reflect on why change is so necessary in health care right now, and the implications of that constant, complex change to our daily existence.

Why Is Change So Necessary?

The answers to why change is necessary right now are all around us. Read any newspaper, and you'll see articles on problems with healthcare systems and the health of people around us—our ill-prepared plans to deal with the increased numbers of elderly patients with multiple health conditions, the huge increase in Type 2 diabetes in young people, the high rate of obesity, our ability to keep people alive without quality of life, potential deadly outbreaks of new and mutated microorganisms, the imbalance between infinite needs and finite resources, the shortage of nurses and nurse educators, the high rates of medical errors, the rapid growth of new medications and treatment possibilities, genetic research, antibiotic resistance, and . . . shall we keep going?

By the way, as an aside for you educators, we'll share a strategy that we use in many of our courses—assignments to increase students' awareness of local to global health issues that are in the news. We have students find articles from the popular media and discuss their implications for nurses. It is always an eye-opening project because many students perceive nurses as dealing with one patient at a time. We are trying to get them better socialized to the many issues that will force them to be changeable and adaptable in their careers.

The examples we just listed are areas that need change specifically in health-care delivery, but remember that according to the IOM, those changes need to start in the health education arena. We are talking not only about the complex changes in health care; we are also talking about complex educational change. Changes in educational systems may be even harder to realize because of the traditions. As Senge, Scharmer, Jaworski, and Flowers (2004) noted, our present educational system is based on industrial-age assembly-line principles that will not prepare people to deal with tomorrow's realities. Likewise, Gardner (2006) had this to say:

> At the start of the third millennium, we lie at a time of vast changes—changes seemingly so epochal that they may well dwarf those experienced in earlier eras. . . . These changes call for new educational forms and processes. The minds of learners must be fashioned and stretched in . . . ways that have not been crucial—or not as crucial—until now. . . . We must recognize what is called for in this new world—even as we hold on to certain perennial skills and values that may be at risk. (p. 11)

We health educators have a double whammy to deal with; we cannot escape change either in the classroom or in the clinical settings.

What Kinds of Change Are We Talking About?

There have been zillions of books, articles, monographs, and so forth, written on the change process and strategies to implement and deal with change. Those that are relevant to healthcare delivery and education start with descriptions of change that depict the confounding complexity of systems such as ours. Paul Plsek (2003) presented a thoughtful, practical perspective for a conference convened in Washington, DC, by the National Institute for Health Care Management Foundation and the National Committee for Quality Health Care. Plsek focused on change in health care as a complex issue, making a distinction among complex, complicated, and simple issues. Change in health care is complex because the healthcare system is a complex adaptive system. "A complex adaptive system is a collection of individual agents who have the freedom to act in ways that are not always totally predictable, and whose actions are interconnected such that one agent's actions change the context for other agents" (Plsek, 2003).

Models for complex adaptive systems are organic systems such as the human body—in which a change in one part will affect a change in another—and the body must always be viewed as a whole, not a collection of parts. In these systems, although there are feedback mechanisms to maintain the status quo, there is always something changing; there are contradictions and lots of unknowns. Think of what happens with a sore knee. To ease the knee pain, a person changes his gait and gets hip or foot pain, takes medications such as non-steroidal anti-inflammatory drugs for the pain, and has side effects of edema that aggravate hypertension. A simple sore knee now presents a potential cardiac problem. We would do well to keep that image in mind when we start to consider complex system changes.

Other authors have made distinctions between types of complexity: detailed and/or dynamic (Senge, 1990). The latter, dynamic complexity, is what we see in health care—the very nature of the complexity is focused on change. Senge et al. (2004) discussed this as transformational change, which is highly focused on the people involved in the change, not just on what change is made and how. It must focus on who we are. "The changes in which we will be called upon to participate in the future will be both deeply personal and inherently systemic" (p. 2). People transform systems; systems don't transform themselves.

Educational systems and change are equally complex, according to Fullan (1993). "Complexity, dynamism, and unpredictability . . . are not merely things that get in the way. They are normal" (p. 20). Many processes are unknowable in advance, and there is nothing linear about the complexities of educational systems and their change. Making educational change more paradoxical is that change is a continuous theme, but the educational system is essentially conservative. Change in these circumstances cannot occur through isolated reforms; the whole educational system needs to become a "learning organization—expert at dealing with change as a normal part of its work" (Fullan, 1993, p. 4).

Linear thinking about change as going from data to conclusions, mandates to coercion, chaos to order, and so forth, is facile, revealing unrealistic thinking processes for today's changes in these complex systems. Fullan (1993) advocated better thinking as a solution: "The solution lies in better ways of thinking about, and dealing with, inherently unpredictable processes" (p. 19). Among his eight basic lessons for this new paradigm of change are three of our favorites: "You can't mandate what matters. . . . Connection with the wider environment is critical for success . . . [and] every person is a change agent" (pp. 21–22). These lessons emphasize the involvement of everyone in this thinking journey.

Senge (2003) echoed these ideas, reminding us that systems thinking must be a priority when considering change; we live in a global society and must use collective creating. He made a distinction between problem solving and creating. "In problem solving we seek to make something we do not like go away. In creating, we seek to make what we truly care about exist" (Senge, 2003, p. 4). It will require a radical change in our thinking to go beyond the old-fashioned problem solving and take on a creative stance.

In a little while, we'll discuss the changes in thinking that need to accompany the changes in healthcare delivery and education. First, however, we must consider the reactions of people involved in change.

Implications of Living with Constant, Complex Change

What about the implications of living with constant, let alone complex, change? With change comes the certainty of uncertainty, messiness, excitement, challenges, learning, refining self, redefining positions, more interactions among people, and calls for creativity. With change comes the possibility (probability?) of coercion, increased work, fatigue, anger, anxiety, judgments, feelings of inadequacy, and a desire to "run away." It's all pretty scary stuff, right? How can we survive with our wits intact in this kind of changing day-to-day reality? For starters, we have to reflect on how we view change and the kinds of experiences we've had with change in the past. Then we have to look at how that view fits with the thinking needed today.

So, just what have been your experiences with change? Many (most?) clinicians and educators have negative experiences. Changes have been handed down from upper-level administration and management. Before we can settle into one change, another comes along to take its place. Sometimes that happens even before we've settled into the first change! People far removed from the day-to-day implementation of the change developed the plan without our input. Before we feel comfortable with the change, we are being evaluated on how well we are doing with it. The focus is on the end point of the change rather than the process of change. Many changes are instigated to save money. Money-saving changes often have a short-term rather than long-term goal. Many changes seem irrelevant or were tried and found ineffective in other situations. Every time we hear from our manager that something is about to change, we feel anxious!

This hierarchical system, with rapidly increasing frequency of episodic change, has been the norm for nurses for a long time. We need to acknowledge that, reflect on it, think about the feelings it brings up, and then think about how we can deal with it successfully in the future. Maybe we can see ourselves within a metamorphosis frame of mind; we are moving toward our "safety champion" nurse image that we discussed in Chapter 5.

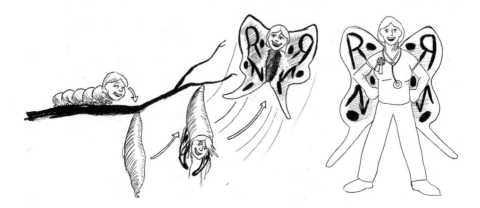

Thinking for Effective Change

The old ways of thinking about change won't work any longer. "As long as our thinking is governed by habit—notably by industrial, 'machine age' concepts such as control, predictability, standardization, and 'faster is better'—we will continue to re-create institutions as they have been, despite their increasing disharmony with the larger world" (Senge et al., 2004, p. 5).

As we consider the CT dimensions that are our model in this book, once again, we can look at all 17 and see how integral they are to the change process. We have addressed all of them in Chapters 5, 6, 7, 8, and 9 in which we've discussed changes inherent in thinking about the five competencies. However, here we'd like to examine six dimensions that are especially important in dealing with the complex, dynamic change that is needed and inevitable. We will focus on *contextual perspective, creativity, intuition, inquisitiveness, reflection,* and *transforming knowledge.* It's not that the others aren't used or important; it's just that these six are particularly useful in helping us initiate and deal with change.

We aren't really going to separate these six very much either because they are so interrelated. What we've done instead is list 15 patterns of change in thinking and learning that, from our review of literature and collective experience, require an amalgamation of these six dimensions. See **Box 11-2**.

BOX 11-2	**Emergent, Necessary Patterns of Change in Thinking and Learning**

1.	From ... Passivity	to ...	Engagement/presence
2.	From ... Answers	to ...	Questions
3.	From ... Separate thinking and doing	to ...	Thinking and doing together
4.	From ... Destinations	to ...	Journeys
5.	From ... Reactive learning	to ...	Proactive learning
6.	From ... Mechanistic Models	to ...	Living system models
7.	From ... Dichotomous thinking	to ...	Relativistic thinking
8.	From ... Thinking of pieces	to ...	Thinking of wholes
9.	From ... Alone/separated	to ...	Connected/systems
10.	From ... Reduction	to ...	Complexity
11.	From ... Matching existing patterns	to ...	New patterns
12.	From ... Linear	to ...	Maps/knots/shapes
13.	From ... Constant success	to ...	Failure possibilities
14.	From ... Valuing only objectivity	to ...	Being open to intuition
15.	From ... Reviewing	to ...	Reflecting

Sources: Fullan, 1993; Plsek, 2003; Plsek & Greenhalgh, 2001; Porter-O'Grady, 2003; Senge, 1998; Senge et al., 2004.

Emergent, Necessary Patterns of Change in Thinking and Learning

Today's reality just doesn't fit with yesterday's thinking patterns. We are not dealing with a machine; we are dealing with a complex system of human beings that is intertwined with many other systems, all in a state of constant flux. As Senge et al. (2004) and Plsek (2003) noted, much of our thinking about organizations has come from the industrial age and a mechanistic mentality that favors assembly lines. Modern systems like health care don't work that way; they are adaptive, with complex feedback mechanisms (**Figure 11-1**). If we want to successfully change health care, we have to approach it more like a living organism system than a machine. (Remember our knee example earlier in this chapter.) Of course, as soon as we move to the living system metaphor, we can see that, in contrast to machine systems, there is very little predictability and a whole lot of potential chaos. As clinicians and educators, not only do we need to initiate change ourselves, but we also must survive changes instigated by others. For that, we've developed the 15 patterns of change in thinking and learning in Box 11-2. We added learning because today's systems are learning environments, not just places to do things.

From Passivity to Engagement/Presence

We have to see that this inevitable change will affect us, but we also have to see that we will affect that change as well. It is not a one-way street, but a two-way

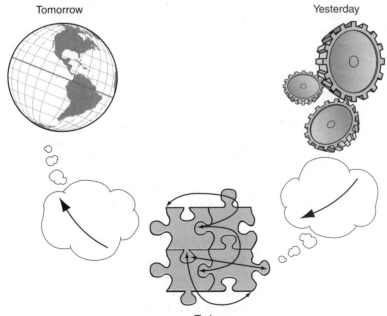

FIGURE 11-1 Realities of thinking.

street. No longer can we sit back and let someone tell us what to do. We have a long tradition of learning and thinking in this passive mode. Educators keep presenting lectures; students keep reading, underlining, memorizing, and spitting back. Clinicians, toward the end of this chapter, we tell the story of a nurse who epitomized engagement in introducing and working through a change. If you don't already have an active approach to your job, think about what it would take to make you more engaged in thinking about changes that are necessary and how you might instigate those changes. Look back to Chapter 4 at the suggestions for reflection in action to increase your engagement. Educators, also look back to Chapter 4 and think about your teaching styles (Box 4-6 on p. 85). Are you promoting passive or active learning? If you are continuing this passive tradition, you are not helping students prepare for the reality they will face. You have to risk getting some bad evaluations while trying different active strategies because students are pretty stuck in their passive learning modes. Most have come through passive educational systems in which they've been taught that there is one "right" answer.

From Answers to Questions

Because change is constant with many issues, unknown until they evolve, there are fewer answers, especially simple ones, and for sure, there is not just one right answer. Senge (1998) said, "Genuine inquiry starts when people ask questions to which they do not have an answer" (section 4). Focusing on questions keeps the door to change open. Remember our discussion of problem-based learning in Chapter 4? The core of that approach is starting with a problem or a question to guide learning (Rideout, 2001). Creative people ask questions: How can I represent the best aesthetic placement of these flowers? Why is this happening? What will this patient need to adapt at home? Later in this chapter, we tell one nurse's story of innovative practice that started with a question: Why are we seeing deep sternal infections postoperatively?

We tend to focus more on answers because it's neater. Think of how much better most people feel after they've straightened up their homes, closets, workbenches, or desks. For a brief period, we have a sense of order in what is increasingly a disorderly world. Questioning takes us down a path of ambiguity because it allows for the possibility that the world isn't perfect. But, of course, the world isn't perfect, especially healthcare practice and education. We really do need to change things, so let's get rid of that desire for perfection, step out into the uncertainty, and question everything, especially those things for which we don't already have answers.

From Separate Thinking and Doing to Thinking and Doing Together

A class activity that we have used for many years at the start of our CT course is to have students draw their "thinking caps." You may want to try this strategy; it's a great CT discussion initiator. After the initial, "What do you want?" questions, students get enough reassurance to draw their caps. The results are quite interesting.

Some talk about putting on a "hat" and going someplace quiet and peaceful to think. They tend to have neat hats with brims. Other students have pictures of things that could only be called "hats" by the most creative; they have all kinds of things going on at once, and they discuss how everything is open and accessible. Secretly we think, "Ah, they'll be better able to adapt to thinking in nursing," but we never say that, of course; we wait for them to see that as the semester progresses, and they broaden their thinking as they see their peers' hats and hear them described.

Now, why do you think we see the latter group of students as being more adaptable to nurse thinking? It's because their thinking is all tied up with their doing, their emotions, things in their lives. They don't picture their thinking in neat, safe, clean spaces; therefore, thinking in the midst of the chaos of healthcare situations will not be a shock to them, and they will likely have an easier time doing *reflection* in practice.

You might want to reflect on when and how you do your thinking. Do you tend to sit back and do it after the fact, or while you're actively doing something?

From Destinations to Journeys

This is similar to moving from answers to questions because it's about uncertainty and ambiguity. We tend to think about our end points. *Things will be better once I get the kitchen fixed; we'll have more money once the kids have finished school; I'll get some order back in my life once the semester ends.* This kind of thinking actually sets us up for frustration because, of course, in today's complex world, almost nothing goes into a neat box on which we can write "finished." Just ask people about projects they have that have never gotten finished; ask them how they feel about them. You'll find some who say, "This is just how life is; I always have things unfinished, and I've learned to live with it." Others are bothered by the lack of closure and try endlessly to close boxes.

Healthcare service and education will never be "finished" with their changes because every change will affect something else that will have to change. New technology will come along and redefine even the simple things that we have firmly in place, and we'll have to open boxes all too frequently. Accept that—start to look more at the journey than the destination—and you'll be less crazy in this world.

If you want a hard lesson in the journey-versus-destination thinking, write an article or a book, and you'll realize how hard it is to let it go as a finished product. As soon as you send it off to the publisher, you read something that you wish you had addressed. That, of course, is why you should always cite authors in the past tense. There's a good chance they might not say today what they said last year!

From Reactive Learning to Proactive Learning

This, too, is related to the first patterns we discussed—to move from passivity to engagement and from answers to questions—but we feel that it's worth describing in these alternate terms to make sure this whole idea comes through. Senge et al. (2004) described reactive learning as "governed by 'downloading' habitual ways of thinking, of continuing to see the world within the familiar categories we're comfortable with. . . . At best, we get better at what we have always done" (p. 6). They made a distinction between "reactive" and "deeper" learning, but we've chosen to call the other end of the pattern "proactive" learning, which we think becomes "deeper" because learners are much more involved in seeking knowledge and putting it into a better workable frame for themselves.

How much of what you read is due to someone telling you to read it or someone recommending it to you? How does that compare with what you read because you are curious enough to go digging something out yourself? How many of you, when you were students, read the recommended readings in addition to the required ones? Ahem, did we strike a nerve there?

When you meet someone new, how much do you ask about what they do and try to learn from them? We have a friend, Connie, and everywhere she goes, she asks tons of questions of everyone she meets. If you happen to be tagging along, you might get antsy as she gets deeper and deeper into conversations, oblivious to time. She is very bright and knows a lot about a lot of things and has worked as a writer/reporter for many years. We're not sure if this is a chicken or egg thing—if she became a writer because she was so curious and wanted to share her knowledge, or if she became that way from being assigned to stories. It's probably a bit of both—just a good match. What she is, without a doubt, is a proactive learner—so much so that she made a guilt-free decision not to finish her doctoral dissertation because it became too narrow a focus for her, and she didn't want to endorse that type of learning!

So where are you compared with Connie? Most of us are more reactive. We go along with the reactive-learning model of mainstream education, and many of us promote reactive learning in our students. It's tough to give up the power of teacher teaching to the power of the learner's learning, but we educators have to move more in that direction if we are to coach active, creative innovators in health care. Remember Fullan's (1993) lesson number 1: You can't mandate what matters. Learners need to come to their learning proactively to be invested in what they are learning and achieve deeper understanding as a result.

From Mechanistic Models to Living Systems Models

We discussed this earlier when we described the types of change needed today. What about the thinking involved in this change of perspective? This is "running like clockwork." We have a "well-oiled machine here." Even though we use such metaphors, do we really believe that our healthcare and education systems fit that picture? Probably not. Senge (1999) repeatedly pointed out the need to consider living systems as our model of change in today's complex world. A most important lesson that we have learned from his writings is to consider the impact of compensating feedback mechanisms in living systems and how that differs from the workings of machines. If you've ever dieted to lose weight (and who hasn't?), you can relate. Initially you lose weight, and then you gain a bit and/or level off even when you think you're eating the same way. Your body is hanging on to your "survival" fat and has a starvation feedback signal. Some of us try to reset that thermostat periodically, some with more success than others, by changing our eating and activity patterns. Much of the resistance to change that we observe is the system trying to conserve itself or something within itself. If we don't recognize the process or what it is trying to conserve, we will continue to be frustrated with "resistance to change."

Senge (1990, 1998) used the example of a hot room with a thermostat. You enter, and, without knowledge of the thermostat, you open the windows to cool things off. Soon it gets warmer again. If you want change, you have to get to the thermostat and reset it or turn off the furnace. Think about that image the next time you wonder why your group is hanging on to something and doesn't want to change; figure out where the furnace is or figure out how to reset the thermostat. Translate that to what the group is hanging on to and what will change their value of that.

From Dichotomous Thinking to Relativistic Thinking

OK, this is all about *contextual perspective*, right? Is there anyone still out there who sees things clearly in terms of right or wrong, blue or yellow, yes or no? We'd like to think that all of you would say, "Well, that depends." And that's the answer that goes "chi-ching" on the relativistic side. Of course, we know that all clinicians and educators don't say that, and those who do acknowledge that they only do it sometimes. Hey, have you taken a multiple-choice test lately? Better yet, have you given one? What do you do with the student who is arguing with this line: "Well, what about if this . . . ?"

One of the great education ironies in nursing is that we try and try to promote relativistic thinking in students so they'll look at the whole context of a clinical situation, but then we test them with dichotomous exams that have rigid right or wrong answers. Because we still have to prepare students for multiple-choice licensure exams, even those of us who hate such exams feel pressure to allow some practice with them. We've gotten around our discomfort with this dichotomous approach by allowing students to challenge questions and answers. "If you can show in writing that your answer is as good as mine, you get credit for that question." It's not the best lesson in relativistic thinking, but it lets us sleep at night.

It is very easy to forget context when looking at a problem or planning change. Foster-Fishman, Nowell, and Yang (2007) developed a model for changing systems. At the outset, they declared that "most systems change efforts have not fully attended to the dynamics and properties of the contexts they are attempting to shift" (p. 198). We must look at issues from many perspectives—find out the view of multiple stakeholders—so that we don't delude ourselves that a straight line from intervention to outcome is possible.

From Thinking of Pieces to Thinking of Wholes

It is very easy to focus on the tree in front of you and forget about the forest, but because living systems are so interconnected, it is folly to be too narrow in your view. Think about how short patient stays in the hospital are these days. Recently, in a class of registered nurses, we asked about patient teaching, and several students replied that they rarely do any patient teaching because they worked in intensive care units (ICUs)—that this was something done more by the nurses "on the floors." Needless to say, I raised my eyebrows a bit and asked questions like this: *Don't your patients have family members sitting around? How often are your patients discharged home only a day or two after leaving the ICU? What constitutes patient teaching to you?* Ultimately, the students realized they were working in a very task-oriented way and were not seeing the whole picture of these patients' lives and how this episode of illness fit within it. They realized that there were lots of "little" things that they could and should be teaching to patients and to family members.

How are we going to get past that task orientation that has been such a huge part of our history in nursing? Educators, how can we teach novices who are so focused on tasks to periodically look up and see the whole patient? One idea is to start teaching tasks with more focus on the absolute essential parts so that students can stop using up their RAM with unnecessary details and leave more of their hard drives open for bigger pictures. We can also pepper our check-off routines with "What if . . .?" questions to get them thinking of this task in a large, constantly changing context.

Clinicians, look around you at things like end-of-shift reports and count how many times a larger view of patients' worlds is mentioned. Start modeling that yourself. Put something in your report room to remind nurses of the larger view—a globe or a picture of a family picnic.

From Thinking Alone to Systems Thinking

This theme is especially emphasized in Chapter 7, on interdisciplinary teams. We need to hone our individual thinking skills, but we also have to focus on how we think as groups, and the dynamics of systems thinking. In their systems change model, Foster-Fishman et al. (2007) noted the importance of thinking about system dynamics: "interaction characteristics . . . the role of feedback . . . delays between actions and consequences, and how unexpected consequences from actions can create new conditions or problems" (p. 200). The complexity of subjectivity within systems cannot be ignored.

Carole Estabrooks (2003) presented a view of nurses within communities of practice. On first reading, we feared that we would have trouble getting nurses to move to new thinking approaches, such as EBP. However, her remarks proved worthy of reflection beyond our first reactions. Here's what she found: "Increasingly, we are aware that nurses rely more on knowledge generated within their communities of practice than on knowledge generated by research. In particular, we have found that 'social interactions' and 'experience' are the two most important sources of knowledge for nurses . . . learning is social" (pp. 60–61). From that perspective, group thinking is perhaps already in place in nursing practice. Estabrooks acknowledged that this social learning phenomenon needs to be studied more, and we agree with her.

If we assume that Estabrooks is on to something, maybe we're halfway there in increasing our group or systems thinking. Maybe we're closer to systems thinking in nursing than professionals are in some other disciplines. Perhaps we should put our energies into the type of learning and thinking that is occurring in those social interactions. To continue with our EBP example, if a group of nurses is using traditions as a basis for practice, then we need to target that group and encourage some of them to explore EBP. All it takes is an instigation of social interactions around a new evidence report or a question about a practice that all nurses can relate to. This is the place for the clinician who models CT, talks aloud about thinking, and asks lots of questions.

From Reduction to Complexity

We probably have our logical positivist tradition to thank for our penchant for reductionist thinking. Although analysis and reducing problems to discover and learn are definite assets to CT, we have to take care that we put things back together after we've done that reduction. This is an issue that comes up when trying to explain CT. It is so complex that we have to break it down to make it understandable; hence, the 17 dimensions. However, as you can probably see by now, each time we try to address each dimension separately, it is never clean. These dimensions work best in harmony, as a whole where they augment each other.

Educators need to be especially aware of complex new patterns of change; years ago, we were able to teach in a reductionist manner—break everything down so students could understand the pieces. However, students are left with skills that they can't put into use because nothing in the clinical world is reduced in that way. Educators must help students put the pieces back together to see the enormous complexity that is the setting for these reduced skills.

This "putting the pieces together" would occur in what Gardner (2006) called the "synthesizing mind." Anyone who has tried to write a scholarly paper can appreciate how difficult synthesis is. Pulling something together to create a "new view" acknowledges the complexity but attempts to make it clear. Gardner called synthesis a "considerable feat" but attempted to define four components of the synthesis process: "a goal . . . a starting point . . . selection of strategy, method and approach . . . and drafts and feedback" (pp. 51–52). Perhaps we can use these components to help deal with the complexity.

From Matching Existing Patterns to New Patterns

When we see something new, we tend to interpret and store it in the established patterns in our brains. It's easier to remember something when it's in the form of a familiar pattern (Hart, 1983). An old pattern might be used to process and store something you hear your manager say—"I want everyone to be involved in coming up with ideas for improvement." If the usual style of change on your unit is hierarchical, with edicts handed down from above, that old pattern for registering the manager's remark might be, "That means we should all be nice and go along with things." It is very hard to throw off old patterns and make new ones. It means standing back and looking at things with "different" eyes. It doesn't necessarily mean throwing away the old patterns; it might be easier sometimes just to change the shape of the existing ones.

Plsek (2003) gave a great example of creative thinking in new connections of patterns to help us teach patients better. We know that repetition helps learning; we know that elderly patients and those under stress often forget things we teach them; we know that if we could tape-record what we tell patients, they could go back and listen to it again; we know that most people have telephone answering machines. The new pattern, then, is to put all those existing patterns together and come up with a plan to record our teaching on patients' home answering machines while we teach them face-to-face. We just ask them if we can call their homes and record the teaching session. Then, when they get home, they can listen to it as often as needed.

These ideas are often called thinking outside the box; some people are better at it than others. In today's world of change, we all must get outside our boxes and open ourselves to new patterns. To tease your brain a bit, look at **Box 11-3**; see if you can figure out these puzzles. The first one was brought home from school by one of our sons, and we're not sure who created it. We both had trouble with it, even though it's very simple, because we have moved to thinking patterns in

---

BOX 11-3	**Brain Teasers to Help Develop and Use New Brain Patterns**

The First Example:

1

11

21

1211

111221

What is the next line?

The Second Example (Perkins, 1994):

$2 + 7 - 118 = 129$

Add one straight line to the mathematical statement above to make it true instead of false. There are at least three solutions.

which numbers are things we count, add, subtract, multiply with, and so forth. We don't look at numbers as words, and that's the key to figuring out that pattern. Have you figured it out yet? The next line is 312211—three ones, two twos, and one one. Start at the top now and say the words instead of seeing the numbers; one one—two ones—one two and one one, and so on.

The second example is from a wonderful book by Harvard's David Perkins (1994) on learning to think by looking at art. In a chapter called "Making Looking Broad and Adventurous," he presented that number puzzle. Once again, one has to get away from usual patterns and assumptions to see the possible solutions. The first solution is to put a vertical line through the equal sign. Did you just say, "Duh"? The second solution is to put a line starting at the left end of the top part of the equal sign and extend it diagonally up to the right. This creates the sign meaning "less than or equal to" and makes the statement true also. The third solution is different; with one line on the plus sign, you make it into a 4, and then the equation becomes 247 – 118 = 129. As Perkins explained, we tend not to cut across categories in our minds. We tend to see things in habitual patterns.

From Linear to Maps/Knots/Shapes

There is nothing linear about the thinking necessary for initiating and dealing with change in complex adaptive systems. Looking for straight lines just sets us up for frustration. Linear thinking does not allow us to be contextual and see the whole. We don't even have neat circles and ovals with today's thinking; we have varying shapes such as knots, where things are so interconnected that it's hard to separate the pieces.

There are many resources in nursing today advocating mind or concept maps as learning mechanisms (e.g., Mueller, Johnston, & Bligh, 2002; Novak, 1998; Wheeler & Collins, 2003). We have been using them for clinical courses in place of columnar care plans, in CT classes to show nonlinear thinking, and in nursing research courses as a way to study—for many years. Increasingly, students are more accepting of them as a way to learn, but we still have students who balk at them. They want linear formats—columns and outlines—because that's what they've used for years. But for others, it has become very liberating because their brains can now focus more naturally on the whole along with the parts in a matrix pattern instead of straight lines.

From Constant Success to Failure Possibilities

If you are going to be innovative, you must risk failure, and that's that. Now, think about that in today's society, which values success over all else, and you'll see the difficulties in moving toward this kind of thinking. A few years ago, there was a news item about physicist Stephen Hawking admitting that he was wrong about black holes (Pogatchnik, 2004). He has now revised his theory that had been considered flawless since the 1980s. It was great to see that news item, not because he failed, but because he was so matter-of-fact about his "failure." He exhibited *intellectual integrity*. Great ideas don't just appear wrapped up neatly;

they develop over time, with experimentation and repeated failures preceding their success. This is another area in which Senge (1998) is adamant: Innovation is a process of failure, and true learning doesn't occur when we train people to avoid failure. There's a story about Thomas Edison, who, in response to a reporter who asked about his failed results while inventing the light bulb, replied, "Results? Why, man, I have gotten lots of results! If I find 10,000 ways something won't work, I haven't failed. I am not discouraged, because every wrong attempt discarded is often a step forward" ("Brainy Quote," 2009).

Gardner (2006) saw those using their creative minds as being dissatisfied and different from others, and often failing. "Creators fail the most frequently and, often, the most dramatically. Only a person who is willing to pick herself up and 'try and try again' is likely to forge creative achievements" (p. 83). Sounds like *perseverance* too, doesn't it?

Think about the last time you gave someone positive feedback for failing. Have you ever done that? Maybe it's time we started doing that so that our creative folks keep creating.

From Valuing Only Objectivity to Being Open to Intuition

You'll note that we have a qualifying adjective there—"only"; we don't want to imply that we shouldn't value objectivity, but we have to be careful that we don't ignore intuition in our attempts to overcome bias and be objective. As you know by now, *intuition* was identified and defined in our consensus research on CT in

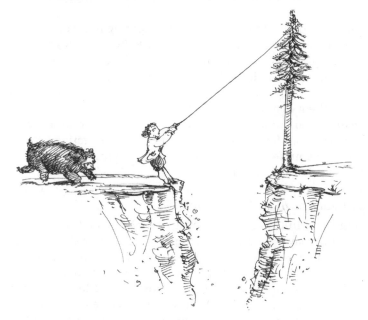

Risk Taking

nursing (Scheffer & Rubenfeld, 2000) as an "insightful sense of knowing without conscious use of reason" (p. 358). Polanyi (1964) described it years ago as "tacit knowing." It has been studied extensively in nursing, the most notable being Benner and Tanner's (1987) work. Effken (2001), after an extensive review of literature, placed intuition in an ecological psychology framework, allowing us to look beyond cognitive or perceptual processes to "the information provided by the patient and the context of care" (p. 252).

Viewing *intuition* in this way links it with *contextual perspective*, making it valuable in living systems environments. Intuitive responses take in a broader view of events, and that's what we need today. Rosanoff (1999) saw deeper intuitive responses as valuable in today's healthcare world, where quick decisions are called for. She suggested strategies to promote *intuition*—stop and look inside for your intuitive response, practice being attentive to intuitive responses, and keep a journal of your intuitive responses to see how accurate they are. She even suggested starting meetings by asking members to look at the agenda, record their thoughts and feelings, and then share them. This probably would enhance intuitive responses if those directions were couched in intuitive-sounding words, such as "your first gut reactions," "immediate hunches," and so forth. Senge (1996) suggested a similar process of meeting check-ins and check-outs focused on the thinking of participants.

From Reviewing to Reflection

The final pattern of change in thinking needed today is perhaps self-evident. If you have read the preceding pages in one sitting, go back now and review what you read. After you've done that, reflect on what you've read. How are reviewing and reflection different? Reviewing can be done fairly passively, but reflection can't. You have to put your personal self into reflection because it's deeper thinking. The Delphi study consensus group defined *reflection* as "contemplation upon a subject, especially one's assumptions and thinking for the purposes of deeper understanding and self-evaluation" (Scheffer & Rubenfeld, 2000, p. 358).

That deeper understanding and self-evaluation is where you need to be to prepare for the challenges of today's and tomorrow's healthcare delivery and education. The old thinking will not work; you need to evaluate yourself and your present thinking patterns and contemplate what you need to do to transform them to meet present and future needs.

At this point, we'd like to share with you a nurse's story. Although she doesn't describe her thinking that much, it's quite easy to see how her thinking fits with the transformations we have described. What do you think?

How One Nurse's Thinking Helped Her Meet the 5 IOM Competencies

Marcia Hegstad is a clinical nurse specialist for diabetes at a large teaching hospital in Michigan. We mentioned her briefly in Chapter 8. She is the epitome of a nurse who demonstrates all five of the IOM competencies. She wouldn't describe it in those terms, but it is easy to see patient-centered care, working in interdisciplinary teams, using EBP, using informatics, and improving quality in her story. She is very matter-of-fact in reporting this great work; we get the feeling that she sees it as "normal" patient care, but we were gleeful hearing a report of such excellence. After you read her story, we'll look at her thinking. Here she discusses a project to use the best evidence in glycemic control with diabetics undergoing cardiac surgery (M. Hegstad, personal communication, December 2, 2008):

I started this somewhere around 1997 for two reasons. I was asked by the heart surgeons to assist in the management of blood glucose of several patients close together. We had several postcardiac surgery patients re-admitted to the ICU with deep sternal wound infections. I noticed in the literature that there were reports of the relationship between hyperglycemia and post-op infections. It really bothered me, and I decided to look at some charts and saw that these patients had hyperglycemia post-operatively.

Around the same time I got a call from a graduate student who was interested in doing a thesis about controlling infections in heart patients. I told her it was "weird" that she had called me because I had just been looking at this. She told me about an article by Zerr and Furnary in the Annals of Thoracic Surgery *(Zerr, Furnary, Grunkemeier, Bookin, Kanhere, & Starr, 1997) that had compelling information about a definite relationship between post-op hyperglycemia and deep sternal infections. These authors had reduced their patients to a less than 200 glucose for the first 3 days post-op and had decreased infections.*

I did a retrospective chart audit and saw that the patients with infections had glucose readings above 200 within the first 72 hours after surgery. I went to the cardio-thoracic surgeons who said they didn't like the infections either and they wanted to do something about this. I told them about the article. We teamed up the endocrinology, SICU, and step-down staff and developed protocols for post-op insulin drips. Then we talked to an anesthesiologist about this. We called Anthony Furnary who said he moved the insulin drips into the OR and had essentially eradicated these infections. The anesthesiologist's eyes nearly popped out of his head and we moved it to the OR. We targeted glucose at 200 and patients did very well. We had months with no deep sternal infections.

I was able to track these data through the Infection Control Department, which has a tracking system for infections, so getting the data was pretty simple. The Anesthesiology Department looked at records with me and could see the patterns.

When we started this project, there wasn't much evidence except to keep glucose below 200. Furnary is now keeping patients between 100 and 150 instead of 200. (See Furnary et al., 2003.) Less than 200 was good for preventing deep sternal infections, but he reported that superficial infections are also controlled with even lower glucoses. We keep them between 125 and 175 now. We'll probably move to keeping them even lower but we have to remember that, during surgery, we have direct technology to see blood pressure, heart rate, etc.

on a monitor but we have to do more to monitor blood sugar and we have to be sensitive to this technology issue.

This has been an endless process of encouraging, monitoring, giving feedback, and so forth. There are so many people involved, such as endocrinologists, physician assistants, surgeons, anesthesiologists, OR perfusionists, and nurses in ICU and step-down units. It has been great interdisciplinary team work. This work has been picked up by another hospital; I'm not sure they're using the protocols just as we developed them or if they've adapted them.

This is obviously a condensed version of these years of work, omitting numerous meetings with diverse teams of providers, gathering information, discussions, trials, revisions, and so forth. She used the best available evidence, but because it was still scarce at the start of the project, the team proceeded with caution. As the evidence grew, so did their plan (see, for example, Clement et al., 2004; Furnary et al., 2003; Furnary, Zerr, Grunkemeier, & Starr, 1999; Zerr et al., 1997). Her use of the available informatics in tracking data allowed her and her team to see patterns. This endeavor, initiated by a nurse who was concerned enough about patients' conditions to launch a huge change of practice, resulted in significant quality improvement. We think that the IOM team should salute her for illustrating what they are trying to get others to achieve.

Look at the hints to Marcia's thinking in this story and compare them with the patterns of change we've been discussing. She certainly was engaged; she focused on questions, not just answers, and combined thinking and doing. She admits this project is not yet completed—a journey, not a destination. She was proactive in her learning; no one told her to do this. She acknowledged the complexities of her system. There certainly were few dichotomous statements; she was looking at a whole, not just pieces. She clearly did her thinking with others, not just on her own. There were no attempts to gloss over the complexities. She saw new patterns and did not take a linear approach to the project. The project has taken several years, so we doubt that every step along the way has been without failures. Marcia's beginning statements imply an *intuitive* response as she questioned practice. She clearly has *reflected* on this, and if you could have heard her talk, as we did, you'd know *intuitively* that she is a constantly *reflective*, humble person.

PAUSE _____

and Ponder

The Hard Work of Thinking

If we thought yesterday's thinking was hard, based on today's thinking, we can project tomorrow's thinking to be even harder.

Do you think that's true? Certainly the context is getting more and more complex. However, it could get easier. Remember when we tried to use CT in the context of yesterday's view of systems as mechanistic and it didn't fit? CT fits better with systems that are nonlinear and dynamic—complex adaptive systems. Today critical thinkers are still considered troublemakers in some systems; however, that is changing, and clinicians and educators with CT abilities are gaining acceptance and are being held up as people who have superior survival skills. If you're sitting there saying we've gone a bit wifty again, you might want to reconsider, because we think we're on track, and there are many who seem to agree.

Reflection Cues

- This chapter is the companion "bookend" to Chapter 4 that encloses the five chapters on CT and the IOM competencies, plus one on assessment (Chapter 10).
- The overwhelming message in discussions of the five competencies is change—change in healthcare delivery and education.
- New conceptualizations of change are needed for today's complex world.
- Realistic models for change in health care and education come from living, adaptive systems, not the older mechanistic models.
- Today's systems are dynamically complex; change is constant, and each part of the system that changes influences all other parts of the system.
- Old thinking patterns will not work with the reality of today and the near future.
- Fifteen patterns of change in thinking are described: passivity to engagement; answers to questions; separate thinking and doing to thinking and doing together; destinations to journeys; reactive to proactive learning; mechanistic to living system models; dichotomous to relativistic thinking; pieces to wholes; alone to systems; reduction to complexity; matching existing patterns to new patterns; linear to maps/knots/shapes; constant success to failure possibilities; valuing only objectivity to being open to intuition; and reviewing to reflecting.
- One nurse's story of changing care of surgical patients with diabetes illustrates the five IOM competencies and new patterns of thinking.
- Critical thinkers will fit better with systems that are complex and adaptive.

References

Benner, P., & Tanner, C. (1987). Clinical judgment: How expert nurses use intuition. *American Journal of Nursing, 87,* 23–31.

Brainy Quote. (2009). Retrieved March 12, 2009, from http://www.brainyquote.com/quotes/authors/t/thomas_a_edison.html

Clement, S., Braithwaite, S. S., Magee, M. F., Ahmann, A., Smith, E. P., Schafer, R. G., et al. (2004). Management of diabetes and hyperglycemia in hospitals. *Diabetes Care, 27,* 553–591.

Effken, J. A. (2001). Informational basis for expert intuition. *Journal of Advanced Nursing, 34,* 246–255.

Estabrooks, C. A. (2003). Translating research into practice: Implications for organizations and administrators. *Canadian Journal of Nursing Research, 35*(3), 53–68.

Foster-Fishman, P. G., Nowell, B., & Yang, H. (2007). Putting the system back into systems change: A framework for understanding and changing organizational and community systems. *American Journal of Psychology, 39,* 197–215. doi:10.1007/s10464-007-9109-0

Fullan, M. (1993). *Change forces: Probing the depths of educational reform.* Bristol, PA: Falmer Press.

Furnary, A. P., Gao, G., Grunkemeier, G. L., Wu, X. X., Zerr, K. J., Bookin, S. O., et al. (2003). Continuous insulin infusion reduces mortality in patients with diabetes undergoing coronary artery bypass grafting. *Journal of Thoracic and Cardiovascular Surgery, 125,* 1007–1021.

Furnary, A. P., Zerr, K. J., Grunkemeier, G. L., & Starr, A. (1999). Continuous intravenous insulin infusion reduces the incidence of deep sternal wound infection in diabetic patients after cardiac surgical procedures. *Annals of Thoracic Surgery, 67,* 352–362.

Gardner, H. (2006). *Five minds for the future.* Boston: Harvard Business School Press.

Hart, L. A. (1983). *Human brain and human learning.* New York: Longman.

Institute of Medicine. (2003). *Health professions education: A bridge to quality.* Washington, DC: National Academies Press.

Mueller, A., Johnston, M., & Bligh, D. (2002). Joining mind mapping and care planning to enhance student critical thinking and achieve holistic nursing care. *Nursing Diagnosis, 13*(1), 24–27.

Novak, J. D. (1998). *Learning, creating, and using knowledge: Concept maps as facilitative tools in schools and corporations.* Mahwah, NJ: Erlbaum.

Perkins, D. N. (1994). *The intelligent eye: Learning to think by looking at art.* Los Angeles: J. Paul Getty Trust.

Plsek, P. (2003, January). *Complexity and the adoption of innovation in health care.* Paper presented at the conference Accelerating Quality Improvement in Health Care Strategies to Speed the Diffusion of Evidence-based Innovations, by National Institute for Health Care Management Foundation and National Committee for Quality Health Care, Washington, DC. Retrieved November 10, 2008, from http://www.nihcm.org/~nihcmor/pdf/Plsek.pdf

Plsek, P. E., & Greenhalgh, T. (2001). The challenge of complexity in health care. *British Medical Journal, 323,* 625–628. Retrieved November 10, 2008, from http://bmj.bmjjournals.com/cgi/content/full/323/7313/625

Pogatchnik, S. (2004, July 22). Physicist's black holes theory turns inside out. *Detroit Free Press.*

Polanyi, M. (1964). The logic of tacit inference. In M. Grene (Ed.), *Knowing and being: Essays by Michael Polanyi* (pp. 138–158). Chicago: University of Chicago Press.

Porter-O'Grady, T. (2003). Innovation and creativity in a new age for health care. *Journal of the New York State Nurses Association, 34*(2), 4–8.

Rideout, E. (2001). *Transforming nursing education through problem-based learning.* Sudbury, MA: Jones and Bartlett.

Rosanoff, N. (1999). Intuition comes of age: Workplace applications of intuitive skill for occupational and environmental health nurses. *AAOHN Journal, 47,* 156–162.

Scheffer, B. K., & Rubenfeld, M. G. (2000). A consensus statement on critical thinking in nursing. *Journal of Nursing Education, 39,* 352–359.

Senge, P. M. (1990). *The fifth discipline: The art and practice of the learning organization.* New York: Doubleday.

Senge, P. M. (1996, Fall). The ecology of leadership. *Leader to Leader, 2*, 18–23. Retrieved November 10, 2008, from http://www.leadertoleader.org/knowledgecenter/journal.aspx? ArticleID=137

Senge, P. M. (1998, Summer). The practice of innovation. *Leader to Leader, 9*, 16–22. Retrieved November 9, 2008, from http://www.leadertoleader.org/knowledgecenter/journal.aspx? ArticleID=159

Senge, P. M. (1999). *Leadership in living organizations.* Retrieved December 4, 2008, from http://www.solonline.org/PeterSenge/articles/

Senge, P. M. (2003). Creating desired futures in a global society. *Reflections, 5*(1). Retrieved November 10, 2008, from http://www.reflections.solonline.org

Senge, P. M., Scharmer, C. O., Jaworski, J., & Flowers, B. S. (2004). Awakening faith in an alternative future. *Reflections, 5*(7), 1–11. Retrieved November 9, 2008, from http://www. reflections.solonline.org

Waldman, J. D., Smith, H. L., & Hood, J. N. (2003). Corporate culture: The missing piece of the healthcare puzzle. *Hospital Topics, 81*(1), 5–14.

Wheeler, L. A., & Collins, S. K. R. (2003). The influence of concept mapping on critical thinking in baccalaureate nursing students. *Journal of Professional Nursing, 19*(96), 339–346.

Zerr, K. J., Furnary, A. P., Grunkemeier, G. L., Bookin, S., Kanhere, V., & Starr, A. (1997). Glucose control lowers the risk of wound infection in diabetics after open heart operations. *Annals of Thoracic Surgery, 63*, 356–361.

Critical Thinking Inventory

Critical Thinking Habits of the Mind

Confidence—"**Assurance of one's reasoning abilities.**" (Scheffer & Rubenfeld, 2000, p. 358)[1]

1. How do you justify your thinking to someone who questions your conclusions?
2. Do you ever think aloud, or do you wait to speak until you have your ideas firmly in place? Why?
3. In what situations are you easily swayed from your thinking by someone else's opinion?

Contextual Perspective—"**Considerate of the whole situation, including the relationships, background, and environment that are relevant to some happening.**"

1. Describe how you approach an ambiguous situation.
2. How often, and under what circumstances, do you ask questions that start with "But what if . . . ?" or "It depends . . . "?
3. When you tell a story, do you tend to include background information, or do you keep more strictly to the point? Why?

Creativity—"**Intellectual inventiveness used to generate, discover, or restructure ideas; imagining alternatives.**"

1. Describe something you did in the past month that required innovative thinking. Why do you think it was innovative?
2. Do you tend to approach a situation the way other people do, or are your interpretations often different from others'? Give an example.
3. If your boss told you to "think outside the box," how would you change your usual thinking process?

---

[1]All quoted material for this appendix is from Scheffer & Rubenfeld, 2000, p. 358.

Flexibility—"Capacity to adapt, accommodate, modify, or change thoughts, ideas, and behaviors."

1. When your practice routines are interrupted, how does your thinking help you adapt?
2. How much of your mind is open to change and how much is closed?
3. What has to occur for you to change your mind about something important?

Inquisitiveness—"An eagerness to know by seeking knowledge and understanding through observation and thoughtful questioning in order to explore possibilities and alternatives."

1. What is your motivation for questioning information provided by an authoritative source, such as a person, an article, or a book?
2. On a continuum from *extremely curious* to *not curious*, where would you place yourself and why?
3. How do you distinguish the thinking differences between information seeking and inquisitiveness?

Intellectual Integrity—"Seeking the truth through sincere, honest processes, even if the results are contrary to one's assumptions and beliefs."

1. How do you deal with ideas and information that conflict with your thinking?
2. How do you feel about debate on issues, as opposed to having everyone agree? Why?
3. When you feel strongly about something, do you also try to see the situation from the opposite point of view? How do you get your thinking to achieve that?

Intuition—"Insightful sense of knowing without conscious use of reason."

1. How often do you have "gut" feelings, a "sixth sense," or a premonition? Describe how you respond to those feelings.
2. Describe how your hunches emerge in your thinking.
3. How do you explain your intuitive behavior to those who might question your choices?

Open-mindedness—"A viewpoint characterized by being receptive to divergent views and sensitive to one's biases."

1. How do you recognize when you have made assumptions, as opposed to basing your conclusions on data collected with your five senses (sight, sound, touch, smell, taste)?
2. What are your assumptions (about cultures, health, illness, time, eating, exercise, economic status, education, and so forth), and how do they affect the questions that you ask or don't ask, or the conclusions that you draw?
3. Why would others describe you as judgmental or nonjudgmental?

Perseverance—"**Pursuit of a course with determination to overcome obstacles.**"

1. Describe a challenging situation, the obstacles involved, and how your thinking allowed you to stick with the task.
2. Describe your thinking when you have to decide whether to pursue a task or move on.
3. How would others describe your ability to persevere?

Reflection—"**Contemplation on a subject, especially one's assumptions and thinking for the purposes of deeper understanding and self-evaluation.**"

1. Which of the 17 dimensions of critical thinking are your strongest? Your weakest? Why do think this?
2. What helps and what hinders your ability to reflect on your thinking before, during, and after an event or activity?
3. Describe how the following emotional states affect your thinking: love, hate, loneliness, frustration, sorrow, ecstasy, anxiety, and embarrassment.

Critical Thinking Skills

Analyzing—"**Separating or breaking a whole into parts to discover their nature, function, and relationships.**"

1. Describe your thinking when you need to deal with a complex issue, such as writing a major research paper or presenting a staff development workshop.
2. How would you describe your thinking to a nursing student or a new nurse who needs to learn how to analyze a patient situation?
3. What goes on in your mind when situations seem overwhelming?

Applying Standards—"**Judging according to established personal, professional, or social rules or criteria.**"

1. How do you decide if something is "right" or "wrong"?
2. When you are working with someone who is not doing his or her job as you think it should be done, what standards are you thinking about, and what do you usually do about it?
3. How do you decide which authority is the highest, and why?

Discriminating—"**Recognizing differences and similarities among things or situations and distinguishing carefully as to category or rank.**"

1. How do you decide what information is missing when you are problem-solving so you can better "zero-in" on the real problem?
2. How did you learn to distinguish the nuances of assessment that allow you to customize/individualize patient care?
3. Describe the thinking you use to help a nursing student or new nurse make differential nursing diagnoses.

Information Seeking—"Searching for evidence, facts, or knowledge by identifying relevant sources and gathering objective, subjective, historical, and current data from those sources."

1. What are your five primary sources for finding accurate information? Have you changed those sources over the past year? If so, how?
2. What format do you prefer for information input—hearing, seeing, a combination of those, or another? How does your preferred method influence the accuracy of your data collection?
3. Describe a typical time frame and process that you used when you searched for information, such as an Internet search.

Logical Reasoning—"Drawing inferences or conclusions that are supported in or justified by evidence."

1. Describe how you have solved a problem using one or all of the following approaches: sequential, random, inspirational, or something different. How effective is your approach?
2. When someone asks, "Why did you conclude that?" how do you describe the thinking behind your conclusion?
3. How do you decide when you have enough information to draw a conclusion?

Predicting—"Envisioning a plan and its consequences."

1. Describe how you project potentially positive and negative consequences of your decisions/actions, and the decisions/actions of others.
2. How often during the day do you think, "What will happen if . . . ?" Under what circumstances do you ask yourself that question?
3. When caring for patients, how far into the future, on average, do you think? How does the healthcare setting (acute care, long-term care, home care, etc.) impact your thinking into the future?

Transforming Knowledge—"Changing or converting the condition, nature, form, or function of concepts among concepts."

1. Describe two situations, one in which you demonstrate abstract thinking, and one in which you demonstrate concrete thinking. Which is your predominant mode of thinking? Why do you think that?
2. Describe a situation in which you learned something new and thought about how you would use that information in different situations.
3. Describe an event in which you have drawn on knowledge from several different sources and "blended" that knowledge to deal with a problem.

Reference

Scheffer, B. K., & Rubenfeld, M. G. (2000). A consensus statement on critical thinking in nursing. *Journal of Nursing Education, 39*(8), 352–359.

Index

Page numbers followed by *b* refer to boxes.